Ajmer Singh Grewal
Neelam Singh
Swati Verma
Chaitanay Vinayak Narayan
Ashutosh Kumar Verma
Editors

Receptor-Targeted Therapies in Diabetes Mellitus

From Pathophysiology to Innovative Treatments

nova
Medicine & Health
New York

DOI: https://doi.org/10.52305/ZDKJ7385

Additional color graphics may be available in the e-book version of this book.

Library of Congress Cataloging-in-Publication Data

ISBN: 979-8-89530-587-4 (Hardcover)
ISBN: 979-8-89530-653-6 (eBook)

Published by Nova Science Publishers, Inc. † New York

Contents

Preface

The prevalence of diabetes mellitus, a complex and chronic metabolic disorder, has surged worldwide, presenting both scientific and clinical challenges. The multifaceted nature of diabetes, encompassing both type 1 and type 2 diabetes, highlights a critical need to explore innovative therapeutic strategies that extend beyond conventional treatments. With recent insights into molecular biology and pharmacology, receptor-targeted therapies have emerged as a promising avenue for managing diabetes mellitus. This edited book, „Receptor-Targeted Therapies in Diabetes Mellitus: From Pathophysiology to Innovative Treatments," provides a comprehensive exploration of receptor-based approaches to diabetes treatment, synthesizing cutting-edge research on molecular targets with novel therapeutic interventions.

The book begins with an introductory overview of diabetes mellitus, examining the biochemical and cellular mechanisms underlying the disease and its progression, which sets the stage for further discussions on targeted therapies. It then evaluates current treatment modalities for diabetes, both pharmacological and non-pharmacological, highlighting the limitations of existing options and the need for new approaches to enhance patient outcomes. Among the central topics, free fatty acid receptor 4 (FFAR4/GPR120) is examined for its role in metabolic regulation and potential therapeutic applications in diabetes, with a focus on recent discoveries and research gaps. The insulin receptor's importance for glucose homeostasis is covered, as well as its role in hypothalamic regulation and implications for diabetic neuropathy, emphasizing its modulation in achieving metabolic balance. Another pivotal section of the book delves into glucagon-like peptide-1 receptors (GLP-1R), key agents in boosting insulin secretion and offering therapeutic potential in both type 1 and type 2 diabetes. The sodium-glucose cotransporter-2 (SGLT2) is discussed extensively, covering its role in glucose homeostasis, the application of SGLT2 inhibitors for glycemic control, and the identification of natural inhibitors with therapeutic promise. SIRT1, as an essential glucose metabolism regulator, is also explored, highlighting strategies for modulating its activity through pharmacological and natural agents. The book further examines AMP-activated protein kinase (AMPK) as a master regulator of cellular energy, evaluating its potential as a target to maintain energy balance and reduce diabetes-related complications. The role of muscarinic acetylcholine receptors (mAChRs) in insulin secretion, fructose 1,6-bisphosphatase in glucose regulation, and the therapeutic impact of neurotransmitter and G protein-coupled receptors are each explored, providing insights into novel diabetes treatments. GAD65, as a biomarker for early diabetes diagnosis, is discussed for its relevance in identifying latent autoimmune diabetes in adults (LADA) and enhancing early intervention. Additionally, alpha-glucosidase inhibitors are evaluated as effective in managing postprandial glucose levels. The emerging role of melatonin receptors in diabetes is explored, bridging chronobiology and metabolic health for novel therapeutic insights, while the inhibition of pyruvate kinase M2 is presented as a unique approach to diabetes management. Finally, 11β-hydroxysteroid dehydrogenase type 1 (11β-

HSD1) is highlighted as a promising target for glucose metabolism regulation. The final chapter, encapsulates the current advancements in receptor-targeted therapies and highlights future directions in this field. It reflects on the potential of emerging receptor-based strategies and the prospects for developing more precise, personalized diabetes treatments.

This book aims to offer valuable insights to researchers, clinicians, and students seeking to understand and advance receptor-targeted therapies in diabetes management. Each chapter provides an in-depth look at specific receptors and their roles in the pathophysiology and treatment of diabetes, fostering a deeper understanding of the molecular foundations of this complex disease and opening new avenues for innovative treatment approaches.

We extend our sincere appreciation to all contributing authors for their meticulous efforts and research contributions. We hope this compilation serves as a valuable resource for advancing therapeutic approaches in diabetes.

Ajmer Singh Grewal
Neelam Singh
Swati Verma
Chaitanay Vinayak Narayan
Ashutosh Kumar Verma
Editors

Chapter 1

Introduction to Diabetes Mellitus: Pathophysiology

Puneet Gupta[1]
Ishu Garg[2,*]
Devbrath Tripathi[2]
Radha Goel[3]
and Jasmine[1]
[1]Amity Institute of Pharmacy, Amity University, Noida, Uttar Pradesh, India
[2]Sardar Bhagwan Singh University, Balawala, Dehradun, Uttarakhand, India
[3]Lloyd Institutes of Management and Technology, Greater Noida, Uttar Pradesh, India

Abstract

Diabetes mellitus (DM) is a complex metabolic disorder characterized by chronic hyperglycemia and its associated complications. It encompasses several types, including type 1, type 2, and gestational diabetes, each with distinct etiological and pathophysiological mechanisms. Type 1 DM is primarily an autoimmune condition, marked by the destruction of pancreatic β-cells, while type 2 DM results from insulin resistance and β-cell dysfunction influenced by genetic predisposition and lifestyle factors. Gestational diabetes is associated with hormonal changes during pregnancy. The pathophysiology of DM involves intricate processes such as oxidative stress, inflammatory pathways, and disruptions in insulin signaling, all of which impair glucose homeostasis. These mechanisms contribute to long-term complications, including diabetic nephropathy, retinopathy, and neuropathy. Advances in nanotechnology and gene therapy present promising opportunities for treatment, underscoring the importance of a thorough understanding of DM pathophysiology to optimize clinical outcomes and enhance the quality of life for affected individuals. This chapter provides a comprehensive overview of the types of DM, emphasizing their unique pathophysiological mechanisms, risk factors, and clinical manifestations. It also examines diabetes-related complications and diagnostic methods, offering insights into established therapeutic approaches aimed at improving disease management and patient outcomes.

Keywords: diabetes, pathophysiology, nanotechnology, gene therapy, insulin

---

* Corresponding Author's Email: atharvrai10@gmail.com

In: Receptor-Targeted Therapies in Diabetes Mellitus
Editors: Ajmer Singh Grewal, Neelam Singh, Swati Verma et al.
ISBN: 979-8-89530-587-4

Abbreviations

AGEs	Glycation end products
Aβ	Amyloid-β
CRP	C-reactive protein
CVD	Cardiovascular diseases
DM	Diabetes mellitus
GAD	Glutamic acid decarboxylase
GDM	Gestational diabetes mellitus
GWAS	Genome-wide association studies
HbA1c	Glycated hemoglobin
HNF	Hepatic transcription factor
IA2	Insulinoma-associated protein 2
IDF	International Diabetes Federation
IST	Insulin signal transduction
JAML	Junctional adhesion molecule-like protein
JNKs	Janus kinase pathways
LADA	Latent autoimmune diabetes in adults
MEF2	myocyte enhancer factor-2
MODY	Maturity-onset diabetes of the young
NAFLD	Nonalcoholic fatty liver disease
PAI-1	Plasminogen activator inhibitor-1
T1DM	Type 1 DM
T2DM	Type 2 DM
T3DM	Type 3 DM
T4DM	Type 4 DM
TNF-α	Tumor necrosis factor-alpha

Introduction

Diabetes mellitus (DM), a chronic hyperglycemic endocrine condition, is considered a persistent disorder of carbohydrate, fat, and protein metabolism. The pancreatic metabolic hormones insulin and glucagon regulate glucose metabolism and blood glucose levels by controlling processes such as glycolysis, glycogenolysis, glycogenesis, and gluconeogenesis (Jiang and Zhang, 2003). The disease primarily arises when the pancreas fails to meet the body's demand for anabolic insulin, causing continuous fluctuations in blood glucose levels (Del Prato, 2005). This can result from either a deficiency or absence of insulin or, in rare cases, insulin resistance. DM involves a variety of modifiable and non-modifiable risk factors. Modern lifestyle habits, such as smoking, alcohol consumption, obesity, and irregular physical activity, contribute significantly to the development of diabetes. Additionally, factors such as sex, age, race, and ethnicity can variably influence the body's homeostasis, functionality, and metabolism, further contributing to the onset of diabetes (Mozaffarian et al. 2009). Elevated oxidative stress and impaired mitochondrial function, often due to toxic arsenic exposure or selenium deficiency (lower GPx-1 activity), can adversely affect β-cell activity. Autoimmunity and genetic factors, such as chromosomal abnormalities and mutations, also play crucial roles in DM pathology, as seen across different types of diabetes (Bonini and Sargis, 2018). Statistical analyses indicate that a sedentary lifestyle could increase the prevalence of diabetes to an estimated 366 million cases among the elderly by 2030 (Khursheed et al. 2019). The International Diabetes Federation (IDF) reported that India had approximately 40.9 million diabetic individuals in 2010, with projections suggesting this number could rise to 69.9 million by 2025 (Goyal et al. 2010). Furthermore, the IDF stated that in 2021, 537 million adults aged 20–79 years worldwide had diabetes, with a predicted increase to 783 million by 2045 (Diaz-Valencia et al. 2015). According to WHO data, 8.5% of individuals aged 18 and older had diabetes in 2014, and the disease causes approximately 1.5 million deaths annually, with 48% of these occurring before the age of 70. In comparison, the IDF reported 6.7 million diabetes-related deaths in 2021. Additionally, diabetes is associated with 460,000 kidney-related deaths and accounts for roughly 20% of deaths caused by cardiovascular diseases (CVD) (Antar et al. 2023). This chapter aims to provide a comprehensive overview of the types of diabetes mellitus, emphasizing their unique pathophysiological mechanisms, risk factors, and clinical manifestations.

Types of Diabetes

DM has been classified enormously and counts for numerous types (Figure 1) which are briefed below (Diaz-Valencia et al. 2015).

Based on Insulin Dependency

- *Type 1 DM (T1DM):* The loss of pancreatic islet β-cells, coupled with the development of T1DM-associated autoantibodies, often with a hereditary basis that can complicate early detection, leads to an insulin-dependent chronic autoimmune disease commonly manifesting in juveniles. This condition can be further classified into idiopathic and fulminant types, both of which are not a consequence of autoimmunity (Diaz-Valencia et al. 2015). The idiopathic type is less severe than the autoimmune form, with clinical features including episodic ketoacidosis and insulin insufficiency. In contrast, the fulminant type is characterized by rapid-onset ketoacidosis following hyperglycemia and undetectable serum C-peptide levels, even at elevated blood glucose levels (≥288 mg/dL). This subtype progresses exceptionally quickly, leading to complete β-cell destruction with no residual insulin production (ElSayed et al. 2023).
- *Type 2 DM (T2DM):* The insulin-independent, hyperglycemic condition often observed in middle-aged individuals results from a complex interplay of genetic and lifestyle factors, such as obesity, with a key feature being defective insulin secretion (Galicia-Garcia et al. 2020). In this condition, β-cell function is either partially impaired or preserved, with no significant loss. Additionally, anti-parietal-cell antibodies are absent, and blood insulin levels may be low, normal or even excessive. The first phase of insulin secretion is disrupted, and the glucose-stimulated insulin

response is inadequate. Patients also exhibit an elevated proinsulin-to-insulin (C-peptide) ratio (Petersen and Shulman, 2018; Dufurrena et al. 2017).

Hybrid Forms of Diabetes

- *Latent autoimmune diabetes in adults (LADA):* Latent autoimmune diabetes in adults (LADA), as it is clinically known, shares characteristics with type 2 diabetes mellitus (T2DM), particularly the presence of pancreatic autoantibodies associated with autoimmune diabetes (Dufurrena et al. 2017).
- *Ketosis-prone T2DM:* This unique clinical condition, observed primarily in specific ethnic groups, is characterized by episodic ketosis and severe insulin deficiency, resembling type 1 diabetes mellitus (T1DM) or diabetic ketoacidosis (Williams et al. 2016). While no genetic evidence or markers of autoimmunity have been identified, glucose toxicity in acute and phasic β-cell failure is proposed as the underlying mechanism for the condition (Mauvais-Jarvis et al. 2004).

Special Cases

- *Type 3 DM (T3DM):* With the progression of type 2 diabetes mellitus (T2DM), an invariably insulin-resistant environment may contribute to the neuropathogenic condition known as type 3 diabetes mellitus (T3DM), which is associated with Alzheimer's disease (AD). The relationship between T3DM, T2DM, and AD involves the toxicity of amyloid-β (Aβ) precursor protein processing and the impaired clearance of Aβ (Mauvais-Jarvis et al. 2004).
- *Type 4 DM (T4DM)/ gestational DM (GDM):* Even neonates are at risk of developing diabetes later in middle age (Hollander et al. 2007). Gestational diabetes mellitus (GDM) is associated with various risk factors, including a family history of diabetes, obesity, advanced maternal age, polycystic ovary syndrome, a sedentary lifestyle, and exposure to environmental pollutants (Hollander et al. 2007).

Genetic Diabetes Types

- *Genetic defects of the β-cell/maturity-onset diabetes of the young (MODY):* MODY is associated with abnormal monogenic β-cell functioning, inherited as an autosomal dominant trait. It is linked to mutations in genes encoding hepatic transcription factors, such as HNF-1, HNF-4, HNF-1α, and the enzyme glucokinase.
- *Genetic defects in insulin action and receptors*: Even in the presence of mutant insulin, the poor binding of these molecules to insulin receptors may result in mild or even normal glucose metabolism. Additional signs of genetic disorders include cystic ovaries, virilization, and acanthosis nigricans (Thomas and Philipson, 2015).

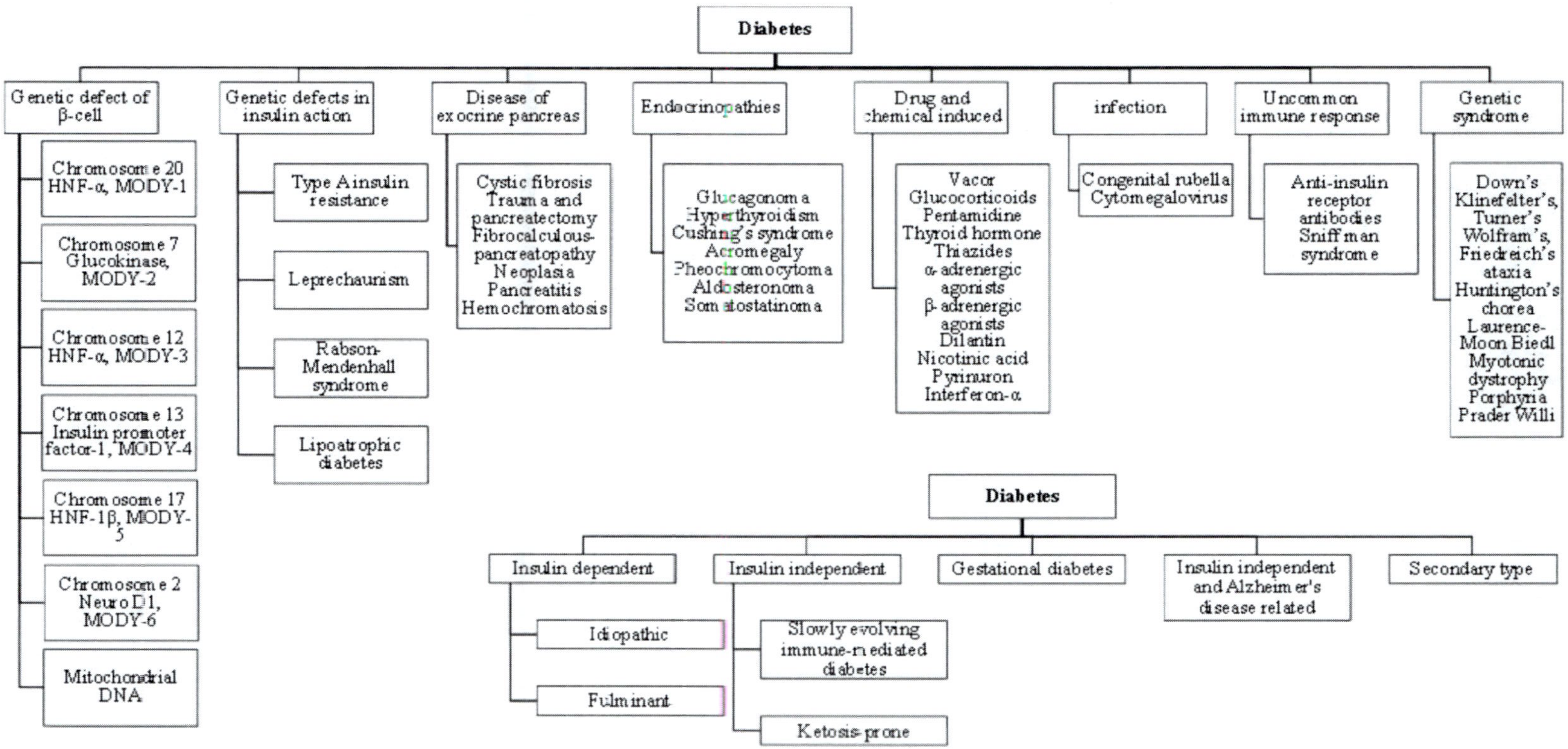

Figure 1. Types of DM.

Exocrine-Endocrine Type of Diabetes

- *Diseases of the exocrine pancreas:* DM can be triggered by even minor pancreatic injury or infection, such as pancreatitis, pancreatic cancer, trauma, or pancreatectomy (Popoviciu et al. 2023).
- *Endocrinopathies:* Endocrine and neurotransmitter-related pathologies, such as acromegaly, glucagonoma, pheochromocytoma, and Cushing's syndrome, can cause diabetes and exacerbate the condition in individuals with pre-existing insulin secretion defects. Additionally, somatostatinomas and aldosterone-induced hypokalemia contribute to the development and progression of diabetes (Popoviciu et al. 2023).

Immune System and Antibodies Related Diabetes

- *Stiff-man syndrome:* Individuals with autoimmune disorders affecting the central nervous system have higher levels of glutamic acid decarboxylase (GAD) autoantibodies and are more likely to develop diabetes (Rakocevic and Floeter, 2012).
- *Anti-insulin receptor antibody-related diabetes*: Antibodies that prevent the insulin receptor from binding to insulin can cause diabetes. However, in rare cases, these antibodies may act as insulin agonists, potentially leading to hypoglycemia. Individuals with autoimmune diseases often experience the onset of this disorder (Petersen et al. 2022).
- *Infections:* Viral infections, such as coxsackievirus B, congenital rubella, and mumps, can attack the pancreas and destroy β-cells, triggering diabetes, especially in individuals with genetic and autoimmune predispositions, leading to further β-cell destruction (Petersen et al. 2022).
- *Drug/chemical induced diabetes*: Certain drugs and toxins can interfere with insulin secretion. In addition to thyroid hormones, diazoxide, β-adrenergic agonists, and α-interferon are also known to contribute to the development of diabetes (ElSayed et al. 2023).

Pathophysiology of Diabetes Mellitus

Glucose homeostasis in the body is a multi-hormonal regulatory mechanism, primarily involving insulin and glucagon. Insulin, released from the β-cells of the islets of Langerhans in response to elevated glucose concentrations, helps decrease blood glucose levels. It does this by inhibiting glucose production through the liver's glucose and glycogen cycles or by enhancing glucose metabolism in the liver, muscle, and fat tissues (Okur et al. 2017). In contrast, glucagon is secreted by the α-cells of the islets of Langerhans when glucose levels are low. It acts as an insulin antagonist, stimulating liver glucose and glycogen cycles. Cortisol and catecholamines also act as glucagon agonists. Additionally, amylin, co-secreted with insulin, functions as an insulin metabolic antagonist by slowing gastric emptying and increasing glucose absorption. Insulinotropic polypeptides, such as glucose-dependent insulinotropic peptides and glucagon-like peptides, are incretins that originate from the gut and assist in insulin production and release (Hieronymus and Griffin, 2015). Furthermore, glucose absorption and distribution are regulated by membrane-bound glycoprotein glucose transporters, specifically the sodium-glucose co-transporter and the facilitative glucose transporter (GLUT) (Ojha et al. 2019). Various other hormones also play a role in regulating glucose homeostasis, as discussed in the section on the pathophysiology of secondary diabetes mellitus. A detailed overview of diabetes mellitus pathophysiology is provided in Figure 2.

Pathophysiology of T1DM

The etiology of T1DM is an autoimmune condition primarily focused on β-cell destruction, associated with both environmental and genetic factors that trigger autoimmune responses. The pathophysiology of T1DM includes the detection of autoantibodies, β-cell death, dysglycemia, and ultimately hyperglycemia accompanied by symptoms (Insel et al. 2015). T1DM is associated with the development of autoantibodies that target insulin, protein tyrosine phosphatase-like molecules (insulinoma-associated protein 2 [IA2 and IA2β]), and 65 kDa glutamic acid decarboxylase, as a result of exposure to β-cell autoantigens months or years before symptoms appear (Ziegler et al. 1999). Children with MHC protein-encoding HLA class II haplotypes, HLA DR3 DQ2 and HLA DR4 DQ8, on chromosome 6 are more prone to developing autoantibodies and T1DM, with incidence peaking at 1-2 years of age. The risk is further complicated by the presence of multiple HLA DRB1 alleles in humans. Genome-wide association studies (GWAS) have identified more than 50 non-HLA genetic factors that contribute to T1DM risk, including genetic polymorphisms in PTPN22 and INS (Ojha et al. 2019). The insufficient production of regulatory T-cells and the inadequate elimination of damaging β-cell antigen-reactive T-cells are influenced by HLA class II and INS polymorphisms (Bell et al. 1980). The first β-cell-targeting autoantibodies, such as anti-insulin or anti-GAD65, typically appear in early childhood, while it is rare for IA2 or ZNT8 autoantibodies to appear first (Krischer et al. 2015). The presence of IA2 as a later autoantibody increases the risk of progressing to stage 3 disease (Krischer et al. 2015). Additionally, the three amino acid-related ZNT8 variants typically emerge later, during stages 1 and 2 (Lampasona et al. 2009). The process affecting the pancreas begins with cognate interactions between T-cells and B-cells, leading to the formation of islet-targeting autoantibodies in response to auto-antigen presentation by dendritic cells and the subsequent activation of CD4+ and CD8+ T-cells. Viral infections, environmental exposures, and the HLA DR3 DQ2 and HLA DR4 DQ8 haplotypes are responsible for triggering this response (Roep and Peakman 2012). T-cells preferentially recognize post-translationally modified peptides from β-cells, which corresponds to a loss of tolerance to β-cell auto-antigens (McGinty et al. 2015). Nevertheless, no correlation was found between T-cell or B-cell infiltration and β-cell-targeting autoantibodies, and even islet cells were found to express higher levels of HLA class I protein (McGinty et al. 2015).

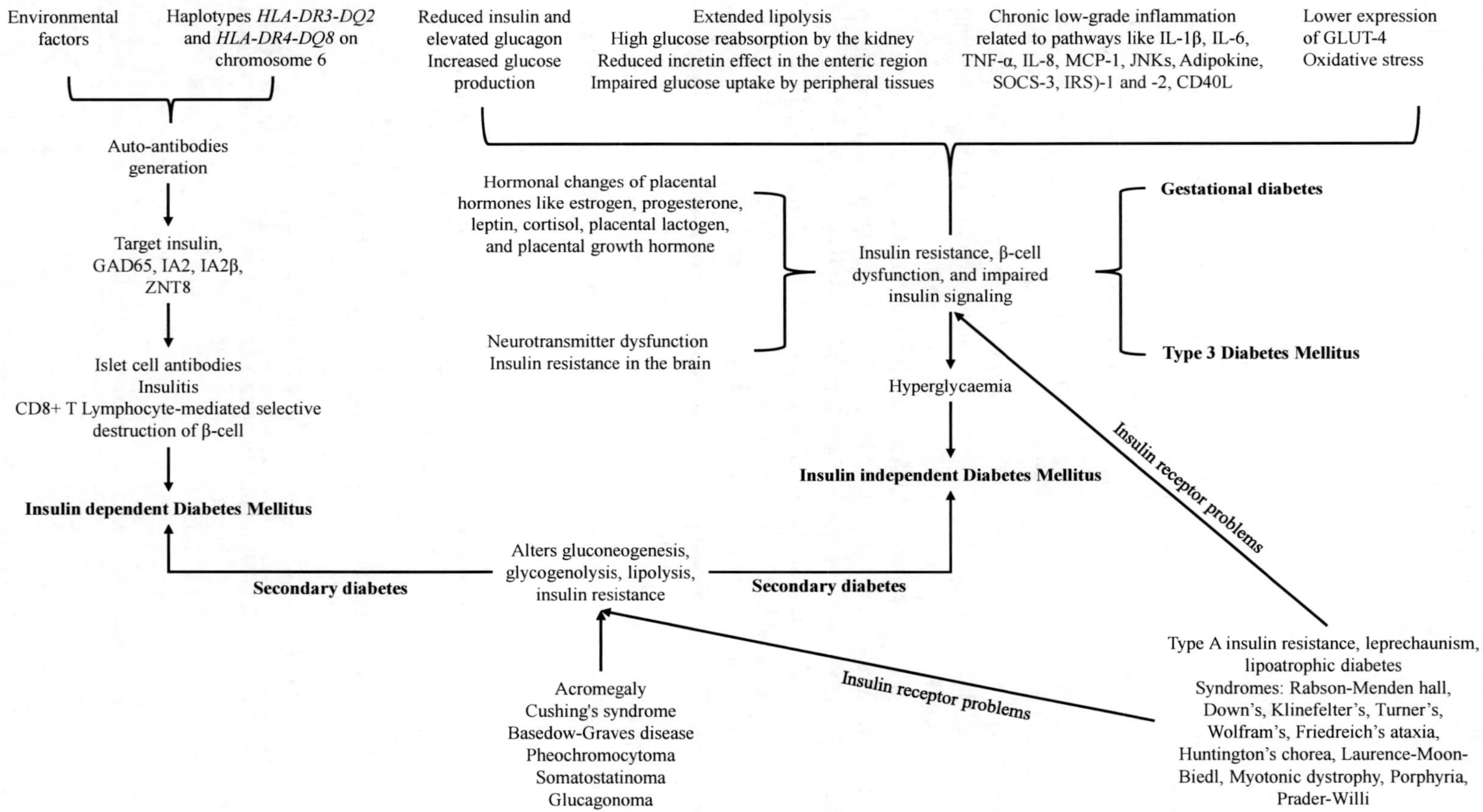

Figure 2. Pathophysiology of DM.

Pathophysiology of T2DM

Insulin-independent T2DM is associated with reduced insulin secretion and elevated glucagon secretion by the pancreas (McGinty et al. 2015). However, the resistance is compensated for by an increase in insulin secretion from the β-cells (Demir et al. 2021). But at the advanced stage, the pancreatic function reserve becomes insufficient, leading to collapse, dedifferentiation, or apoptosis of β-cells. This results in cytotoxic dysfunction, which worsens T2DM (Mlinar et al. 2007). Insulin resistance, β-cell dysfunction, and impaired insulin signaling are all linked to chronic low-grade inflammation. IL-1β contributes to the dysfunction and apoptosis of β-cells, stimulated by free fatty acids, endocannabinoids, and amyloid polypeptides. IL-6 and tumor necrosis factor-alpha (TNF-α), produced by adipocytes (the endocrine cells of adipose tissue), initiate pancreatic islet apoptosis, impair insulin action, and promote insulin resistance and β-cell dysfunction (Mlinar et al. 2007). Janus kinase (JNK) pathways and TNF-α are involved in the production of pro-inflammatory cytokines, as well as impaired glucose metabolism and insulin resistance (Rani et al. 2016). While adiponectin enhances insulin sensitivity, suppresses liver glucose synthesis, promotes fatty acid oxidation in muscles, and exhibits anti-inflammatory qualities, its effects are diminished by IL-6, which is linked to insulin resistance and increased production of pro-inflammatory cytokines. Additionally, the adipokine leptin regulates energy homeostasis and contributes to insulin resistance (Rani et al. 2016). The resistin hormone, secreted by white adipose tissue, is also involved in insulin resistance (Ukkola and Santaniemi 2002). The lower expression of GLUT-4, a significant molecular mechanism of insulin resistance induced by oxidative stress, occurs due to the suppression of transcriptional regulators such as NF-κB, PPAR-γ, nuclear factor-1, p85, CEB/Ps, myocyte enhancer factor-2 (MEF2), and hypoxia-inducible factors-alpha (HIF-α) (Tebay et al. 2015). The associated factors and by-products, including p38 MAPK, PKC, JNK/SAPK, hexosamine, and sorbitol, inhibit the expression of GLUT-4 (Yaribeygi et al. 2020). Akt (also known as PKB), AMPK, mTOR, and GSK-3 are other serine/threonine kinases that can disrupt insulin signaling. Oxidative stress increases insulin resistance by downregulating the activity of free radicals, including GSK-3, IRS, IRS-1, and Akt (Tebay et al. 2015).

Pathophysiology of T4DM/GDM

GDM occurs due to hormonal changes during pregnancy, as placental hormones and placental growth hormone reduce cellular insulin sensitivity (Prentki and Nolan, 2006). This results in increased endogenous glucose production and fat breakdown, leading to elevated blood glucose and free fatty acid concentrations (Berberoglu, 2019). β-cell dysfunction can occur at multiple levels, including pro-insulin production, post-translational modifications, granule storage, blood glucose detection, and the complex mechanisms behind granule exocytosis. In GDM, insulin-stimulated glucose uptake decreases by 54%, even though insulin receptor abundance remains unchanged. Instead, insulin signaling is impaired due to reduced tyrosine phosphorylation or increased serine/threonine phosphorylation (Prentki and Nolan, 2006). Neurohormonal dysfunction further affects GDM by altering adiposity and glucose utilization through leptin and adiponectin (Di Cianni et al. 2003). Placental insulin resistance raises plasma leptin levels, which peak in GDM, contributing to hyperleptinemia and fetal macrosomia

(Catalano et al. 1991; Di Cianni et al. 2003). Additionally, the syncytiotrophoblast produces low adiponectin levels, impairing insulin signaling, amino acid transport, and fetal growth. The endocrine role of adipose tissue, through adipokines, pro-inflammatory mediators, and oxidative stress, disrupts IRS-1 and GLUT-4 function, leading to T2DM-like alterations in glucose metabolism. Iron and homocysteine further increase oxidative stress in GDM (Prentki and Nolan, 2006).

Pathophysiology of Secondary DM

Diabetes that develops as a side effect of another illness is known as secondary diabetes. Insulin resistance and β-cell function are influenced by various factors, including hormone excess or deficiency (Scaroni et al. 2017). The primary endocrinopathies that affect blood sugar regulation and body mass index in secondary diabetes include acromegaly, Cushing's syndrome, Basedow-Graves' disease (hyperthyroidism), pheochromocytoma, somatostatinoma, and glucagonoma. These conditions directly and indirectly affect gluconeogenesis, glycogenolysis, and lipolysis, contributing to insulin resistance (Nishi, 2018). The lipolytic effect of acromegaly decreases insulin-mediated glucose uptake by inhibiting glucose transporters in adipose tissue and suppresses glucose production in the liver (Popoviciu et al. 2023). Cushing's syndrome enhances glucagon action and inhibits glycogenogenesis. Muscle tissue induces insulin resistance by disrupting the insulin-signaling cascade, stimulating proteolysis, and causing muscle mass loss (Popoviciu et al. 2023). Abdominal obesity exacerbates insulin resistance and further impacts the synthesis and release of adipokines, contributing to impaired glucose metabolism. In pancreatic cells, thyroid hormones stimulate glucagon secretion and enhance hepatic glucose production by upregulating GLUT-2 expression, stimulating lipolysis, and promoting hepatic gluconeogenesis (Nishi, 2018). Additionally, conditions like primary aldosteronism, glucagonoma, and somatostatinomas alter glucose tolerance. Somatostatinomas, in particular, inhibit glucagon secretion, growth hormone (GH), and other hormones capable of increasing blood sugar levels (Scaroni et al. 2017).

Clinical Manifestations and Diagnosis

Insulin resistance caused by metabolic abnormalities can affect the liver, skeletal muscles, and adipose tissue differently. Individuals with high blood sugar may exhibit symptoms such as increased hunger, polydipsia, dysuria, weight loss, and visual disturbances, particularly in cases of complete insulin deficiency or in children. In the early stages of type II diabetes, symptoms are often absent. In T1DM, insulitis is diagnosed when two or more auto-antibodies are present. The progression from stage 1 to stage 2 is characterized by dysglycemia, detectable through oral glucose tolerance tests, loss of first-phase insulin release, and increased glycated hemoglobin (HbA1c) levels. Stage 3 is identified by inflammation in pancreatic islets, which impairs glucose sensing and insulin secretion by β-cells. This stage is diagnosed through fine-needle biopsy, pancreatic tail resection, or tissue sample analysis in patients with ketoacidosis. Diabetes Mellitus inflammatory pathology is further evidenced by elevated levels of TNF-α, pro-inflammatory markers, interferon-γ (IFN-γ), and plasminogen activator inhibitor-1 (PAI-

1), which are linked to abnormalities in lipid and carbohydrate metabolism. Clinical findings in insulin-resistant T2DM patients show reduced expression and localization of GLUT-4. Secondary diabetes is diagnosed based on the underlying primary disease, often determined through changes in blood serum hormonal levels and other specific diagnostic tests. For instance, acromegaly is diagnosed through serum IGF-1 screening, oral glucose tolerance tests, serum growth hormone (GH) levels, and MRI of the pituitary. Fasting glucose, oral glucose tolerance, and HbA1c tests are the primary diagnostic tools for DM. Glucose in the blood binds to hemoglobin, and higher blood glucose levels result in more hemoglobin being coated with glucose. The fasting blood sugar test involves testing a blood sample before breakfast. An oral glucose tolerance test measures blood glucose levels over two hours following sugar intake. According to diagnostic criteria, individuals with fasting plasma glucose ≥126 mg/dL (7 mmol/L) or HbA1c ≥6.5% during an oral glucose tolerance test are classified as diabetic (Zhao et al. 2023). GDM is diagnosed using the O'Sullivan test, where a fasting patient is given 50g of glucose, and blood tests are conducted every hour. Plasma glucose levels exceeding 1500 mg/dL indicate GDM (Zhao et al. 2023).

Complications

Acute Complications

- *Diabetic ketoacidosis*: A severe complication of T1DM arises from insulin deficiency, disrupted glucose metabolism, and acid-base imbalances, resulting in elevated blood glucose levels and ketone production. This condition can lead to cerebral edema, acute respiratory distress syndrome, and sepsis (Kanikarla-Marie and Jain, 2016). The underlying abnormal physiology is characterized by increased levels of glucagon, growth hormone, and catecholamines, placing the body in a catabolic state. This results in hyperglycemia, hyperketonemia, hyperosmolarity, and electrolyte imbalances. The impaired intracellular transport of glucose leads to elevated free fatty acid (FFA) levels in the bloodstream. Upon reaching the mitochondria, these FFAs undergo oxidation, producing ketone bodies such as beta-hydroxybutyrate, acetone, and acetoacetate (Kanikarla-Marie and Jain, 2016).
- *Hyperosmolar hyperglycemic state*: This severe condition, marked by profound hyperglycemia, hyperosmolality with hypernatremia, and dehydration without ketosis, is commonly observed in patients with type 2 diabetes mellitus (T2DM). It results from relative insulin deficiencies and differs from diabetic ketoacidosis, as it involves minimal lipolysis and ketogenesis (Kanikarla-Marie and Jain, 2016).

Macrovascular Chronic Complications

- *CVD:* Advanced glycation end products (AGEs), stimulated by the RNA-binding protein QKI-7, contribute to endothelial dysfunction and the activation of vascular smooth muscle cells in hyperglycemia. Dysregulated calcium signaling, induced by AGEs and hyperglycemia, leads to heart failure and reduced expression and activity of sarcoplasmic/endoplasmic reticulum Ca2+ ATPase2a. This process is further exacerbated by sarcolipin and epigenetic modifications mediated by histone deacetylases (McCormick et al. 2010).

- *Diabetic cerebrovascular:* Intracranial large and small vessel disease, caused by cerebral vascular complications of T2DM and nutritional metabolic abnormalities, primarily begins with inflammatory atherosclerosis. Hyperglycemia damages blood vessel endothelium through oxidative stress, uric acid, cytokines, and adhesive inflammatory cells such as T-lymphocytes, mononuclear leukocytes, C-reactive protein (CRP), IL-6, and IL-17. This leads to the narrowing or complete occlusion of vessels. Additionally, matrix metalloproteinase-9 (MMP-9) damages the basement membrane and accelerates unstable plaque rupture within the vessels. The resulting thrombosis can enter the brain's small vessels, leading to cerebral infarction (McCormick et al. 2010). Hyperglycemia-induced lactate production exacerbates brain acidosis by increasing anaerobic glucose metabolism, inhibiting mitochondrial respiration, and contributing to vasogenic edema, a hyperthrombotic state, and reduced cerebral blood flow (McCormick et al. 2010).

Microvascular Chronic Complications

- *Diabetic nephropathy:* DM leads to severe interstitial inflammation, contrast-induced nephropathy, urinary tract infections, and acute kidney injury, all of which exacerbate lipotoxicity, oxidative stress, and hyperglycemic memory (Zelniker and Braunwald, 2020). Diabetic kidneys exhibit impaired podocyte function and a thickened glomerular basement membrane, resulting in tubulointerstitial fibrosis, glomerulosclerosis, and reduced kidney function, which manifest as albuminuria and a decreased glomerular filtration rate. This condition is further aggravated by the involvement of growth factor-beta-1 (TGF-β1), JAK-STAT signaling, sphingomyelin phosphodiesterase acid-like 3b (SMPDL3b), junctional adhesion molecule-like protein (JAML), VEGF-B, and mTORC1 (Zelniker and Braunwald, 2020).
- *Diabetic retinopathy:* The condition is characterized by dysfunction of the retina's endothelial cells and pericytes (Whitehead et al. 2019). Hyperglycemia, advanced glycation end products (AGEs), and oxidative stress disrupt the tight junctions between endothelial cells in the retinal blood vessels. Consequently, pericytes detach and undergo apoptosis, signifying the onset of diabetic retinopathy. These changes increase the permeability of the blood-retina barrier, allowing harmful substances to leak in and exacerbate the condition. Pathways such as Notch 1, Notch 3, hypoxia-inducible factor-1-alpha (HIF-1α), and vascular endothelial growth factor-1 (VEGF-1) signal the internalization and phosphorylation of vascular endothelial cadherin, further weakening the tight junctions. Diabetic retinopathy is marked by persistent inflammation, elevated levels of oxidized lipoproteins, AGEs, and free radicals. Pro-inflammatory cytokines, prostaglandin E2, IL-1β, and NLRP3 contribute to vascular leakage, endothelial cell apoptosis, and capillary degeneration (Whitehead et al. 2019).
- *Diabetic neuropathy:* The condition affects the sensory nerve endings in the limbs, causing pain, burning sensations, tingling, and numbness. In later stages, it progresses

to the motor nerve endings of the lower extremities, leading to imbalance and loss of sensation. It typically spreads from the central parts of the body to the outermost areas (Pham et al. 2015). Both insulin deficiency and resistance in sensory nerves significantly contribute to the development of diabetic neuropathy, as insufficient insulin signaling reduces nerve regeneration capacity, impairs neurochemical synthesis, and causes mitochondrial dysfunction. Hyperglycemia leads to Schwann cell dysfunction, resulting in disrupted myelin, compromised axon conduction, and impaired nerve regeneration, which further exacerbates diabetic neuropathy. This condition also affects molecular targets such as MAPK, the p75 neurotrophin receptor, neurotrophic factor-3, and β-nerve growth factor, further contributing to the progression of diabetic neuropathy (Pham et al. 2015).

Others

- *Liver cirrhosis:* Hepatogenous diabetes results from the cirrhosis-induced decline in liver function. By aggravating immunodepression and accelerating liver fibrosis and inflammation, possibly due to insulin resistance and increased adipokine production, diabetes contributes to liver failure. The metabolic syndrome associated with type 2 diabetes, obesity, and dyslipidemia leads to nonalcoholic fatty liver disease (NAFLD), which includes cirrhosis, fibrosis, and simple steatosis. Additionally, visceral obesity, hypertriglyceridemia, and insulin resistance promote the development of complex nonalcoholic steatohepatitis (NASH) by impairing the liver's ability to effectively metabolize lipids (Chitturi et al. 2002).
- *Impaired cytokine production and compromised immune system:* DM results in excessive blood sugar and insufficient insulin, which can weaken the immune system. In individuals with T1D and T2D, monocytes and peripheral blood mononuclear cells produce fewer cytokines. Since IL-6 plays a role in both adaptive immunity and pathogen defense, cytokine inhibition may impair the immune response in hyperglycemic individuals (Tesch, 2010).

Conclusion

Diabetes mellitus remains a complex and multifaceted disorder that requires a comprehensive understanding of its pathophysiology, clinical management, and emerging therapeutic options. Early diagnosis, effective glycemic control, and prevention of complications are essential components of providing optimal care for individuals with diabetes. Additionally, it is crucial to protect diabetes patients from the potential negative effects of inappropriate, ineffective, or unnecessary pharmacological treatments, which can often delay the desired outcomes and prolong hyperglycemic exposure.

References

Antar, S. A., Ashour, N. A., Sharaky, M., Khattab, M., Ashour, N. A., Zaid, R. T., Roh, E. J., Elkamhawy, A., & Al-Karmalawy, A. A. (2023). Diabetes mellitus: Classification, mediators, and complications; A gate to identify potential targets for the development of new effective treatments. *Biomedicine & Pharmacotherapy*, 168, 115734.

Bell, G. I., Pictet, R., & Rutter, W. J. (1980). Analysis of the regions flanking the human insulin gene and sequence of an Alu family member. *Nucleic Acids Research*, 8(18), 4091–4110.

Berberoglu, Z. (2019). Pathophysiology of gestational diabetes mellitus. *European Medical Journal*, 7(1), 97-106.

Bonini, M. G., & Sargis, R. M. (2018). Environmental toxicant exposures and type 2 diabetes mellitus: Two interrelated public health problems on the rise. *Current Opinion in Toxicology*, 7, 52–59.

Catalano, P. M., Tyzbir, E. D., Roman, N. M., Amini, S. B., & Sims, E. A. H. (1991). Longitudinal changes in insulin release and insulin resistance in nonobese pregnant women. *American Journal of Obstetrics & Gynecology*, 165(6), 1667–1672.

Chitturi, S., Abeygunasekera, S., Farrell, G. C., Holmes-Walker, J., Hui, J. M., Fung, C., Karim, R., Lin, R., Samarasinghe, D., Liddle, C., Weltman, M., & George, J. (2002). NASH and insulin resistance: Insulin hypersecretion and specific association with the insulin resistance syndrome. *Hepatology*, 35(2), 373–379.

Del Prato, S. (2005). Pathophysiology of insulin action in humans. In M. Serrano Ríos, J. F. Caro, R. Carraro, & J. A. Gutiérrez Fuentes (Eds.), *The Metabolic Syndrome at the Beginning of the XXI Century* (pp. 179–197). Madrid: Elsevier España.

Demir, S., Nawroth, P. P., Herzig, S., & Üstünel, B. E. (2021). Emerging targets in type 2 diabetes and diabetic complications. *Advanced Science*, 8(18), 2100275.

Di Cianni, G., Miccoli, R., Volpe, L., Lencioni, C., & Del Prato, S. (2003). Intermediate metabolism in normal pregnancy and in gestational diabetes. *Diabetes/Metabolism Research and Reviews*, 19(4), 259–270.

Diaz-Valencia, P. A., Bougnères, P., & Valleron, A.-J. (2015). Global epidemiology of type 1 diabetes in young adults and adults: A systematic review. *BMC Public Health*, 15(1), 1–15.

Dufurrena, Q., Amjad, F. M., Scherer, P. E., Weiss, L. M., Nagajyothi, J., Roth, J., Tanowitz, H. B., & Kuliawat, R. (2017). Alterations in pancreatic β cell function and Trypanosoma cruzi infection: Evidence from human and animal studies. *Parasitology Research*, 116(3), 827–838.

ElSayed, N. A., Aleppo, G., Aroda, V. R., Bannuru, R. R., Brown, F. M., Bruemmer, D., Collins, B. S., Hilliard, M. E., Isaacs, D., Johnson, E. L., Kahan, S., Khunti, K., Leon, J., Lyons, S. K., Perry, M. L., Prahalad, P., Pratley, R. E., Seley, J. J., Stanton, R. C., Gabbay, R. A., on behalf of the American Diabetes Association. (2022). 2. Classification and diagnosis of diabetes: Standards of care in diabetes—2023. *Diabetes Care*, 46(Supplement_1), S19–S40.

Galicia-Garcia, U., Benito-Vicente, A., Jebari, S., Larrea-Sebal, A., Siddiqi, H., Uribe, K. B., Ostolaza, H., & Martín, C. (2020). Pathophysiology of type 2 diabetes mellitus. *International Journal of Molecular Sciences*, 21(17), 6275.

Goyal, A., Raina, S., Kaushal, S. S., Mahajan, V., & Sharma, N. L. (2010). Pattern of cutaneous manifestations in diabetes mellitus. *Indian Journal of Dermatology*, 55(1), 39.

Hieronymus, L., & Griffin, S. (2015). Role of amylin in type 1 and type 2 diabetes. *The Diabetes Educator*, 41(1_suppl), 47S-56S.

Hollander, M. H., Paarlberg, K. M., & Huisjes, A. J. M. (2007). Gestational diabetes: A review of the current literature and guidelines. *Obstetrical & Gynecological Survey*, 62(2), 125.

Insel, R. A., Dunne, J. L., Atkinson, M. A., Chiang, J. L., Dabelea, D., Gottlieb, P. A., Greenbaum, C. J., Herold, K. C., Krischer, J. P., Lernmark, Å., Ratner, R. E., Rewers, M. J., Schatz, D. A., Skyler, J. S., Sosenko, J. M., & Ziegler, A. G. (2015). Staging presymptomatic type 1 diabetes: A scientific statement of JDRF, the Endocrine Society, and the American Diabetes Association. *Diabetes Care*, 38(10), 1964–1974.

Jiang, G., & Zhang, B. B. (2003). Glucagon and regulation of glucose metabolism. *American Journal of Physiology-Endocrinology and Metabolism*, 284(4), E671–E678.

Kanikarla-Marie, P., & Jain, S. K. (2016). Hyperketonemia and ketosis increase the risk of complications in type 1 diabetes. *Free Radical Biology and Medicine*, 95, 268–277.

Khursheed, R., Singh, S. K., Wadhwa, S., Kapoor, B., Gulati, M., Kumar, R., Ramanunny, A. K., Awasthi, A., & Dua, K. (2019). Treatment strategies against diabetes: Success so far and challenges ahead. *European Journal of Pharmacology*, 862, 172625.

Krischer, J. P., Lynch, K. F., Schatz, D. A., Ilonen, J., Lernmark, Å., Hagopian, W. A., Rewers, M. J., She, J. X., Simell, O. G., Toppari, J., Ziegler, A. G., Akolkar, B., Bonifacio, E., & TEDDY Study Group. (2015). The 6-year incidence of diabetes-associated autoantibodies in genetically at-risk children: The TEDDY study. *Diabetologia*, 58(5), 980–987.

Lampasona, V., Petrone, A., Tiberti, C., Capizzi, M., Spoletini, M., di Pietro, S., Songini, M., Bonicchio, S., Giorgino, F., Bonifacio, E., Bosi, E., Buzzetti, R., & Non Insulin Requiring Autoimmune Diabetes (NIRAD) Study Group. (2009). Zinc transporter 8 antibodies complement GAD and IA-2 antibodies in the identification and characterization of adult-onset autoimmune diabetes: Non-insulin requiring autoimmune diabetes (NIRAD) 4. *Diabetes Care*, 33(1), 104–108.

Mauvais-Jarvis, F., Sobngwi, E., Porcher, R., Riveline, J. P., Kevorkian, J. P., Vaisse, C., Charpentier, G., Guillausseau, P. J., Vexiau, P., & Gautier, J. F. (2004). Ketosis-prone type 2 diabetes in patients of Sub-Saharan African origin: Clinical pathophysiology and natural history of β-cell dysfunction and insulin resistance. *Diabetes*, 53(3), 645–653.

McCormick, M., Hadley, D., McLean, J. R., Macfarlane, J. A., Condon, B., & Muir, K. W. (2010). Randomized, controlled trial of insulin for acute poststroke hyperglycemia. *Annals of Neurology*, 67(5), 570–578.

McGinty, J. W., Marré, M. L., Bajzik, V., Piganelli, J. D., & James, E. A. (2015). T cell epitopes and post-translationally modified epitopes in type 1 diabetes. *Current Diabetes Reports*, 15(11), 90.

Mlinar, B., Marc, J., Janež, A., & Pfeifer, M. (2007). Molecular mechanisms of insulin resistance and associated diseases. *Clinica Chimica Acta*, 375(1), 20–35.

Mozaffarian, D., Kamineni, A., Carnethon, M., Djoussé, L., Mukamal, K. J., & Siscovick, D. (2009). Lifestyle risk factors and new-onset diabetes mellitus in older adults: The cardiovascular health study. *Archives of Internal Medicine*, 169(8), 798–807.

Nishi, M. (2018). Diabetes mellitus and thyroid diseases. *Diabetology International*, 9(2), 108–112.

Ojha, A., Ojha, U., Mohammed, R., Chandrashekar, A., & Ojha, H. (2019). Current perspective on the role of insulin and glucagon in the pathogenesis and treatment of type 2 diabetes mellitus. *Clinical Pharmacology: Advances and Applications*, 11, 57–65.

Okur, M. E., Karantas, I. D., & Siafaka, P. I. (2017). Diabetes mellitus: A review on pathophysiology, current status of oral medications, and future perspectives. *ACTA Pharmaceutica Sciencia*, 55(1), 61-82.

Petersen, M. C., & Shulman, G. I. (2018). Mechanisms of insulin action and insulin resistance. *Physiological Reviews*, 98(4), 2133–2223.

Petersen, M. C., Graves, J. M., Yao, T., Schomburg, L., Minich, W. B., Parks, D. L., McGill, J. B., & Salam, M. (2022). Insulin receptor autoantibody–mediated hypoglycemia in a woman with mixed connective tissue disease. *Journal of the Endocrine Society*, 6(1), bvab182.

Pham, M., Oikonomou, D., Hornung, B., Weiler, M., Heiland, S., Bäumer, P., Kollmer, J., Nawroth, P. P., & Bendszus, M. (2015). Magnetic resonance neurography detects diabetic neuropathy early and with proximal predominance. *Annals of Neurology*, 78(6), 939–948.

Popoviciu, M. S., Paduraru, L., Nutas, R. M., Ujoc, A. M., Yahya, G., Metwally, K., & Cavalu, S. (2023). Diabetes mellitus secondary to endocrine diseases: An update of diagnostic and treatment particularities. *International Journal of Molecular Sciences*, 24(16), 12676.

Prentki, M., & Nolan, C. J. (2006). Islet β cell failure in type 2 diabetes. *The Journal of Clinical Investigation*, 116(7), 1802–1812.

Rakocevic, G., & Floeter, M. K. (2012). Autoimmune stiff person syndrome and related myelopathies: Understanding of electrophysiological and immunological processes. *Muscle & Nerve*, 45(5), 623–634.

Rani, V., Deep, G., Singh, R. K., Palle, K., & Yadav, U. C. S. (2016). Oxidative stress and metabolic disorders: Pathogenesis and therapeutic strategies. *Life Sciences*, 148, 183–193.

Roep, B. O., & Peakman, M. (2012). Antigen targets of type 1 diabetes autoimmunity. *Cold Spring Harbor Perspectives in Medicine*, 2(4), a007781.

Scaroni, C., Zilio, M., Foti, M., & Boscaro, M. (2017). Glucose metabolism abnormalities in Cushing syndrome: From molecular basis to clinical management. *Endocrine Reviews*, 38(3), 189–219.

Sosenko, J. M., Skyler, J. S., DiMeglio, L. A., Beam, C. A., Krischer, J. P., Greenbaum, C. J., Boulware, D., Rafkin, L. E., Matheson, D., Herold, K. C., Mahon, J., Palmer, J. P., Type 1 Diabetes TrialNet Study Group, & Diabetes Prevention Trial-Type 1 Study Group. (2015). A new approach for diagnosing type 1 diabetes in autoantibody-positive individuals based on prediction and natural history. *Diabetes Care*, 38(2), 271–276.

Tebay, L. E., Robertson, H., Durant, S. T., Vitale, S. R., Penning, T. M., Dinkova-Kostova, A. T., & Hayes, J. D. (2015). Mechanisms of activation of the transcription factor Nrf2 by redox stressors, nutrient cues, and energy status and the pathways through which it attenuates degenerative disease. *Free Radical Biology & Medicine*, 88(Pt B), 108–146.

Tesch, G. H. (2010). Macrophages and diabetic nephropathy. Seminars in Nephrology, 30(3), 290–301.

Thomas, C. C., & Philipson, L. H. (2015). Update on diabetes classification. *Medical Clinics of North America*, 99(1), 1–16.

Ukkola, O., & Santaniemi, M. (2002). Adiponectin: A link between excess adiposity and associated comorbidities? *Journal of Molecular Medicine*, 80(11), 696–702.

Whitehead, M., Osborne, A., Widdowson, P. S., Yu-Wai-Man, P., & Martin, K. R. (2019). Angiopoietins in diabetic retinopathy: Current understanding and therapeutic potential. *Journal of Diabetes Research*, 2019(1), 5140521.

Williams, G. M., Long, A. E., Wilson, I. V., Aitken, R. J., Wyatt, R. C., McDonald, T. J., Wong, F. S., Hattersley, A. T., Williams, A. J., Bingley, P. J., & Gillespie, K. M. (2016). Beta cell function and ongoing autoimmunity in long-standing, childhood onset type 1 diabetes. *Diabetologia*, 59(12), 2722–2726.

Yaribeygi, H., Sathyapalan, T., Atkin, S. L., & Sahebkar, A. (2020). Molecular mechanisms linking oxidative stress and diabetes mellitus. *Oxidative Medicine and Cellular Longevity*, 2020(1), 8609213.

Zelniker, T. A., & Braunwald, E. (2020). Mechanisms of cardiorenal effects of sodium-glucose cotransporter 2 inhibitors: JACC state-of-the-art review. *Journal of the American College of Cardiology*, 75(4), 422–434.

Zhao, X., An, X., Yang, C., Sun, W., Ji, H., & Lian, F. (2023). The crucial role and mechanism of insulin resistance in metabolic disease. *Frontiers in Endocrinology*, 14, 1149239.

Ziegler, A. G., Hummel, M., Schenker, M., & Bonifacio, E. (1999). Autoantibody appearance and risk for development of childhood diabetes in offspring of parents with type 1 diabetes: The 2-year analysis of the German BABYDIAB study. *Diabetes*, 48(3), 460–468.

Chapter 2

Current Treatment Approaches for Diabetes Mellitus

Suparna Majumder[1]
Ankita Das[2]
Tuhin Manna[1]
Kartik Chandra Guchhait[1]
Amiya Kumar Panda[3]
and Chandradipa Ghosh[1,*]
[1]Department of Human Physiology, Vidyasagar University, Midnapore, West Bengal, India
[2]Department of Physiology, Vidyasagar College for Women, Kolkata, West Bengal, India
[3]Department of Chemistry, Vidyasagar University, Midnapore, West Bengal, India

Abstract

Diabetes mellitus (DM) is a complex metabolic disorder characterized by elevated blood glucose levels due to the body's inability to produce or effectively utilize insulin. If left untreated or poorly managed, this chronic hyperglycemic condition can lead to long-term complications, including damage to various organs, which may result in cardiovascular diseases, nerve damage (neuropathy), kidney disease (nephropathy), and vision impairment (retinopathy). This chapter provides a comprehensive overview of current treatment approaches for DM, focusing on both type 1 and type 2 diabetes. It highlights the current treatment strategies, including lifestyle interventions, personalized medicine, pharmacological treatments such as insulin therapy and oral hypoglycemics, herbal treatments, and surgical options like bariatric surgery. Emerging therapies, including stem cell therapy and artificial pancreas technology, are also explored for managing the long-term detrimental effects of DM.

Keywords: diabetes mellitus, type 1 diabetes mellitus, type 2 diabetes mellitus, hyperglycemia, artificial pancreas, stem cell therapy

* Corresponding Author's Email: ch_ghosh@mail.vidyasagar.ac.in

In: Receptor-Targeted Therapies in Diabetes Mellitus
Editors: Ajmer Singh Grewal, Neelam Singh, Swati Verma et al.
ISBN: 979-8-89530-587-4

Abbreviations

AP	Artificial pancreas
BPD/DS	Biliopancreatic diversion with duodenal switch
CDMP	Chronic disease management program
DM	Diabetes mellitus
DPP-4 inhibitors	Dipeptidyl peptidase-4 inhibitors
DSME	Diabetes self-management education system
GLP-1	Glucagon-like peptide-1
HbA1c	Glycosylated haemoglobin
ITx	islet transplantation
MSCs	Mesenchymal stem cells
NAP	Neural-Net Artificial Pancreas
PAK	Pancreas after kidney transplant
PTA	Pancreas transplant alone
RYGB	Roux-en-Y gastric bypass
SG	Sleeve gastrectomy
SGLT2 inhibitors	Sodium Glucose Cotransporter-2 inhibitors
SPK	Simultaneous pancreas and kidney transplant
SU	Sulfonylureas
T1DM	Type 1 diabetes mellitus
T2DM	Type 2 diabetes mellitus

Introduction

Diabetes mellitus (DM) is an intricate and chronic metabolic health issue affecting millions of people worldwide. Global estimates suggest that over half a billion individuals have diabetes, accounting for more than 10.5% of people over 18 years old (Sun et al. 2021). It is defined as persistent hyperglycemia caused by either a lack of insulin synthesis, reduced insulin action, or a combination of both conditions (DiMeglio et al. 2018). This condition encompasses several disorders, the most common of which are type 1 DM (T1DM) and type 2 DM (T2DM), each with its distinct set of pathophysiological causes, clinical symptoms, and treatment options. T1DM is primarily caused by an autoimmune response, in which the body mistakenly attacks and destroys insulin-producing β-cells in the pancreas. This autoimmune imbalance results in a severe insulin deficit, requiring lifelong exogenous insulin treatment (Long & Buckner, 2022). T1DM often appears unexpectedly in adolescence or early childhood, though it can develop at any age. In contrast, T2DM is associated with insulin resistance, which occurs when the body's cells become less responsive to the effects of insulin. This insulin resistance often leads to a subsequent loss of β-cell function, ultimately resulting in inadequate insulin production (Galicia-Garcia et al. 2020). T2DM is closely associated with lifestyle factors such as obesity, lack of exercise, and poor nutrition, and its onset is often slow, typically occurring in adults. However, an increase in cases among younger populations is being observed. Gestational diabetes occurs during pregnancy, while monogenic diabetes is caused by genetic defects that affect β-cell function. Diabetes management involves various scientific approaches aimed at keeping blood sugar levels within an acceptable range to prevent or delay health complications. The treatment options differ according to the type of diabetes and the patient's individual characteristics. The objective of this chapter is to provide an in-depth understanding of DM management, with a focus on distinguishing treatment approaches for type 1 and type 2 diabetes. This chapter explores both traditional and innovative therapeutic strategies, including lifestyle modifications, personalized medicine, pharmacological interventions (such as insulin therapy and oral hypoglycemics), herbal remedies, and surgical options, such as bariatric surgery. Additionally, the chapter addresses emerging treatments, including stem cell therapy and artificial pancreas technology, which offer promising advancements in minimizing the chronic complications associated with DM.

Current Treatment Approaches

Lifestyle Interventions

Lifestyle modification is key to maintaining the metabolic changes associated with diabetes in the long run, and these modifications must include both physical activity and nutritional interventions. Modifications in the form of DSME (diabetes self-management education), counseling, physical activity, and psychological and social care are typically implemented. However, it is essential to first address the glycemic index through medical interventions, and lifestyle modifications should only be recommended after successful management of diabetes through comprehensive diagnosis and post-discharge medications (Haas et al. 2014). Studies have shown that lifestyle modification plays a significant role in lowering HbA1c, body weight, and the glycemic index, while reducing treatment costs and improving the quality of life (Deakin et al. 2005). A report by the National Health and Nutrition Examination Survey revealed that leading an active lifestyle (through physical activity or exercise for at least 60 minutes per day) and adopting good eating habits can lower the risk of diabetes and related cardiovascular diseases (Sisson et al. 2010). Physical activity is essential for preventing diabetes. It indirectly increases insulin sensitivity and helps prevent other diabetes-related complications. Moderate physical activities such as walking, household chores, swimming, playing, and dancing enhance both physical and mental strength. Therefore, combining lifestyle modifications with pharmacotherapy can significantly reduce the complications of diabetes.

Pharmacological Treatments

Pharmacological or pharmaco-therapeutic treatment for DM should be tailored to the specific type of diabetes. T1DM and gestational diabetes require insulin therapy, with T1DM necessitating lifelong insulin replacement (Sibony et al. 2023). Insulin preparations vary in terms of action duration and are administered at different stages, including rapid-acting, intermediate-acting, and long-acting insulins, as well as premixed options and subcutaneous insulin injections for effective delivery. Treatment typically begins with a lower dose, gradually increasing to achieve optimal control (Thota & Akbar, 2024). The American Diabetes Association also advocates for lifestyle modifications alongside metformin monotherapy as an initial approach to diabetes management. Effective diabetes treatment must address multiple aspects beyond glycemic control, including cardiovascular risk reduction, and should be individualized based on patient needs, risk factors, and health status. The goal is to provide a comprehensive approach to managing the condition and improving long-term outcomes.

Insulin Therapy

Normal insulin production is impaired in diabetic patients, leading to elevated blood sugar levels. However, not all patients with T2DM require insulin, whereas patients with T1DM need a daily supply of insulin for their entire life. The treatment process, however, differs from individual to individual. Some patients may need two or more doses of insulin each day, using various methods such as pumps, pens, injections, or inhalers. Additionally, selecting the appropriate type of insulin is crucial, as it helps customize an effective and safe insulin therapy for T1DM patients. Since insulin is a prescribed medication, patients should consult a physician before beginning any insulin therapy to gain a clear understanding of the appropriate form of insulin, potential side effects, and how to administer insulin injections correctly. Patients must also monitor their blood sugar levels daily, as taking too high or too low a dose of insulin can lead to several side effects. It is essential for patients to stick to their prescribed treatment schedule, taking each dose at the same or correct time every day (Nkonge et al. 2023). If any complications arise during therapy, patients should immediately consult their physician to make suitable adjustments to the treatment. The timing of insulin injections is critical, as blood sugar levels can drop rapidly, leading to hypoglycemia, which could result in unconsciousness. Insulin therapy may cause weight gain and hypoglycemia in individuals with T1DM. On the other hand, individuals with T2DM or gestational diabetes may never require insulin therapy and can manage their condition with non-insulin medications and lifestyle modifications.

Oral Hypoglycemic Agents

The choice of oral drug therapy for T2DM is highly complex, as numerous drugs are available on the market for treatment. Selecting the best combination of drugs is critical for physicians, depending on clinical judgment. This selection becomes particularly important for patients undergoing long-term treatment, as their response to medications can change over time. Sulfonylureas (SUs) stimulate the β-cells of the pancreas to produce insulin. They act on SU receptors on pancreatic beta cells, which open calcium channels and ultimately lead to insulin secretion from the pancreas. These drugs also improve insulin sensitivity and reduce hepatic glucose production. A common side effect associated with SUs is hypoglycemia, as insulin release is not regulated by blood glucose levels. First-generation SUs includes tolbutamide, chlorpropamide, tolazamide, and acetohexamide, while second-generation SUs include glimepiride, glipizide, glibenclamide, and gliclazide. Biguanides, such as metformin, have insulin-sensitizing properties. Metformin is considered the first choice for treating T2DM, as it is efficient, safe, and cost-effective (Garber et al. 2017). It helps reduce glucose production in the liver and improves insulin sensitivity (An & He, 2016). Additionally, metformin positively affects various physiological parameters, including hemostasis, oxidative stress, lipid profiles, endothelial function, and fat redistribution. Metformin is available as a single-pill option with a fixed dosage or in combination with other glucose-reducing agents, such as thiazolidinediones and sulfonylureas. Some patients may experience gastric intolerance with metformin formulations, which can often be improved by switching to extended-release or other formulations. Patients with chronic kidney disease are advised to avoid metformin and its formulations, as they may increase the risk of lactic acidosis (Inzucchi, 2016). Therefore, in these patients, it is advisable to assess renal function using an estimated glomerular filtration rate (eGFR) instead of solely relying on serum creatinine levels. DPP-4 inhibitors promote the enzymatic breakdown of incretin hormones, such as glucose-dependent insulinotropic polypeptide and GLP-1, by lowering serum DPP-4 levels. This, in turn, enhances pancreatic insulin production while inhibiting glucagon release from the pancreas. These agents (such as alogliptin or pioglitazone) can be administered as monotherapy or in combination with biguanides. Studies have shown that they reduce HbA1c levels and have blood pressure-lowering effects (Zhang & Zhao, 2016). DPP-4 inhibitors are generally considered safe and well tolerated, with a low risk of hypoglycemia. However, if severe joint pain or pancreatitis is reported, the treatment should be discontinued. Since most DPP-4 inhibitors are eliminated through urine, clinical trials and dosage adjustments should be conducted for patients receiving treatment with saxagliptin or alogliptin. SGLT2 inhibitors reduce hyperglycemia and promote urinary glucose excretion by acting on the kidneys. Normally, the kidneys reabsorb almost all filtered glucose, but evidence suggests that patients with T2DM show increased SGLT2 expression, leading to higher blood glucose levels and increased glucose reabsorption. SGLT2 inhibitors counteract this by increasing urinary glucose excretion by 50%, which helps lower hyperglycemia (Abdul-Ghani et al. 2013). These can also be used in combination with other hypoglycemic agents due to their non-insulin-dependent mode of action. Thiazolidinediones act by activating intracellular receptors, which increases insulin sensitivity in muscle. Their effects take longer to become evident. Body weight gain and subcutaneous fat deposition are among the side effects of thiazolidinediones. They can also be used in combination with sulfonylureas and biguanides. Examples include rosiglitazone and pioglitazone.

Non-Insulin Injectable Medications

Non-insulin injectable medications include glucose-dependent insulinotropic polypeptide and GLP-1. Both act as incretin hormones that increase insulin release from the pancreas after intravenous glucose injection. They also reduce glucagon secretion from the pancreas and delay gastric emptying, which ultimately leads to suppressed appetite and reduced body weight. These medications mimic the action of human GLP-1 but with more stable pharmacodynamic properties. GLP-1 receptor agonists, such as exenatide and lixisenatide (short-acting), are less similar to the human GLP-1 molecule, while dulaglutide and albiglutide (long-acting) are more closely aligned. Studies have shown that GLP-1 receptor agonists significantly reduce HbA1c in patients receiving pharmacological therapy (Madsbad, 2016). When GLP-1 receptor agonists are used in combination with insulin or other insulin-stimulating drugs like sulfonylureas, they may cause gastrointestinal disorders. Therefore, patients with gastrointestinal diseases are typically not recommended GLP-1 receptor agonist therapy. Patients with a family history of thyroid carcinoma or endocrine neoplasia are also advised against using GLP-1 receptor agonists. However, no clear association between these conditions and GLP-1 receptor agonist therapy has been established in any studies. Therapy should be discontinued if acute pancreatitis is suspected in patients receiving GLP-1 receptor agonist treatment. Renal function should also be monitored if the patient experiences adverse gastrointestinal reactions after treatment.

Surgical Interventions

Surgical interventions in DM are complicated due to the high prevalence of specific complications associated with the disease, such as cardiovascular issues, obesity-related conditions, and diabetic foot pathologies. Surgical procedures in diabetic patients are generally considered high-risk due to challenges related to surgery and anesthesia, which may impair hyperglycemia and ketoacidosis, resulting in prolonged hospital stays and the need for meticulous metabolic control to reduce complications (Cali & Pérez, 2023). However, early diagnosis of diabetic foot complications, including infections, ulcers, and Charcot arthropathy, may necessitate surgical intervention with care to mitigate adverse outcomes. Surgical options range from conservative surgeries to amputations and reconstructive procedures, each tailored to the individual patient's profile (Roberts et al. 2024). Hybrid surgical interventions, particularly in patients with combined arterial lesions, have shown improved outcomes in terms of arterial bed capacity and surgical results, emphasizing the importance of advanced diagnostic tools and novel surgical techniques (Didenko, 2018). Currently, bariatric surgery and pancreatic transplantation are considered valuable options for minimizing DM related complications and morbidity.

Bariatric Surgery

This surgical method, primarily aimed at weight loss, has demonstrated significant benefits in diabetes control. In many cases, it has led to rapid and sustainable remission of T2DM. It is a well-established fact that individuals who undergo bariatric surgery reduce their use of diabetic medications and insulin intake. Multiple cases have reported an 87% reduction in oral medications and around a 79% decrease in insulin requirements post-operatively (Affinati et al. 2019). The key objective of this surgery is to achieve significant and long-term weight loss, which in turn alleviates obesity-related comorbidities like T2DM. Bariatric procedures can be broadly classified into: i) restrictive, ii) malabsorptive, or a combination of both. Restrictive procedures, such as sleeve gastrectomy (SG), involve reducing two-thirds of the stomach size along the stomach curvature to limit food intake, followed by stitching the stomach's open edges to form a tubular or banana shape. This is an irreversible process that involves laparoscopic techniques. Although SG is currently the most commonly performed bariatric surgery due to its effectiveness and lower complication rates (Poghosyan & Baratte, 2022), it is not very effective in treating T2DM. Roux-en-Y gastric bypass (RYGB) is a malabsorptive procedure that involves rerouting the intestines to decrease nutrient absorption. A new connection is created between the upper part of the stomach and the small intestine, which results in reduced nutrient absorption in the gut (Pucci & Batterham, 2019). Additionally, gut hormone levels are altered by the surgery resulting in a complete reset of hunger and satiety levels. RYGB remains the reference procedure because it addresses both weight loss and metabolic complications, making it particularly effective for patients with T2DM. Lately, another type of bariatric surgery, biliopancreatic diversion with duodenal switch (BPD/DS) has gained popularity due to its higher efficacy. BPD/DS is a multiple step procedure and in the first step SG is performed, which results in permanent stomach size reduction. This is followed up by change is small intestine and stomach connection. An alimentary limb is created by connecting ileum of small intestine with stomach. In the final step, residual intestinal segments are joined so that digestive fluids from the gallbladder and pancreas can enter the newly formed alimentary limb (Conner & Nottingham, 2024). In comparison to SG and RYGB, BPD/DS is more effective in weight loss as well as T2DM. Meta-analysis study reveals that bariatric surgery could reduce mortality by 59% in T2DM obese adults and increased life expectancy of 5 years (Syn et al. 2021). Bariatric surgery can be performed with recommendations of The International Diabetes Federation Task in case of individuals with BMI of 30-35 and subsequent failure of conventional T2DM Additionally, gut hormone levels are altered by the surgery, resulting in a complete reset of hunger and satiety levels. Roux-en-Y gastric bypass (RYGB) remains the reference procedure because it addresses both weight loss and metabolic complications, making it particularly effective for patients with T2DM. Recently, another type of bariatric surgery, biliopancreatic diversion with duodenal switch (BPD/DS), has gained popularity due to its higher efficacy. BPD/DS is a multi-step procedure. In the first step, sleeve gastrectomy (SG) is performed, resulting in permanent stomach size reduction. This is followed by a change in the connection between the small intestine and stomach. An alimentary limb is created by connecting the ileum of the small intestine with the stomach. In the final step, the residual intestinal segments are joined so that digestive fluids from the gallbladder and pancreas can enter the newly formed alimentary limb (Conner & Nottingham, 2024). In comparison to SG and RYGB, BPD/DS is more effective in both weight loss and T2DM management. A meta-analysis reveals that bariatric surgery can reduce mortality by 59% in obese adults with T2DM and increase life expectancy by five years (Syn et al. 2021). Bariatric surgery can be performed based on recommendations from The International Diabetes Federation Task Force in cases of individuals with a BMI of 30-35 and subsequent failure of conventional T2DM therapies.

Pancreatic Transplantation

Pancreatic transplantation has emerged as a key therapeutic option for patients with T2DM. It aims to restore endogenous insulin secretion, achieving long-term normoglycemia and preventing severe hypoglycemia and other secondary complications. Pancreatic transplantations are generally categorized into three types: pancreas transplant alone (PTA), simultaneous pancreas and kidney transplant (SPK), and pancreas after kidney transplant (PAK). SPK is the most common procedure, particularly for individuals with end-stage renal disease, while PTA is recommended for non-uremic patients experiencing unstable diabetes. This procedure has significantly improved patient outcomes and graft survival rates, facilitated by advances in surgical techniques, immunosuppressive therapies, and refined criteria for patient and donor selection. One-year patient survival rates exceed 96%, with pancreas graft survival rates surpassing 90% for SPK and 86% for solitary transplants (Gruessner & Gruessner, 2023; Maria & Anna, 2023). Despite these advancements, the requirement for lifelong immunosuppression remains a substantial challenge due to the associated risks of infections and malignancies. Pancreatic islet transplantation (ITx) has also gained traction as a less invasive alternative, particularly for managing recurrent hypoglycemia in diabetes patients. ITx isolates islets from a donor pancreas and infuses them into the recipient's liver. This approach has shown high success rates in maintaining normoglycemia, although multiple infusions are often required (Robertson, 2023; Wolanin et al. 2023). However, long-term insulin independence is rarely achieved with ITx, and the procedure still requires immunosuppression (Maria & Anna, 2023; Robertson, 2023). Studies have shown that ITx can significantly reduce hypoglycemia and improve glycemic control, but the median graft survival is approximately 5.9 years, with insulin independence rates declining significantly over time (Maria & Anna, 2023). Additionally, ITx has been used for patients with chronic pancreatitis undergoing pancreatectomy, where auto-islet transplantation can be performed without the need for immunosuppression (Robertson, 2023). Pancreas transplantation is also being explored for the treatment of exocrine disorders, with patient and graft survival rates comparable to those observed in diabetic patients (Gruessner et al. 2024). Despite its complexities and associated risks, pancreas transplantation remains the only long-term treatment for diabetes that consistently restores euglycemia, halts, or reverses secondary complications. This, in turn, significantly improves the quality of life for recipients.

Emerging and Experimental Therapies

Apart from the previously discussed therapies, new-generation treatments have emerged alongside the existing medications for T2DM. Stem cell therapy (SCT) and artificial pancreas technologies have garnered significant attention and are considered promising future prospects in diabetes management strategies.

Stem Cell Therapy

SCT is emerging as a promising approach for treating T2DM, a condition characterized by insulin resistance and impaired insulin secretion. Mesenchymal stem cells (MSCs) have garnered particular interest due to their ability to differentiate into insulin-producing cells. Once transformed into insulin-secreting cells, MSCs enhance insulin sensitivity and reduce chronic inflammation (Ochyra & Łopuszyńska, 2024). Additionally, MSCs improve diabetes-related complications, such as kidney, heart, eye, and nerve damage, and accelerate wound healing. However, challenges remain in producing fully mature pancreatic β cells from stem cells. Further research is needed to optimize differentiation protocols and ensure the reliability and efficacy of these therapies. The positive outcomes of SCT in post-stroke diabetic patients also suggest broader applications for regenerative medicine in diabetes management (Vinski & Vinski, 2024). While current findings are promising, extensive research is required to establish standardized guidelines and address the technical, ethical, and regulatory challenges associated with SCT in diabetes (Cui et al. 2023). Overall, SCT represents a novel and potentially transformative approach to managing T2DM, offering hope for improved glycemic control and reduced complications in patients unresponsive to conventional treatments (Avogaro & Fadini, 2024).

Artificial Pancreas Technology

Artificial pancreas (AP) technology, initially developed for T1DM, is now increasingly used in the management of T2DM Renowned for its effectiveness in improving glucose control and reducing the burden of intensive insulin therapy, AP systems combine continuous glucose monitors and insulin pumps with advanced regulatory algorithms to automate insulin delivery. This integration helps maintain glucose levels within target ranges with minimal manual intervention (Nwokolo & Hovorka, 2023). Recent research highlights the benefits of AP technology for T2DM patients, particularly those requiring multiple daily insulin injections. For instance, a crossover study using a single-hormone AP system (insulin-only) in T2DM patients demonstrated significant improvements in glucose management (Nwokolo & Hovorka, 2023). Additionally, the Neural-Net AP (NAP), a novel system embedding insulin delivery algorithms into a neural network, has shown performance comparable to traditional model-predictive control algorithms but with lower computational demands. This suggests its potential for broader application in T2DM (Kovatchev et al. 2024). By incorporating multimedia data such as physical activity and meal information, AP systems can further personalize care, enhancing their effectiveness, particularly for elderly patients (Kalita et al. 2024). However, challenges persist, including data gaps caused by device errors or patient non-compliance (Kalita et al. 2024). Despite these hurdles, the clinical adoption of AP systems for T2DM is in its early stages. Currently, hybrid closed-loop systems, which require user-initiated prandial insulin delivery, represent the most advanced AP technology available. Fully closed-loop and dual-hormone systems remain under investigation, showing promise for improved efficacy and safety (Nwokolo & Hovorka, 2023). The integration of AP technology into T2DM care marks a significant advancement. Ongoing research is focused on optimizing these systems to ensure broader adoption and more effective management of diabetes.

Management of Diabetes Complications

Effective management of T2DM complications requires a holistic strategy that integrates both pharmacological and non-pharmacological interventions. Programs such as the Chronic Disease Management Program (CDMP) emphasize the significance of comprehensive education and counseling by medical professionals for optimal disease control (Hyun et al. 2023). A multidisciplinary approach including lifestyle modifications, regular risk assessments, and the use of advanced disease-modifying medications like SGLT2 inhibitors and GLP-1 receptor agonists is essential to enhance the overall well-being of individuals with diabetes (Abu-Alfa et al. 2023). Despite recent therapeutic advancements, global glycemic control remains suboptimal, particularly in regions such as the Asia-Pacific, where resource variability and diverse patient needs necessitate a balanced strategy that combines effective glucose management with cardio-renal risk reduction (Chan et al. 2023). The rising prevalence of T2DM has further exacerbated the burden of cardiovascular and microvascular complications, underscoring the importance of incorporating newer antihyperglycemic agents. These drugs not only optimize glycemic control but also reduce the risk of hypoglycemia and address cardiovascular risk factors such as dyslipidemia and hypertension (Napoli et al. 2020; Tsoutsouki et al. 2020). Innovative diabetes technologies, including continuous glucose monitoring systems and automated insulin delivery devices, offer enhanced glycemic management for patients requiring insulin therapy, enabling them to achieve target glucose levels more effectively (Daly & Hovorka, 2021). Furthermore, patient adherence to self-management practices has been shown to significantly lower the risk of microvascular complications such as nephropathy and neuropathy, highlighting the critical role of consistent self-care in managing T2DM (Mehravar et al. 2016). Altogether, these approaches underscore the importance of a comprehensive, personalized, and multidisciplinary strategy for managing T2DM and mitigating its associated complications.

Conclusion

DM is a chronic condition characterized by numerous risk factors and severe macrovascular and microvascular complications that significantly affect an individual's physical and mental well-being. The landscape of diabetes research and treatment is continually evolving, with the goal of improving the prognosis, diagnosis, treatment, and management of its various forms. A comprehensive understanding of the pathophysiology of both Type 1 and Type 2 diabetes is essential for effective treatment. Recent advancements in diabetes care have enhanced strategies for managing insulin resistance and secretion. However, the adequacy of current treatments in fully addressing underlying metabolic deficiencies remains an area of ongoing investigation. Recent studies have explored the genetic basis, signal transduction pathways, and cellular mechanisms of diabetes, providing valuable insights. Moreover, the development of precise and personalized therapeutic targets offers promising opportunities for more effective treatments, representing a significant step forward in diabetes care.

References

Abdul-Ghani, M. A., DeFronzo, R. A., & Norton, L. (2013). Novel hypothesis to explain why SGLT2 inhibitors inhibit only 30-50% of filtered glucose load in humans. *Diabetes*, 62(10), 3324–3328.

Abu-Alfa, A. K., Atallah, P. J., Azar, S. T., Dagher, E. C., Echtay, A. S., El-Amm, M. A., Hazkial, H. G., Kassab, R. Y., Medlej, R. C., Mohamad, M. A., & Lebanese Consortium for Early, Comprehensive Management of Type 2 Diabetes (LCECMD). (2023). Recommendations for Early and Comprehensive Management of Type 2 Diabetes and Its Related Cardio-Renal Complications. *Diabetes Therapy*, 14(1), 11–28.

Affinati, A. H., Esfandiari, N. H., Oral, E. A., & Kraftson, A. T. (2019). Bariatric Surgery in the Treatment of Type 2 Diabetes. *Current Diabetes Reports*, 19(12), 156.

An, H., & He, L. (2016). Current understanding of metformin effect on the control of hyperglycemia in diabetes. *The Journal of Endocrinology*, 228(3), R97-106.

Avogaro, A., & Fadini, G. P. (2024). Stem Cell Therapy in Diabetes. In *Textbook of Diabetes* (pp. 1137–1143). John Wiley & Sons, Ltd.

Cali, C., & Pérez, W. (2023). Consideraciones anestésicas en la diabetes mellitus: Revisión narrativa. *INSPILIP*, 7(21), Article 21.

Chan, S. P., Lim, L. L., Chan, J. C. N., & Matthews, D. R. (2023). Adjusting the Use of Glucose-Lowering Agents in the Real-World Clinical Management of People with Type 2 Diabetes: A Narrative Review. *Diabetes Therapy*, 14(5), 823–838.

Conner, J., & Nottingham, J. M. (2024). *Biliopancreatic Diversion with Duodenal Switch.* In StatPearls. StatPearls Publishing. http://www.ncbi.nlm.nih.gov/books/NBK563193/

Cui, Y. K., Shemet, Y. A., & Ziablitsev, S. V. (2023). The Use of Stem Cells in the Treatment of Diabetes. *Medical Science of Ukraine (MSU)*, 19(1), Article 1.

Daly, A., & Hovorka, R. (2021). Technology in the management of type 2 diabetes: Present status and future prospects. *Diabetes, Obesity and Metabolism*, 23(8), 1722–1732.

Deakin, T. A., McShane, C. E., Cade, J. E., & Williams, R. (2005). Group based training for self-management strategies in people with type 2 diabetes mellitus. *Cochrane Database of Systematic Reviews*, 2, CD003417.

Didenko, S. (2018). Hybrid surgical interventions in occlusive stenotic lesions of distal arteries in patients with diabetes mellitus. *Emergency Medicine*, (3.90), 86–89.

DiMeglio, L. A., Evans-Molina, C., & Oram, R. A. (2018). Type 1 diabetes. *The Lancet*, 391(10138), 2449-2462.

Galicia-Garcia, U., Benito-Vicente, A., Jebari, S., Larrea-Sebal, A., Siddiqi, H., Uribe, K. B., Ostolaza, H. and Martín, C., (2020). Pathophysiology of type 2 diabetes mellitus. *International Journal of Molecular Sciences*, 21(17), 6275.

Garber, A. J., Abrahamson, M. J., Barzilay, J. I., Blonde, L., Bloomgarden, Z. T., Bush, M. A., Dagogo-Jack, S., DeFronzo, R. A., Einhorn, D., Fonseca, V. A., Garber, J. R., Garvey, W. T., Grunberger, G., Handelsman, Y., Hirsch, I. B., Jellinger, P. S., McGill, J. B., Mechanick, J. I., Rosenblit, P. D., & Umpierrez, G. E. (2017). Consensus statement by the American Association of Clinical Endocrinologists and American College of Endocrinology on the comprehensive type 2 diabetes management algorithm–2017 executive summary. *Endocrine Practice*, 23(2), 207-238.

Gruessner, R. W., & Gruessner, A. C. (2023). Transplantation of the Pancreas. In *The Pancreas: An Integrated Textbook of Basic Science, Medicine, and Surgery*, Wiley, pp. 1323-1332.

Gruessner, R. W. G., Laftavi, M. R., Pankewycz, O., & Gruessner, A. C. (2024). Pancreas Transplantafion for the Treatment of Pancreafic Exocrine Disorders. *Journal of Surgery*, 4(1), 1158.

Haas, L., Maryniuk, M., Beck, J., Cox, C. E., Duker, P., Edwards, L., Fisher, E. B., Hanson, L., Kent, D., Kolb, L., McLaughlin, S., Orzeck, E., Piette, J. D., Rhinehart, A. S., Rothman, R., Sklaroff, S., Tomky, D., Youssef, G., & 2012 Standards Revision Task Force. (2014). National standards for diabetes self-management education and support. *Diabetes Care*, 37 Suppl 1(Suppl 1), S144-S153.

Inzucchi, S. E. (2016). *FDA drug safety communication: FDA revises warnings regarding use of the diabetes medicine metformin in certain patients with reduced kidney function.* U.S. Food and Drug Administration. https://www.fda.gov/drugs/drug-safety-and-availability/fda-drug-safety-communication-fda-revises-warnings-regarding-use-diabetes-medicine-metformin-certain. Accessed August 3, 2023.

Kalita, D., Sharma, H., & Mirza, K. B. (2024). Continuous Glucose, Insulin and Lifestyle Data Augmentation in Artificial Pancreas Using Adaptive Generative and Discriminative Models. *IEEE Journal of Biomedical and Health Informatics*, 28(8), 4963–4974.

Kovatchev, B., Castillo, A., Pryor, E., Kollar, L. L., Barnett, C. L., DeBoer, M. D., Brown, S. A., & for the NAP Study Team. (2024). Neural-Net Artificial Pancreas: A Randomized Crossover Trial of a First-in-Class Automated Insulin Delivery Algorithm. *Diabetes Technology & Therapeutics*, 26(6), 375–382.

Madsbad, S. (2016). Review of head-to-head comparisons of glucagon-like peptide-1 receptor agonists. *Diabetes, Obesity & Metabolism*, 18(4), 317–332.

Maria, G., & Anna, T. (2023). C191Pancreas Transplantation. In A. Abd-Elsayed & A. Abd-Elsayed (Eds.), *Advanced Anesthesia Review* (p. 0). Oxford University Press.

Mehravar, F., Mansournia, M. A., Holakouie-Naieni, K., Nasli-Esfahani, E., Mansournia, N., & Almasi-Hashiani, A. (2016). Associations between diabetes self-management and microvascular complications in patients with type 2 diabetes. *Epidemiology and Health*, 38, e2016004.

Napoli, R., Formoso, G., Piro, S., Targher, G., Consoli, A., & Purrello, F. (2020). Management of type 2 diabetes for prevention of cardiovascular disease. An expert opinion of the Italian Diabetes Society. *Nutrition, Metabolism and Cardiovascular Diseases*, 30(11), 1926–1936.

Nkonge, K. M., Nkonge, D. K., & Nkonge, T. N. (2023). Insulin Therapy for the Management of Diabetes Mellitus: A Narrative Review of Innovative Treatment Strategies. *Diabetes Therapy*, 14(11), 1801–1831.

Nwokolo, M., & Hovorka, R. (2023). The Artificial Pancreas and Type 1 Diabetes. *The Journal of Clinical Endocrinology & Metabolism*, 108(7), 1614–1623.

Ochyra, Ł., & Łopuszyńska, A. (2024). The use of stem cells in the treatment of diabetes mellitus and its complications—Review. *Journal of Education, Health and Sport*, 74, 51736.

Poghosyan, T., & Baratte, C. (2022). Bariatric surgery techniques. La Revue du Praticien, 72(2), 160-163.

Pucci, A., & Batterham, R. L. (2019). Mechanisms underlying the weight loss effects of RYGB and SG: Similar, yet different. *Journal of Endocrinological Investigation*, 42(2), 117–128.

Roberts, R. H. R., Davies-Jones, G. R., Brock, J., Satheesh, V., & Robertson, G. A. (2024). Surgical management of the diabetic foot: The current evidence. *World Journal of Orthopedics*, 15(5), 404–417.

Robertson, R. P. (2023). Brief Review: Pancreatic Islet Transplantation for Type 1 Diabetes in Humans. *OBM Transplantation*, 7(2), Article 2.

Sisson, S. B., Camhi, S. M., Church, T. S., Tudor-Locke, C., Johnson, W. D., & Katzmarzyk, P. T. (2010). Accelerometer-determined steps/day and metabolic syndrome. *American Journal of Preventive Medicine*, 38(6), 575–582.

Sun, H., Saeedi, P., Karuranga, S., Pinkepank, M., Ogurtsova, K., Duncan, B. B., Stein, C., Basit, A., Chan, J. C., Mbanya, J. C. and Pavkov, M. E., (2022). IDF Diabetes Atlas: Global, regional and country-level diabetes prevalence estimates for 2021 and projections for 2045. *Diabetes Research and Clinical Practice*, 183, 109119.

Syn, N. L., Cummings, D. E., Wang, L. Z., Lin, D. J., Zhao, J. J., Loh, M., Koh, Z. J., Chew, C. A., Loo, Y. E., Tai, B. C., Kim, G., So, J. B. Y., Kaplan, L. M., Dixon, J. B., & Shabbir, A. (2021). Association of metabolic-bariatric surgery with long-term survival in adults with and without diabetes: A one-stage meta-analysis of matched cohort and prospective controlled studies with 174 772 participants. *The Lancet*, 397(10287), 1830–1841.

Thota, S., & Akbar, A. (2024). *Insulin*; StatPearls [Internet]; StatPearls Publishing: Treasure Island, FL, USA. http://www.ncbi.nlm.nih.gov/books/NBK560688/.

Vinski, D. S., & Vinski, N. C. (2024). The Miracle of Stem Cell Therapy for Post-Stroke Patients with Type 2 Diabetes. *Journal of World Science*, 3(1), 8–15.

Sibony, R. W., Segev, O., Dor, S., & Raz, I. (2023). Drug Therapies for diabetes. *International Journal of Molecular Sciences*, 24(24), 17147.

Wolanin, M., Stachyra, B., Stawikowski, C., Zielonka, B., Osińska, A., Wolanin, I., Madej, K., Dengler, B., Kowalczyk, I., & Krawiec, P. (2023). Pancreatic Islet Transplantation in Patients suffering from Type 1 diabetes - Indications, methods, possible risks and future directions: A literature review. *Journal of Education, Health and Sport*, 32(1), Article 1.

Zhang, X., & Zhao, Q. (2016). Effects of dipeptidyl peptidase-4 inhibitors on blood pressure in patients with type 2 diabetes: A systematic review and meta-analysis. *Journal of hypertension*, 34(2), 167–175.

Chapter 3

Free Fatty Acid Receptors: Metabolic Regulation and Therapeutic Implications

Manasvi Saini[1]
and Ria Kaushik[2,*]
[1]College of Pharmacy, Shivalik Campus, Dehradun, Uttrakhand, India
[2]Parmarth College of Pharmacy, Hapur Bypass, Acheja, Uttar Pradesh, India

Abstract

FFAR4, also known as GPR120, is a G-protein-coupled receptor activated by long-chain fatty acids that play a crucial role in metabolic regulation. This receptor is predominantly expressed in tissues involved in energy balance, including the intestines, adipose tissue, and macrophages. Activation of FFAR4 influences various metabolic pathways, promoting anti-inflammatory effects, enhancing insulin sensitivity, and increasing energy expenditure. These effects are mediated through multiple signaling pathways, such as the inhibition of the NLRP3 inflammasome and the modulation of the PI3K/Akt and MAPK pathways. FFAR4 is a promising therapeutic target for managing metabolic disorders, including Type 2 diabetes, non-alcoholic fatty liver disease (NAFLD), and obesity. FFAR4 agonists have shown potential in preclinical and clinical studies by improving insulin sensitivity, reducing inflammation in adipose tissue, and supporting weight loss. Current research delves into the mechanisms underlying these metabolic benefits and evaluates the therapeutic potential of FFAR4-targeted interventions. Future studies aim to develop selective and potent FFAR4 agonists, investigate tissue-specific effects, and conduct long-term safety and efficacy assessments in clinical settings, paving the way for novel treatments for metabolic disorders.

Keywords: G-protein-coupled receptors, nucleotide-binding oligomerization domain-like receptors, phosphoinositide 3-kinase

* Corresponding Author's Email: riakaushik01@gmail.com

In: Receptor-Targeted Therapies in Diabetes Mellitus
Editors: Ajmer Singh Grewal, Neelam Singh, Swati Verma et al.
ISBN: 979-8-89530-587-4

Abbreviations

7-TM receptors	7-Transmembrane domain receptors
ALS	Amyotrophic Lateral Sclerosis
AMPK	AMP-Activated Protein Kinase
CCK	Cholecystokinin
CYP450	Cytochrome P450 Enzyme Family
FDA	Food and Drug Administration
FFARs	Free fatty acid receptors
GIP	Glucose-Dependent Insulinotropic Polypeptide
GIPR	Glucose-Dependent Insulinotropic Polypeptide Receptor
GIT	Gastrointestinal Tract
GLP-1	Glucagon-Like Peptide-1
GLP-1R	Glucagon-Like Peptide-1 Receptor
GLUT	Glucose Transporter
GPCRs	G-protein-coupled receptors
GSIS	Glucose-Stimulated Insulin Secretion
HupA	Huperzine A
IGF-1	Insulin-Like Growth Factor-1
IL-6	Interleukin-6
IRS	Insulin Receptor Substrate
mTOR	Mechanistic Target of Rapamycin
NAFLD	Non-alcoholic fatty liver disease
NF-κB	Nuclear Factor Kappa B
NO	Nitric Oxide
OXM	Oxyntomodulin
PCR	Polymerase Chain Reaction
PD	Parkinson's Disease
PDE	Phosphodiesterase
PFAS	Per- and Polyfluoroalkyl Substances
PI3K	Phosphoinositide 3-Kinase
PKA	Protein Kinase A
SSRI	Selective Serotonin Reuptake Inhibitor
STC-1	Murine Enteroendocrine Cell Line STC-1
TMD	Transmembrane Domain
TNF-α	Tumor Necrosis Factor Alpha

Introduction

G-protein-coupled receptors (GPCRs) are membrane-bound receptors composed of a single polypeptide chain that act as molecular messengers, relaying external signals into the cell to initiate cellular responses (Bryne et al. 2014). Due to their critical signaling roles, GPCRs are considered promising therapeutic targets in modern drug research (Zhou & Wild, 2019). It is estimated that humans have around 850 GPCRs, each with specific expression patterns linked to distinct cell types or tissues, and serving various physiological and therapeutic functions (Gottesman-Katz et al. 2021). GPCRs are also known as 7-transmembrane domain receptors (7-TM receptors), heptahelical receptors, or serpentine receptors, and they play a vital role in cellular processes, with approximately 370 of them identified as potential drug targets. Mutations in human GPCRs are rare. Free fatty acid receptors (FFARs), a subgroup of GPCRs, have gained attention as potential treatments for obesity and Type 2 diabetes due to their ability to sense fatty acids (Eleazu et al. 2018). Among this group, GPR40 (FFAR1) and GPR120 (FFAR4) are particularly notable therapeutic targets for diabetes and metabolic conditions (Eleazu et al. 2018). Many dietary molecules or metabolites function as nutrition sensors by binding to "class A" or rhodopsin-like GPCRs. Specifically, GPR40 and GPR120, renamed FFAR1 and FFAR4, respectively, are activated by long-chain fatty acids, which serve as primary endogenous activators of these receptors (Reimann et al. 2012). FFAR1 has been validated as a therapeutic target for regulating blood glucose levels, while studies in rodent models suggest that FFAR4 may help modulate glucose levels and improve insulin sensitivity (Ghislain & Poitout, 2017). Recent research indicates expanding FFAR4 studies to areas beyond metabolic disorders, including pulmonary function and resistance to platinum-based chemotherapies. FFAR4/GPR120, part of the rhodopsin GPCR family, is emerging as a key therapeutic target for metabolic diseases, inflammation, and cancer (Milligan et al. 2017). Several patents on potential FFAR4-targeted chemotypes have been published by various companies, many of which were filed after 2013 (Formicola et al. 2015). GPCRs located in pancreatic beta cells, such as those for GLP-1, GIP, glucagon, somatostatin, pancreatic polypeptide, cholecystokinin, peptide YY, oxyntomodulin, and ghrelin, play essential roles in regulating peptide secretion (Urban et al. 2007). Fatty acid GPCRs, including short-chain FFARs (GPR41, GPR43), medium-chain FFARs (GPR84), long-chain FFARs (GPR40, GPR120), and cannabinoid-like receptors (GPR55, GPR119), are increasingly recognized for their roles in modulating peptide secretions. Numerous clinical trials are exploring peptide GPCR-based therapies, including double- and triple-agonist peptides (Moran et al. 2016). This chapter provides an overview of FFAR4 (GPR120) and its role in metabolic regulation. It explores FFAR4's activation by long-chain fatty acids and its expression in energy-regulating tissues, as well as its impact on signaling pathways like PI3K/Akt and MAPK, alongside its anti-inflammatory effects.

Discovery and Evolution of Orphan GPCR

GPR120 was identified and characterized in the early 2000s using genomic and bioinformatics methods aimed at discovering novel GPCRs (Alfonzo-Méndez et al. 2016). Historically, pharmacological research often began by identifying a biologically significant response to a ligand, which then led to the discovery of the receptor responsible for that response (Urban et al. 2007). The identification of the broader GPCR family occurred when it was found that the β2-adrenoceptor shared sequence homology and the characteristic seven-transmembrane structure with rhodopsin. This discovery marked a shift in research approaches and enabled DNA hybridization and PCR-based methods to rapidly identify additional GPCRs (Scholten, 2012). However, many receptors identified through these methods were "orphans", as their ligands remained unknown (Wise et al. 2004). Research on orphan GPCRs took a reverse approach, using the receptor to search for possible ligands instead of starting with the ligand (Ngo et al. 2016). This was done through methods such as sequence homology with known ligands and analyzing the receptor's tissue distribution (So et al. 2020). As more orphan GPCRs were discovered, these approaches became less effective, leading researchers to adopt high-throughput techniques, which entailed screening a large number of known or putative GPCR ligands that interact with the orphan receptors. This reverse pharmacology method has been successful in identifying new therapeutic targets, although the pace of deorphanization has slowed in recent years. Orphan receptor research has also presented unique experimental challenges in validating these receptors as viable therapeutic targets. After pairing an orphan GPCR with its endogenous ligands, detailed characterization is often needed before it can be considered for therapeutic use. Initial screening for deorphanization typically focuses on GPCR activation indicators that are independent of prior signaling pathways, such as receptor internalization, β-arrestin interaction, and Ca2+ mobilization through chimeric or promiscuous G proteins. A key challenge is determining the G protein coupling and signaling pathways the receptor normally activates. Further steps in receptor pharmacology involve understanding how ligands interact with the receptor, which can then inform the development of selective ligands. Another essential aspect of advancing poorly characterized receptors as therapeutic targets is identifying specific diseases or conditions the receptor may help treat. This process typically begins by investigating the receptor's biological role using *in vitro* and *in vivo* models, such as receptor knockdown or knockout studies, and exploring genetic links or polymorphisms that suggest disease associations. Once the receptor's biological functions are understood, potential therapeutic applications for ligands targeting the receptor can be explored and validated through proof-of-concept studies. Free fatty acid-activated GPCRs (FFARs) are a subset of GPCRs that have gained attention as efficient therapeutic targets for various diseases. This group includes three receptors in the FFAR family: FFAR1, FFAR2, and FFAR3, as well as two additional receptors, GPR120 and GPR84.

Structure Elaboration of GPR120

GPR120, located at chromosomal position 10q23.33, was initially identified by Fredriksson et al. through a search of databases for rhodopsin-like G protein-coupled receptors (GPCRs) (Fredriksson et al. 2003). Key active sites within the transmembrane domains (TMD) of GPR120 include Arg 2.64 at the top of TMD2 and Arg 4.65 at the top of TMD4, which may interact with the carboxylate groups of agonists. Animal studies indicate that GPR120-short mice fed a high-calorie diet tend to become obese, develop glucose intolerance, decrease lipogenesis, and show reduced adipocyte differentiation. Moreover, GPR120 expression is increased in the adipose tissue of obese subjects compared to lean controls. A harmful nonsynonymous mutation (p.R270H) has been associated with an elevated risk of obesity by inhibiting the GPR120 signaling pathway, underscoring its crucial role in maintaining energy balance in both rodents and humans (Carullo et al. 2021). The human GPR120 receptor has two identified sequences in the UniProt database: Q5NUL3 and Q5NUL3-2. The primary structural difference between the long isoform, GPR120L (Q5NUL3, consisting of 377 residues), and the short isoform, GPR120S (Q5NUL3-2, comprising 361 residues), is the inclusion of 16 additional amino acids in the third intracellular loop of GPR120L, which may confer distinct signaling properties. This third intracellular loop is critical for G-protein and β-arrestin interactions in rhodopsin-like GPCRs (Watson et al. 2012). Only one variant closely resembles the human equivalent in mice, rats, and cynomolgus monkeys. A pharmacological comparison of the functional activity of human GPR120 receptors and the human splice variant was established in 2009, demonstrating that the pharmacology of both species is similar. This was evidenced by measuring intracellular calcium release in cells expressing these sequences, triggered by free fatty acids (FFAs) and the small molecule GPR120 agonist GW9508 (Table 1) (Moore et al. 2009). GPR120L contains four phospho-labile serine/threonine residues in the additional region of its third intracellular loop. However, the degree and rate of phosphorylation of the two human GPR120 variants after agonism did not differ significantly. Interestingly, evidence suggests that the additional gap in the third loop may contain constitutive phosphorylation sites, indicating that basal phosphorylation of GPR120S is more prominent in the absence of an agonist (Burns et al. 2010). Furthermore, Watson et al. employed calcium mobilization and dynamic mass redistribution (DMR) tests to investigate the signaling and movement of GPR120S and GPR120L within cells. Their research indicated that GPR120L's third intracellular loop can couple with β-arrestin but loses its ability to trigger intracellular calcium and DMR responses. Distinct tissues exhibit unique pathways for signal transduction through the GPR120 receptor. In adipose tissue and enteroendocrine cells of the gastrointestinal tract, the Gq/G11 pathway predominates. In contrast, GPR120 activation in macrophages reduces inflammation by forming scaffolds with β-arrestin.

Table 1. Expression and function of FFAR4 in different tissues and cells (Liu et al. 2015)

Tissues	Cell/cell line	Functions
Adipose tissue	3T3-L1, M1-like Macrophage	Stimulating glucose uptake, angiogenesis, and adipogenesis, anti-inflammation; ameliorate adipose inflammation and insulin resistance
Digestive tract	K cell STC-1 cell, Glutag cell	Secreting GIP Secreting CCK, GLP-1, and GLP-2
	SSG-1, MGN3-1, GOC	Decrease the secretion of ghrelin
Liver	Macrophage Kupffer cells	Anti-inflammation
	WB-F344	Promote glucose uptake and motile activity
	Huh-7	Lipid droplet formation
Islet	MIN-6, INS-1, BRIN-BDII	Promote cell proliferation and insulin secretion
	Delta cell	Decrease the secretion of somatostatin
Colorectal cancer cells	HCT 116, SW480	Promote proliferation
Bone	ATDC5	Bone Osteoblastic action and accelerates bone growth
	Bone marrow-derived	Anti-apoptosis
	Macrophages	
Heart		Promote glucose uptake
Skeletal muscle		Promote glucose uptake
Lung	Clara cell	Production and/or secretion of surfactant
Hypothalamus	rHypoE-7	Anti-inflammation
Umbilical cord	Human umbilical vein endothelial cells	Anti-inflammation, inhibiting VEGF-induced cell migration
Breast cancer cells	MDA-MB-231 MCF-7	Promote cell proliferation and invasion

This chapter will outline the unique biological roles and current state of GPR120 agonists, supported by both *in vitro* and *in vivo* research. Mice, rats, and the murine enteroendocrine cell line STC-1 are stimulated to secrete incretin hormones and FFAs (Fredriksson et al. 2003). Additionally, FFAs have been shown to inhibit apoptosis induced by serum deprivation through GPR120 in STC-1 cells (Katsuma et al. 2005). Beyond Gq-dependent pathways, activated GPR120 enhances glucose uptake in adipocytes and promotes anti-inflammatory responses in macrophages via the β-arrestin 2 signaling pathway (Oh et al. 2010). GPR120 mRNA is widely expressed in various cell types, including taste cells (Matsumura et al. 2007), gastric ghrelin cells (Lu et al. 2012), duodenal enteroendocrine I cell (Sykaras et al. 2012), murine K cells (Parker et al. 2009), adipocytes, and macrophages (Cornish et al. 2008), as well as osteoblasts and osteocalcin (Reber et al. 2007). GPR120 is also expressed in several cell lines, such as mouse GLUTag cells (Janssen et al. 2012), the murine enteroendocrine cell line STC-1 (Soto-Guzman et al. 2008), the ghrelin-producing cell line MGN3–1 (Whalley et al. 2011), the human breast cancer cell line MCF-7 (Morgan & Dhayal, 2009), the islet-α cell line αTC1–6 (Navarro-Tito et al. 2008), human RAW 264.7 cells (Morgan et al. 2016), rat β-cell lines (Ahrén, 2009), human MDA-MB-231 breast cancer cells (Fredriksson et al. 2003), and human MCF-7 and MCF10A cells (Lagerström and Schiöth et al. 2008).

Pharmacology of GPCRs

GPCRs form the largest superfamily of integral membrane proteins in the human body. The human genome encodes approximately 400 non-odorant GPCRs, which respond to various stimuli, including hormones, neurotransmitters, ions, lipids, photons, and peptides (Fredriksson et al. 2003). Due to their crucial role in mediating signals from extracellular ligands to trigger intracellular responses, GPCRs have emerged as highly effective drug targets. It is estimated that about 30% of currently used drugs act on GPCRs (Hopkins et al. 2002). Despite this success, only around 30 of the more than 400 non-odorant GPCRs have been targeted by existing medications, indicating a wealth of untapped opportunities in GPCR-related drug development. Historically, pharmaceutical research on GPCRs began by investigating biological responses to ligands and subsequently identifying the corresponding receptors (Hudson et al. 2011). However, this approach evolved after the discovery that the β2-adrenoceptor and rhodopsin shared sequence similarities. This revelation enabled researchers to swiftly identify new GPCRs using techniques such as DNA hybridization and PCR. Nevertheless, many of these newly discovered receptors were classified as "orphan" receptors due to the absence of known ligands (Dixon et al. 1986). The study of orphan GPCRs reversed the traditional pharmacological approach, with researchers now focusing on identifying ligands for these receptors rather than the other way around. Early investigations relied on sequence homology between orphan receptors and known GPCRs, along with their tissue distribution, to predict potential ligands (Civelli, 2012; Chung et al. 2008). Furthermore, orphan GPCR research presents challenges in validating these receptors as viable therapeutic targets. Even after identifying an endogenous ligand for an orphan GPCR, extensive work is required to develop the receptor into a drug target. Initial steps typically involve assays for GPCR activation, including receptor internalization, β-arrestin association, and Ca^{2+} mobilization, to elucidate the signaling pathways utilized by the receptor (Frooninckx et al. 2012). Subsequent studies focus on understanding ligand-receptor binding dynamics, facilitating the development of selective ligands (Alexander et al. 2011). In addition to grasping receptor pharmacology, researchers must also predict and confirm the diseases and conditions that the receptor could potentially treat. This process often employs methods such as receptor knockdown or knockout in cellular or animal models, investigating disease associations through genomics, and exploring the biological functions of the receptor *in vitro* and *in vivo*. The challenges involved in deorphanizing and characterizing GPCRs as drug targets vary for each receptor. However, there is much to be learned from how similar challenges were addressed in earlier research. One group of GPCRs that has attracted considerable interest as potential drug targets includes those activated by FFAs, such as FFAR1, FFAR2, FFAR3, GPR120, and GPR84 (Tsuda et al. 2017). Research has investigated the therapeutic potential of these FFARs, highlighting both the progress achieved and the challenges that remain to be overcome to fully exploit their clinical value (Milligan et al. 2009).

Research and Therapeutic Potential of FFAR

FFAR1

FAR1, a receptor highly expressed in pancreatic cells and the intestine, has gained attention as a promising therapeutic target due to its crucial role in glucose-stimulated insulin secretion (GSIS) in response to free fatty acids. FFAR1 mediates GSIS, and studies on FFAR1 knockout and transgenic mice suggest it offers a protective effect against toxicity caused by chronic or excessive glucose stimulation in pancreatic cells (Itoh et al. 2003; Mancini and Poitout, 2013). Insulin secretion mediated by FFAR1 involves the depolymerization of F-actin and the activation of protein kinase D1 (PKD1) (Abaraviciene et al. 2013). Beyond insulin regulation, FFAR1 is also present in glucagon-producing pancreatic cells, where it contributes to glucagon secretion. In the intestine, FFAR1 expression has been identified in cells responsible for incretin secretion, such as K cells for gastric inhibitory polypeptide (GIP) and L cells for GLP-1 (Hirasawa et al. 2005). Additionally, FFAR1 is found in intestinal cells that produce cholecystokinin (CCK), further implicating FFAR1 in the indirect regulation of insulin secretion (Oh et al. 2010). Elevated FFAR1 expression in pancreatic cells corresponds with an increased insulin response to glucose, underscoring its dual role in both direct and indirect insulin regulation. Together with GPR120, FFAR1 represents a viable target for diabetes therapy due to its impact on GSIS. However, while numerous ligands for FFAR1 exist, the limited availability of synthetic ligands for GPR120 has constrained the understanding of its physiological roles. Additionally, despite advances in structural research on GPCRs like FFAR1, the lack of structural information on GPR120 (FFAR4) has impeded the rational design of its agonists (Briscoe et al. 2003).

FFAR4

FFAR4, a receptor expressed in the gut, adipose tissue, and taste buds, has emerged as a promising therapeutic target for metabolic disorders. In the gut, FFAR4 is found in intestinal

L-cells, where it promotes the secretion of GLP-1, a hormone crucial for glucose regulation, similar to the role of FFAR1 in these cells. In adipose tissue, FFAR4 helps regulate adipocyte differentiation and GLUT-4 translocation, both of which are vital for efficient glucose uptake. Studies involving GPR120 (FFAR4) knockout mice underscore FFAR4's key role in energy metabolism, and FFAR4 in macrophages has been linked to anti-inflammatory responses (Stuttgen and Sahoo, 2021). FFAR4 is activated by natural long-chain fatty acids, including both saturated and unsaturated types (Christiansen et al. 2015). Many polyunsaturated fatty acids act as dual agonists for FFAR4 and FFAR1, with omega-3 fatty acids such as αLA, DHA, EPA, and pinolenic acid demonstrating notable efficacy. DHA and EPA, for instance, have been used to study FFAR4's functions across various cell types and animal models. Although these fatty acids may also target FFAR1, PPARα, and RXRα, they remain valuable for their ability to form anti-inflammatory mediators like maresin 1 and resolvins (Ulven et al. 2015). EPA has been shown to reduce inflammation in cerebral ischemia models by inhibiting NLRP3 inflammasome activation, with this protective effect absent in FFAR1 and FFAR4 double-knockout animals (Serhan et al. 2018). DHA and EPA also increase FFAR4 protein expression and promote RAW264.7 macrophage cell proliferation (Mo et al. 2020). FFAR4 also shows therapeutic promise in immune modulation; DHA supplementation in FFAR4 mutant mice inhibited dendritic cell maturation and increased regulatory T cells, promoting a tolerogenic phenotype. In colitis models, DHA reduced symptoms of chronic colitis and enhanced FFAR4 expression through the TAK1/IKK-α/IκB-α/p65 pathway, suggesting a potential therapeutic approach for Crohn's disease (Han et al. 2017). Additionally, FFAR4 levels are lower in osteoarthritis patients than in healthy controls, and DHA-mediated FFAR4 activation reduced inflammation in chondrocytes and promoted wound healing in mouse models by reducing pro-inflammatory cells (Zhao et al. 2020). Endogenous FFAR4 ligands include branched fatty acid esters like 9-PAHSA, which enhance insulin-stimulated glucose absorption by activating FFAR4, supporting its role in glucose homeostasis (Yore et al. 2014).

Navigating the Challenges and Opportunities of FFAR1 and FFAR4 in Therapy

The physiological and pharmacological roles of receptors like FFAR1 and FFAR4 are becoming clearer, supported by an expanding range of synthetic ligands tested in both *in vitro* and *in vivo* models. Research has shown that FFAR1 couples exclusively with Gq proteins, while FFAR4 interacts with both Gq proteins and arrestin pathways (Salehi et al. 2005). However, the precise connections between these signaling pathways and specific physiological responses are not yet fully understood. For instance, receptor dimerization, a process known to impact ligand affinity, signaling outcomes, and physiological functions, could serve as a regulatory factor, especially since FFARs are often co-expressed in organs such as the immune system, gastrointestinal tract, and pancreas (Hirasawa et al. 2005). Understanding FFAR signaling and function is also complicated by inconsistent data on receptor expression levels. While some studies measure expression at the mRNA level, this does not always correlate with protein expression, highlighting the need for more accurate profiling. Moreover, although antibodies for FFAR1 and FFAR4 are commercially available, GPCR antibodies often require careful validation due to selectivity challenges. In developing targeted therapies, pathway-specific agonists (or biased ligands) could be particularly valuable, as these compounds selectively activate specific signaling pathways over others. This selectivity could be instrumental in isolating beneficial effects from potential side effects, making them promising therapeutic candidates. To advance FFAR1 and FFAR4 ligands as pharmaceutical agents, a screening system focused on individual signaling pathways, alongside comprehensive structure-activity relationship studies, would be essential. Such an approach could enable the separation of desirable effects from undesirable ones, optimizing the therapeutic profiles of these ligands (Salehi et al. 2005).

Conclusion

In conclusion, FFAR4 (GPR120) has garnered significant attention for its role in metabolic diseases, including T2DM and nonalcoholic steatohepatitis. Its widespread expression suggests it may influence a variety of physiological and pathological processes. Tool compounds and genetically engineered mouse models have provided valuable insights into FFAR4 signaling, opening the door to novel therapeutic possibilities, particularly in areas such as cancer and respiratory function. Incretin-based therapies, such as GLP-1 receptor agonists and DPP-4 inhibitors, have already transformed diabetes treatment, and small molecule agonists targeting both insulin-secreting β-cells and GLP-1-producing L-cells hold promising potential for future therapies. FFAR4 plays a central role in regulating energy homeostasis, affecting processes like adipogenesis, glucose metabolism, and anti-inflammatory responses. The identification of endogenous FFAR4 activators, such as PAHSA, along with selective agonists like cpdA, further highlights its therapeutic value, especially in the areas of inflammation and metabolic control.

References

Ahrén, B. (2009). Islet G protein-coupled receptors as potential targets for treatment of type 2 diabetes. *Nature Reviews Drug Discovery*, 8(5), 369–385.

Alexander, S., Mathie, A., & Peters, J. (2011). G protein-coupled receptors. *British Journal of Pharmacology*, 164(S1), S5–S113.

Alfonzo-Méndez, M. A., Alcántara-Hernández, R., & García-Sáinz, J. A. (2016). Novel structural approaches to study GPCR regulation. *International Journal of Molecular Sciences*, 18(1), 27.

Augments Glucose-Stimulated Insulin Secretion and Improves Glucose Tolerance in Normal and Diabetic Mice. *Diabetes*, 58(5), 1067–1076.

Briscoe, C. P., Tadayyon, M., Andrews, J. L., Benson, W. G., Chambers, J. K., Eilert, M. M., Ellis, C., Elshourbagy, N. A., Goetz, A. S., Minnick, D. T., Murdock, P. R., Sauls, H. R., Shabon, U., Spinage, L. D., Strum, J. C., Szekeres, P. G., Tan, K. B., Way, J. M., Ignar, D. M., Wilson, S., & Muir, A. I. (2003). The Orphan G Protein-coupled Receptor GPR40 Is Activated by Medium and Long Chain Fatty Acids. *Journal of Biological Chemistry*, 278(13), 11303–11311.

Burns, R. N., & Moniri, N. H. (2010). Agonism with the omega-3 fatty acids α-linolenic acid and docosahexaenoic acid mediates phosphorylation of both the short and long isoforms of the human GPR120 receptor. *Biochemical and Biophysical Research Communications*, 396(4), 1030–1035.

Byrne, J. H., Heidelberger, R., & Waxham, M. N. (Eds.). (2014). From Molecules to Networks: An Introduction to Cellular and Molecular Neuroscience (3rd ed). Elsevier AP.

Carullo, G., Mazzotta, S., Vega-Holm, M., Iglesias-Guerra, F., Vega-Pérez, J. M., Aiello, F., & Brizzi, A. (2021). GPR120/FFAR4 Pharmacology: Focus on Agonists in Type 2 Diabetes Mellitus Drug Discovery. *Journal of Medicinal Chemistry*, 64(8), 4312–4332.

Chen, Y., Zhang, D., Ho, K. W., Lin, S., Suen, W. C.-W., Zhang, H., Zha, Z., Li, G., & Leung, P. S. (2018). GPR120 is an important inflammatory regulator in the development of osteoarthritis. *Arthritis Research & Therapy*, 20(1), 163.

Chung, S., Funakoshi, T., & Civelli, O. (2008). Orphan GPCR research. *British Journal of Pharmacology*, 153(S1), S339-46.

Christiansen, E., Watterson, K. R., Stocker, C. J., Sokol, E., Jenkins, L., Simon, K., Grundmann, M., Petersen, R. K., Wargent, E. T., Hudson, B. D., Kostenis, E., Ejsing, C. S., Cawthorne, M. A., Milligan, G., & Ulven, T. (2015). Activity of dietary fatty acids on FFA1 and FFA4 and characterisation of pinolenic acid as a dual FFA1/FFA4 agonist with potential effect against metabolic diseases. *British Journal of Nutrition*, 113(11), 1677–1688.

Civelli, O. (2012). Orphan GPCRs and Neuromodulation. *Neuron*, 76(1), 12–21.

Cornish, J., MacGibbon, A., Lin, J.-M., Watson, M., Callon, K. E., Tong, P. C., Dunford, J. E., Van Der Does, Y., Williams, G. A., Grey, A. B., Naot, D., & Reid, I. R. (2008). Modulation of Osteoclastogenesis by Fatty Acids. *Endocrinology*, 149(11), 5688–5695.

Dixon, R. A. F., Kobilka, B. K., Strader, D. J., Benovic, J. L., Dohlman, H. G., Frielle, T., Bolanowski, M. A., Bennett, C. D., Rands, E., Diehl, R. E., Mumford, R. A., Slater, E. E., Sigal, I. S., Caron, M. G., Lefkowitz, R. J., & Strader, C. D. (1986). Cloning of the gene and cDNA for mammalian β-adrenergic receptor and homology with rhodopsin. *Nature*, 321(6065), 75–79.

Eleazu, C., Charles, A., Eleazu, K., & Achi, N. (2018). Free fatty acid receptor 1 as a novel therapeutic target for type 2 diabetes mellitus current status. *Chemo- biological Interactions*, 289, 32–39.

Formicola, R., Pevarello, P., Kuhn, C., Liberati, C., Piscitelli, F., & Sodano, M. (2015). FFA4/GPR120 agonists: a survey of the recent patent literature. *Pharmaceutical patent analyst*, 4(6), 443-451.

Fredriksson, R., Höglund, P. J., Gloriam, D. E. I., Lagerström, M. C., & Schiöth, H. B. (2003). Seven evolutionarily conserved human rhodopsin G protein-coupled receptors lacking close relatives. *FEBS Letters*, 554(3), 381–388.

Fredriksson, R., Lagerström, M. C., Lundin, L.-G., & Schiöth, H. B. (2003). The G-Protein-Coupled Receptors in the Human Genome Form Five Main Families. Phylogenetic Analysis, Paralogon Groups, and Fingerprints. *Molecular Pharmacology*, 63(6), 1256–1272.

Frooninckx, L., Van Rompay, L., Temmerman, L., Van Sinay, E., Beets, I., Janssen, T., Husson, S. J., & Schoofs, L. (2012). Neuropeptide GPCRs in C. elegans. *Frontiers in Endocrinology*, 3, 167.

Ghislain, J., & Poitout, V. (2017). The role and future of FFA1 as a therapeutic target. *Free Fatty Acid Receptors*, 236, 159-180.

Gottesman-Katz, L., Latorre, R., Vanner, S., Schmidt, B. L., & Bunnett, N. W. (2021). Targeting G protein-coupled receptors for the treatment of chronic pain in the digestive system. *Gut*, 70(5), 970–981.

Han, L., Song, S., Niu, Y., Meng, M., & Wang, C. (2017). Eicosapentaenoic Acid (EPA) Induced Macrophages Activation through GPR120-Mediated Raf-ERK1/2-IKKβ-NF-κB p65 Signaling Pathways. *Nutrients*, 9(9), 937.

Hirasawa, A., Tsumaya, K., Awaji, T., Katsuma, S., Adachi, T., Yamada, M., Sugimoto, Y., Miyazaki, S., & Tsujimoto, G. (2005). Free fatty acids regulate gut incretin glucagon-like peptide-1 secretion through GPR120. *Nature Medicine*, 11(1), 90–94.

Hopkins, A. L., & Groom, C. R. (2002). The druggable genome. *Nature Reviews Drug Discovery*, 1(9), 727–730.

Hudson, B. D., Smith, N. J., & Milligan, G. (2011). Experimental Challenges to Targeting Poorly Characterized GPCRs: Uncovering the Therapeutic Potential for Free Fatty Acid Receptors. *In Advances in Pharmacology* (Vol. 62, pp. 175–218). Elsevier.

Itoh, Y., Kawamata, Y., Harada, M., Kobayashi, M., Fujii, R., Fukusumi, S., Ogi, K., Hosoya, M., Tanaka, Y., Uejima, H., Tanaka, H., Maruyama, M., Satoh, R., Okubo, S., Kizawa, H., Komatsu, H., Matsumura, F., Noguchi, Y., Shinohara, T., Hinuma, S., Fujisawa, Y., & Fujino, M. (2003). Free fatty acids regulate insulin secretion from pancreatic beta cells through GPR40. *Nature*, 422(6928), 173–176.

Jacoby, E., Bouhelal, R., Gerspacher, M., & Seuwen, K. (2006). The 7 TM G-Protein-Coupled Receptor Target Family. *ChemMedChem*, 1(8), 760–782.

Janssen, S., Laermans, J., Iwakura, H., Tack, J., & Depoortere, I. (2012). Sensing of Fatty Acids for Octanoylation of Ghrelin Involves a Gustatory G-Protein. *PLoS ONE*, 7(6), e40168.

Katsuma, S., Hatae, N., Yano, T., Ruike, Y., Kimura, M., Hirasawa, A., & Tsujimoto, G. (2005). Free Fatty Acids Inhibit Serum Deprivation-induced Apoptosis through GPR120 in a Murine Enteroendocrine Cell Line STC-1. *Journal of Biological Chemistry*, 280(20), 19507–19515.

Lagerström, M. C., & Schiöth, H. B. (2008). Structural diversity of G protein-coupled receptors and significance for drug discovery. *Nature Reviews Drug Discovery*, 7(4), 339–357.

Liu, H. D., Wang, W., Xu, Z., Liu, C., He, D., Du, L. P., Li, M. Y., Yu, X., & Sun, J. (2015). FFA4 receptor (GPR120): A hot target for the development of anti-diabetic therapies. *European Journal of Pharmacology*, 763, 160–168.

Lu, X., Zhao, X., Feng, J., Liou, A. P., Anthony, S., Pechhold, S., Sun, Y., Lu, H., & Wank, S. (2012). Postprandial inhibition of gastric ghrelin secretion by long-chain fatty acid through GPR120 in isolated gastric ghrelin cells and mice. *American Journal of Physiology-Gastrointestinal and Liver Physiology*, 303(3), G367–G376.

Mancini, A. D., & Poitout, V. (2013). The fatty acid receptor FFA1/GPR40 a decade later: How much do we know? *Trends in Endocrinology & Metabolism*, 24(8), 398–407.

Matsumura, S., Mizushige, T., Yoneda, T., Iwanaga, T., Tsuzuki, S., Inoue, K., & Fushiki, T. (2007). GPR expression in the rat taste bud relating to fatty acid sensing. *Biomedical Research*, 28(1), 49–55.

Abaraviciene, S. M, Muhammed, S. J., Amisten, S., Lundquist, I., & Salehi, A. (2013). GPR40 protein levels are crucial to the regulation of stimulated hormone secretion in pancreatic islets. Lessons from spontaneous obesity-prone and non-obese type 2 diabetes in rats. *Molecular and Cellular Endocrinology*, 381(1–2), 150–159.

Milligan, G., Stoddart, L. A., & Smith, N. J. (2009). Agonism and allosterism: The pharmacology of the free fatty acid receptors FFA2 and FFA3. *British Journal of Pharmacology*, 158(1), 146–153.

Milligan, G., Alvarez-Curto, E., Hudson, B. D., Prihandoko, R., & Tobin, A. B. (2017). FFA4/GPR120: pharmacology and therapeutic opportunities. *Trends in pharmacological sciences*, 38(9), 809-821.

Moore, K., Zhang, Q., Murgolo, N., Hosted, T., & Duffy, R. (2009). Cloning, expression, and pharmacological characterization of the GPR120 free fatty acid receptor from cynomolgus monkey: Comparison with human GPR120 splice variants. *Comparative Biochemistry and Physiology Part B: Biochemistry and Molecular Biology*, 154(4), 419–426.

Moran, B. M., McKillop, A. M., & O' Harte, F. P. (2016). Development of novel ligands for peptide GPCRs. *Current opinion in pharmacology*, 31, 57-62.

Moran, B. M., Flatt, P. R., & McKillop, A. M. (2016). G protein-coupled receptors: Signalling and regulation by lipid agonists for improved glucose homoeostasis. *Acta Diabetologica*, 53(2), 177–188.

Morgan, N. G., & Dhayal, S. (2009). G-protein coupled receptors mediating long chain fatty acid signalling in the pancreatic beta-cell. *Biochemical Pharmacology*, 78(12), 1419–1427.

Mo, Z., Tang, C., Li, H., Lei, J., Zhu, L., Kou, L., Li, H., Luo, S., Li, C., Chen, W., & Zhang, L. (2020). Eicosapentaenoic acid prevents inflammation induced by acute cerebral infarction through inhibition of NLRP3 inflammasome activation. *Life Sciences*, 242, 117133.

Navarro-Tito, N., Robledo, T., & Salazar, E. P. (2008). Arachidonic acid promotes FAK activation and migration in MDA-MB-231 breast cancer cells. *Experimental Cell Research*, 314(18), 3340–3355.

Oh, D. Y., Talukdar, S., Bae, E. J., Imamura, T., Morinaga, H., Fan, W., Li, P., Lu, W. J., Watkins, S. M., & Olefsky, J. M. (2010). GPR120 Is an Omega-3 Fatty Acid Receptor Mediating Potent Anti-inflammatory and Insulin-Sensitizing Effects. *Cell*, 142(5), 687–698.

Parker, H. E., Habib, A. M., Rogers, G. J., Gribble, F. M., & Reimann, F. (2009). Nutrient-dependent secretion of glucose-dependent insulinotropic polypeptide from primary murine K cells. *Diabetologia*, 52(2), 289–298.

Reber, S. O., Birkeneder, L., Veenema, A. H., Obermeier, F., Falk, W., Straub, R. H., & Neumann, I. D. (2007). Adrenal Insufficiency and Colonic Inflammation after a Novel Chronic Psycho-Social Stress Paradigm in Mice: Implications and Mechanisms. *Endocrinology*, 148(2), 670–682.

Reimann, F., Tolhurst, G., & Gribble, F. M. (2012). G-Protein-Coupled Receptors in Intestinal Chemo sensation. *Cell Metabolism*, 15(4), 421–431.

Salehi, A., Flodgren, E., Nilsson, N. E., Jimenez-Feltstrom, J., Miyazaki, J., Owman, C., & Olde, B. (2005). Free fatty acid receptor 1 (FFA1R/GPR40) and its involvement in fatty-acid-stimulated insulin secretion. *Cell and Tissue Research*, 322(2), 207–215.

Serhan, C. N., Chiang, N., & Dalli, J. (2018). New pro-resolving n-3 mediators bridge resolution of infectious inflammation to tissue regeneration. *Molecular Aspects of Medicine*, 64, 1–17.

Scholten, D. J. (2012). Chemokine Receptors CXCR3 and CXCR7: Allosteric Ligand Binding, Biased Signaling, and Receptor Regulation. [PhD-Thesis - Research and graduation internal, Vrije Universiteit Amsterdam].

So, S. S., Ngo, T., Keov, P., Smith, N. J., & Kufareva, I. (2020). Tackling the complexities of orphan GPCR ligand discovery with rationally assisted approaches. In GPCRs (pp. 295-334). *Academic Press.*

Soto-Guzman, A., Robledo, T., Lopez-Perez, M., & Salazar, E. P. (2008). Oleic acid induces ERK1/2 activation and AP-1 DNA binding activity through a mechanism involving Src kinase and EGFR transactivation in breast cancer cells. *Molecular and Cellular Endocrinology*, 294(1–2), 81–91.

Stuttgen, G. M., & Sahoo, D. (2021). FFAR4: A New Player in Cardiometabolic Disease? *Endocrinology*, 162(8), bqab111.

Sykaras, A. G., Demenis, C., Case, R. M., McLaughlin, J. T., & Smith, C. P. (2012). Duodenal Enteroendocrine I-Cells Contain mRNA Transcripts Encoding Key Endocannabinoid and Fatty Acid Receptors. *PLoS ONE*, 7(8), e42373.

Tsuda, N., Kawaji, A., Sato, T., Takagi, M., Higashi, C., Kato, Y., Ogawa, K., Naba, H., Ohkouchi, M., Nakamura, M., Hosaka, Y., & Sakaki, J. (2017). A novel free fatty acid receptor 1 (GPR 40/ FFAR 1) agonist, MR 1704, enhances glucose-dependent insulin secretion and improves glucose homeostasis in rats. *Pharmacology Research & Perspectives*, 5(4), e00340.

Tyndall, J., & Sandilya, R. (2005). GPCR Agonists and Antagonists in the Clinic. *Medicinal Chemistry*, 1(4), 405–421.

Urban, J. D., Clarke, W. P., von Zastrow, M., Nichols, D. E., Kobilka, B., Weinstein, H., Javitch, J. A., Roth, B. L., Christopoulos, A., Sexton, P. M., Miller, K. J., Spedding, M., & Mailman, R. B. (2007). Functional selectivity and classical concepts of quantitative pharmacology. *Journal of Pharmacology and Experimental Therapeutics*, 320(1), 1-13.

Ulven, T., & Christiansen, E. (2015). Dietary Fatty Acids and Their Potential for Controlling Metabolic Diseases Through Activation of FFA4/GPR120. *Annual Review of Nutrition*, 35(1), 239–263.

Watson, S. J., Brown, A. J. H., & Holliday, N. D. (2012). Differential Signalling by Splice Variants of the Human Free Fatty Acid Receptor GPR120. *Molecular Pharmacology*, 81(5), 631–642.

Whalley, N. M., Pritchard, L. E., Smith, D. M., & White, A. (2011). Processing of proglucagon to GLP-1 in pancreatic α-cells: Is this a paracrine mechanism enabling GLP-1 to act on β-cells? *Journal of Endocrinology*, 211(1), 99–106.

Wise, A., Jupe, S. C., & Rees, S. (2004). The identification of ligands at orphan G-protein coupled receptors. *Annu. Rev. Pharmacol. Toxicol.*, 44(1), 43-66.

Yore, M. M., Syed, I., Moraes-Vieira, P. M., Zhang, T., Herman, M. A., Homan, E. A., Patel, R. T., Lee, J., Chen, S., Peroni, O. D., Dhaneshwar, A. S., Hammarstedt, A., Smith, U., McGraw, T. E., Saghatelian, A., & Kahn, B. B. (2014). Discovery of a Class of Endogenous Mammalian Lipids with Anti-Diabetic and Anti-inflammatory Effects. *Cell*, 159(2), 318–332.

Zhou, J., & Wild, C. (2019). GPCR Drug Discovery: Emerging Targets, Novel Approaches and Future Trends. *Current Topics in Medicinal Chemistry*, 19(16), 1363–1364.

Zhao, C., Zhou, J., Meng, Y., Shi, N., Wang, X., Zhou, M., Li, G., & Yang, Y. (2020). DHA Sensor GPR120 in Host Defense Exhibits the Dual Characteristics of Regulating Dendritic Cell Function and Skewing the Balance of Th17/Tregs. *International Journal of Biological Sciences*, 16(3), 374–387.

Chapter 4

Therapeutic Potential of Free Fatty Acid Receptor 4 (FFAR4/GPR120) in Diabetes Mellitus: Insights into Molecular Mechanisms and Future Directions

Jithin Mathew[1,*]
Anson S. Maroky[2]
Srushti Mahesh Bendale[3]
and Yash Sanjay Agarwal[4]
[1]Department of Pharmacology, NGSM Institute of Pharmaceutical Sciences, Nitte (Deemed to be University), Paneer, Mangalore, Karnataka, India
[2]Department of Pharmacology, Devaki Amma Memorial College of Pharmacy, Malappuram, Kerala, India
[3]Department of Pharmacology and Toxicology, National Institute of Pharmaceutical Education and Research (NIPER), S.A.S. Nagar, Mohali, Punjab, India
[4]Department of Pharmaceutical Technology, National Institute of Pharmaceutical Education and Research (NIPER), S.A.S. Nagar, Mohali, Punjab, India

Abstract

Free fatty acid receptor 4 (FFAR4), also known as GPR120, is a G-protein coupled receptor (GPCR) responsive to long-chain fatty acids and has emerged as a promising therapeutic target for diabetes mellitus. Research has identified FFAR4 as a sensor for unsaturated long-chain fatty acids, providing insights into the cellular processes through which these fatty acids promote various beneficial biological effects. These processes include the secretion of peptide hormones in the digestive tract and the maintenance of glucose balance. Activation of FFAR4 has been associated with improved insulin sensitivity and reduced glucagon-like peptide-1 secretion in enteroendocrine cell lines, making it a compelling target for the development of obesity and diabetes treatments. FFAR4 agonists have shown the potential to enhance satiety mechanisms, promote incretin release, reduce inflammatory metabolic responses, and improve insulin effectiveness. As a result, drugs targeting FFAR4 are expected to become available soon. This chapter explores the role of FFAR4 in regulating essential metabolic functions, including adipogenesis, lipid metabolism, and glucose metabolism. It also examines the potential of FFAR4-based

---

* Corresponding Author's Email: jithinmathew051@gmail.com

In: Receptor-Targeted Therapies in Diabetes Mellitus
Editors: Ajmer Singh Grewal, Neelam Singh, Swati Verma et al.
ISBN: 979-8-89530-587-4

therapies for treating obesity and diabetes mellitus, highlighting recent advancements and future directions in this expanding area of metabolic research.

Keywords: therapeutic target, insulin sensitivity, diabetes mellitus, G-protein coupled receptor, glucose homeostasis

Abbreviations

BAT	Brown adipose tissue
COX-2	Cyclooxygenase-2
DHA	Docosahexanoic acid
DM	Diabetes mellitus
DPP-IV	Dipeptidyl peptidase-4
EC50	Half maximal effective concentration
EPA	Eicosapentaenoic acid
FFAR4	Free fatty acid receptor -4
FFAs	Free fatty acids
GIP	Gastric inhibitory protein
GLP-1	Glucagon like peptide-1
GLUT4	Glucose transporter protein type-4
ICL3	Intracellular loop
IP1	Inositol triphosphate-1
IRS-1	Insulin receptor-1
KO	Knockout
LCFA	Long chain fatty acid
LPS	Lipopolysaccharides
OGTT	Oral glucose tolerance test
PGE2	Prostaglandin –E2
PI3K	Phosphotidyl inositol 4,5 bi phosphate
PUFAs	Polyunsaturated fatty acids
T2DM	Type 2 DM
TMDs	Trans membrane domains
TNF-α	Tumor necrosis factor-α
UCP 1	Uncoupling protein-1
WAT	White adipose tissue
WT	Wild type

Introduction

Type 2 diabetes mellitus (T2DM) is a chronic metabolic condition characterized by disrupted insulin secretion, increased hepatic glucose production, and reduced peripheral glucose uptake. The pathophysiology of T2DM is complex, involving not only insulin resistance in adipose tissue and the brain but also elevated glucagon secretion, diminished incretin levels, enhanced renal glucose reabsorption, and other metabolic disturbances. Recent research has identified several novel therapeutic targets in clinical development aimed at addressing these issues. These include agents designed to enhance insulin sensitivity, such as glucocorticoid receptor antagonists, and those targeting hepatic glucose production, including glucagon receptor antagonists, glycogen phosphorylase inhibitors, and fructose-1,6-bisphosphatase inhibitors (Belete et al. 2020). Traditional treatments for T2DM typically involve biguanides, sulfonylureas, thiazolidinediones, and dipeptidyl peptidase-IV (DPP-IV) inhibitors. However, recent advancements have introduced new drug classes, such as sodium-glucose cotransporter 2 (SGLT2) inhibitors, which work by reducing glucose reabsorption in the kidneys, thereby lowering blood sugar levels (Htike et al. 2017). Additionally, glucagon-like peptide-1 (GLP-1) receptor modulators, including exenatide, liraglutide, and lixisenatide, have been developed. These agonists enhance GLP-1 function, a gut hormone released in response to oral glucose intake, which promotes insulin secretion and suppresses glucagon release, thus exerting a glucoregulatory effect (Lee et al. 2019). The FFAR4 receptor is predominantly expressed in the lungs, fat tissue, and intestines. This receptor interacts with extended-chain lipids, particularly omega-3 fatty acids. Stimulation of FFAR4 facilitates the translocation of glucose transporter 4 (GLUT4), leading to heightened glucose uptake in 3T3-L1 adipose tissue cells, playing a crucial role in regulating energy processing. Chronic inflammation, a significant contributor to insulin resistance, is closely associated with T2DM and obesity (Schenk et al. 2008). This chapter explores the potential role of FFAR4 in managing metabolic disorders, examining how advancements in molecular pharmacology and innovative drug discovery approaches can contribute to the treatment of diabetes. It highlights the importance of FFAR4 in developing novel therapeutic strategies for effective diabetes management.

Structural and Pharmacological Profile of FFAR4 (GPR120)

Human GPR120, a notable G-protein-coupled receptor (GPCR) located on chromosome 10q23.33, features seven transmembrane domains (TMDs 1–7). Key active sites include arginine at position 99, located at the top of TMD2, and arginine at position 178, found at the top of TMD4, both of which are crucial for agonist binding and receptor activation. The primary endogenous ligands for GPR120 are polyunsaturated fatty acids (PUFAs), including linoleic acid and docosahexaenoic acid (DHA) (Moore et al. 2009). GPR120 exists in two alternatively spliced forms: one is the shortened variant, comprising 361 amino acids, and the other is the long isoform (GPR120L), with 377 amino acids. The main distinction between these variants is a 16-amino-acid segment present in the third intracellular loop (ICL3) of GPR120L, which influences their signaling characteristics. GPR120S interacts with both Gq/G11 and the β-arrestin pathways, facilitating Ca2+ mobilization. In contrast, GPR120L does not interact with Gq/G11 but still activates the β-arrestin pathway. GPR120S signaling involves inositol triphosphate inhibitors, linking it to Ca2+ signaling through Gαq/11 (Milligan et al. 2015). Both isoforms can recruit β-arrestin proteins, leading to receptor internalization and degradation. They also exhibit rapid ERK1/2 phosphorylation via Gαq/11 signaling, subsequently triggering the transactivation of the epidermal growth factor receptor. Agonist binding induces significant receptor internalization through β-arrestin interaction, involving the phosphorylation of serine and threonine residues located at the intracellular C-terminal end of the receptor (Watson et al. 2012). This phosphorylation, particularly at clusters 1 (Thr347, Thr349, and Ser350) and 2

(Ser357 and Ser361), regulates β-arrestin 2 recruitment, receptor endocytosis, and Akt phosphorylation (Moniri et al. 2016).

FFAR4 Agonists and Their Mechanisms

FFAR4 Agonists

Research has elucidated the signaling events and pharmacological mechanisms of FFAR4 agonists, highlighting their potential as novel therapeutic agents. FFAR4 activation increases intracellular Ca2+ levels, indicating the involvement of Gq and/or G11 G proteins associated with phosphoinositidase C. This has been confirmed by the inability of FFAR4 to induce inositol phosphate production or elevate Ca2+ levels in genetically modified HEK293 cells lacking Gq and G11 (Alvarez et al. 2016). Additionally, FFAR4's role in regulating ghrelin and somatostatin release suggests the involvement of Gi-family G proteins (Engelstoft et al. 2013; Stone et al. 2014). The receptor shows higher mRNA expression in pancreatic delta cells compared to beta cells, suggesting a potential therapeutic bias between Gq/11 and Gi-family G proteins (Segerstolpe et al. 2016). FFAR4 activation by α-linolenic acid enhances GLP-1 and insulin production, indicating a promising approach for improving glucose regulation and managing diabetes (Hirasawa et al. 2005). Omega-3 fatty acids, via GPR120, reduce macrophage migration, leading to a decreased presence of inflammatory macrophages in adipose tissue, as shown in wild-type mice but not in GPR120 knockout mice (Oh et al. 2010). This suggests GPR120's essential role in mediating the inflammation-reducing and insulin-enhancing properties of omega-3 fatty acids. Synthetic agonists like GW9508 and TUG-891 have shown high potency and selectivity towards FFAR4, offering therapeutic potential for metabolic disorders (Hudson et al. 2013). FFAR4, found in tissues such as the intestines, adipose tissue, liver, and pancreatic beta cells, plays a vital role in regulating metabolic processes. Stimulation of FFAR4 boosts glucose metabolism by triggering the release of GLP-1. This, in turn, improves insulin sensitivity, modulates anti-inflammatory pathways, and directly impacts insulin signaling (Oh et al. 2010; Hirasawa et al. 2005). GLP-1, released by enteroendocrine L-cells in response to food intake, boosts insulin secretion, suppresses glucagon release, slows gastric emptying, and promotes satiety, making it a key target for managing T2DM and obesity (Drucker, 2006; Holst, 2007).

Phenyl Propionic Acid Derivatives

The development of TUG-891 involved a streamlined optimization process, starting with GW-9508, a GPR40 agonist with balanced GPR120 activity. This process entailed examining structural analogs of GW-9508 to discover selective GPR120 activators. Initial adjustments included modifying the replacements on the phenyl ring near the carboxylic group in GW-9508 and substituting the N-linker with an O-linker (Figure 1). The optimization revealed that a phenyl group positioned at the meta-site of the terminal ring enhanced efficacy, although it did not improve selectivity for GPR120. In contrast, an ortho-positioned phenyl substituent increased selectivity, as seen with TUG-891 (Briscoe et al. 2006). Further adjustments to the biphenyl moiety affected potency, with TUG-891 featuring a fluorine substituent near the carboxylic group and a methyl substituent on the ortho-terminal phenyl ring. These modifications improved both potency and selectivity for GPR120 compared to its non-methylated counterpart. In a comparative structural model of GPR120 bound with TUG-891 (based on the β2-adrenoceptor crystal structure), the carboxylic acid group formed two hydrogen bonds with Arg99, and the phenylpropionate interacted with Phe304 and Phe311. The biphenyl component was accommodated within a hydrophobic region. Additional research revealed that TUG-891 exhibited pharmacological effects comparable to those of GW-9508 in murine cell models, including enhanced glucose uptake in adipocytes and decreased release of pro-inflammatory mediators (Hudson et al. 2014).

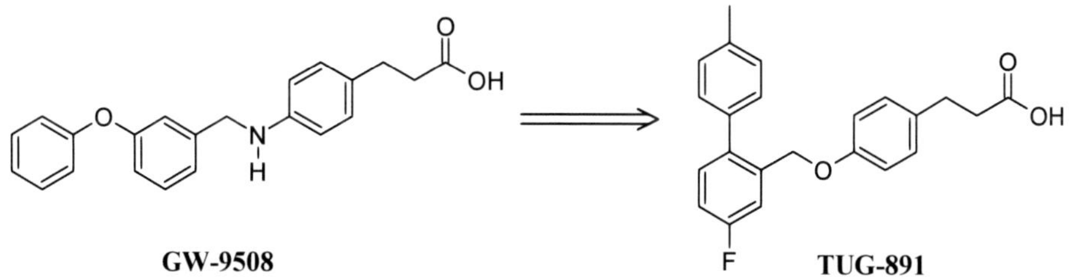

GW-9508
Dual GPR40/120 agonist
GPR40 EC_{50} = 48 nM
GPR120 EC_{50} = 3500 nM

TUG-891
Selective GPR/120 agonist
GPR40 EC_{50} = 65000 nM
GPR120 EC_{50} = 44 nM

Figure 1. From targets of GPR40 to GPR120 receptors: alterations.

Heterocycle-Substituted Phenylpropanoic Acids

Recently, researchers screened a diverse array of compounds featuring various heterocyclic moieties derived from the phenylpropanoic acid backbone to identify potential GPR120 agonists. Zhang et al. (2017) developed and evaluated a new series of isoxazole-based phenylpropanoic acid derivatives, starting with TUG-891. Significant modifications were made to minimize hydrophobicity and enhance the compounds' ability to activate GPR120. Notably, in TUG-891, the meta-fluoro-phenyl group was substituted with a five-membered heterocyclic ring, while the end phenyl group and the phenylpropanoic acid nucleus were retained at positions 3 and 4, respectively. The study involved testing various polar heterocycles, leading to the identification of new active compounds in two calcium flux assays (using human embryonic kidney cells transfected with human GPR120) and β-arrestin assays. Heterocycles such as triazole, tetrazole, and imidazole displayed diminished effects against hGPR120, likely due to their high orientation. In contrast, isoxazole was well-tolerated, demonstrating EC50 values between 81 and 217 nM in calcium assays, though it exhibited moderate stability in microsomal tests (Zhang et al. 2017). Small substituents at the 5-position of isoxazole, such as methyl or ethyl groups, enhanced the potency for hGPR120 compared to analogs without substitutions, while larger substituents reduced potency. The most effective compound in the series featured a 5-CF3 group, 3,5-di-fluoro substitutions within the phenylpropanoic acid component, and an ethyl group para to the terminal ring (compound 1, Figure 2) (Sparks et al. 2014).

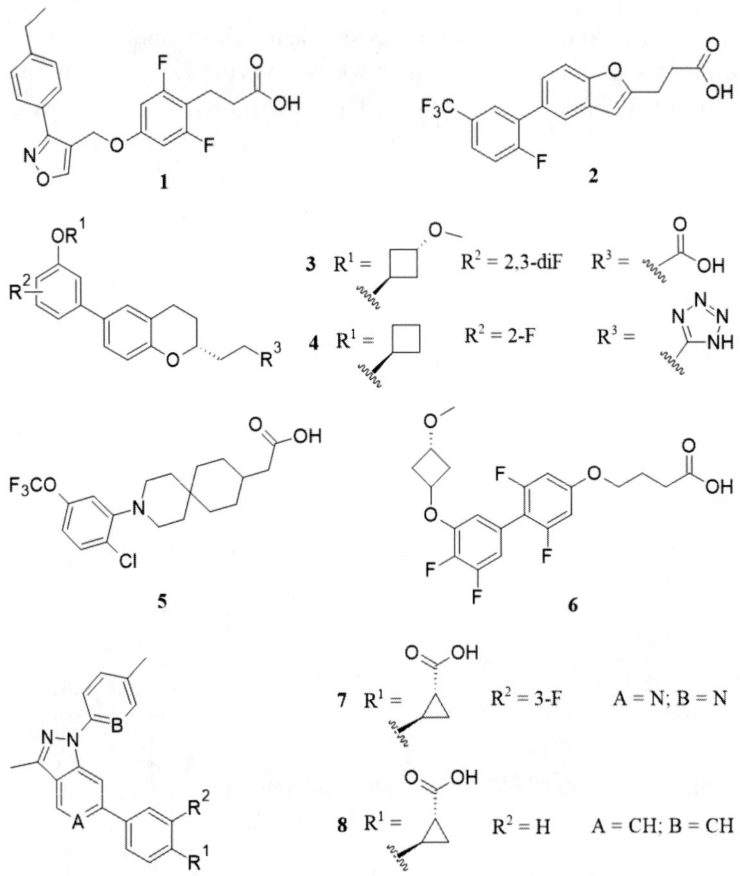

Figure 2. Development of GPR120 agonists from carboxylic acid structures.

Bicyclic Aliphatic Carboxylic Acids

The phenylpropanoic acid backbone has previously shown promise in the development of GPR120 ligands. Building on this, researchers at Merck investigated modifications to this core structure to create more effective agonists. They replaced the phenyl ring of phenylpropanoic acid with a benzofuran core. Through ultrahigh-throughput screening, they identified benzofuran propionic acid derivatives and observed that compounds with fluorine substitutions on the end phenyl ring, attached to the benzofuran core, exhibited enhanced efficacy in IP1 assays conducted on both human and mouse models. These compounds demonstrated EC50 values between 20 and 63 nM in human assays and 7 to 43 nM in mouse assays, significantly lower than the control values of 474 to 487 nM (Winters et al. 2018). Compound 2 displayed strong efficacy against both human and mouse GPR120, with moderate receptor activation of 73% and 75%, respectively. It also showed a 29-fold selectivity for GPR120 over GPR40 and favorable pharmacokinetic properties, including good oral absorption, extended half-life, and effective plasma clearance. Additionally, this compound significantly lowered blood glucose levels in both wild-type and GPR120 knockout mice at doses of 30 and 100 mg/kg. Subsequent optimization involved incorporating a chromane framework, leading to compounds 3 and 4. Despite some modifications resulting in reduced activity in GPR120 assays, these compounds maintained high efficacy and selectivity for GPR120. Notably, compound 3 demonstrated dose-dependent glucose reduction and an excellent pharmacokinetic profile. Further developments included compound 5, featuring a spirocyclic system, which exhibited high GPR120 selectivity and anti-inflammatory effects in obese mice, though it showed high unbound clearance in pharmacokinetic studies. Sheng and colleagues introduced biphenyl butanoic acid derivatives, with compound 6 showing notable GPR120 selectivity and hypoglycemic activity in mice. Molecular modeling of compound 6 revealed key interactions with GPR120, though stability issues were observed. McCoull and colleagues developed biphenyl derivatives with a condensed-pyrazole core, where compounds 7 and 8 exhibited strong GPR120 selectivity, reduced glucose excursions in OGTT tests, and good selectivity over hGPR40. Both compounds demonstrated moderate oral bioavailability and high target specificity (Lombardo et al. 2016). In summary, GPR120 agonists exhibit intricate pharmacological effects with significant implications for metabolic syndromes, particularly non-insulin-dependent diabetes mellitus (NIDDM). Despite extensive research, no GPR120 agonists have yet been approved as hyperglycemic treatments. Currently, the management of T2DM involves dietary control and pharmacological interventions, with insulin treatment reserved as a last resort (Roder et al. 2017). The main classes of drugs used include metformin, which is favored due to its minimal risk of causing hypoglycemia and obesity, though it is associated with gastrointestinal side effects. Sulfonylureas, while effective, increase the risk of hypoglycemia and obesity, while DPP-IV inhibitors improve glycemic control but are linked to a higher incidence of acute pancreatitis and heart failure. These limitations have driven the search for new therapeutic targets, with Free Fatty Acid Receptors (FFARs), particularly GPR40 and GPR120, emerging as promising candidates. GPR120, in particular, has shown potential as a pharmacological target, offering opportunities for the development of new and innovative treatments for T2DM (Ballatore et al. 2013).

FFAR4 in Glucose Homeostasis and Islet Function

Impact of FFAR4 on Islet Function in Langerhans

Activation of FFAR4 by dietary long-chain free fatty acids (FFAs), particularly omega-3s like DHA and EPA, triggers intracellular signaling pathways that raise calcium levels, leading to the release of GLP-1 (Hirasawa et al. 2005). This process has been confirmed in both *in vitro* and *in vivo* studies, demonstrating significant increases in GLP-1 production and subsequent insulin secretion. GLP-1 enhances glucose-dependent insulin release, reducing the risk of hypoglycemia, inhibits glucagon release, and decreases hepatic glucose production. Additionally, GLP-1 slows gastric emptying and enhances satiety, leading to reduced food intake and weight loss, which further improve insulin sensitivity and overall metabolic health (Drucker, 2006; Holst, 2007). Despite the promising preclinical findings, translating the benefits of FFAR4 activation into clinical therapy presents challenges. Developing FFAR4-based treatments requires careful consideration of human metabolic complexity, potential off-target effects, and species differences. The long-term safety and efficacy of FFAR4 agonists need thorough clinical validation (Hudson et al. 2013).

GPR120 Deficiency and Reduced Potentiation of Glucagon Secretion

GPR120 exhibits high expression in the colon, adipose tissue, and pituitary gland, but its presence is less prominent in the pancreatic islets, where its function has not been extensively studied. Evidence indicates that GPR120 is activated by both saturated fatty acids, such as palmitic acid, and unsaturated fatty acids, such as docosahexaenoic acid (DHA). Research shows that GPR120 knockout (KO) islets have significantly reduced glucagon production in response to both palmitate and DHA. Interestingly, islets from GPR40 KO mice also show a similar decrease in long-chain fatty acid (LCFA)-stimulated glucagon release (Suckow et al. 2014). GPR120 was first identified for its involvement in stimulating GLP-1 secretion from the colon in response to the unsaturated long-chain fatty acid alpha-linolenic acid (Matsuzaka & Shimano, 2011). GLP-1, an incretin hormone, enhances insulin secretion and is thought to support cell survival and proliferation in preclinical studies (Danforth, 2000). Recent studies have further implicated GPR120 in the action of omega-3 fatty acids (n-3), demonstrating its involvement in reducing inflammation and mitigating insulin resistance in models of diet-induced diabetes (Oh et al. 2010). In mice, the absence of GPR120 leads to glucose intolerance and obesity. Similarly, a genetic alteration that disrupts GPR120 signaling has been linked to a higher risk of obesity in European populations (Yan et al. 2013). Additionally, reduced GPR120 expression in human islets has been linked to higher HbA1c levels, an indicator of long-term glucose control (Ichimura et al. 2012).

FFAR4 and Lipid Metabolism

Numerous studies highlight the essential role of FFAR4 in regulating adipocyte metabolism. FFAR4 is prominently expressed in adipocytes across different fat tissues, including white adipose tissue (WAT) and brown adipose tissue (BAT), with increased expression observed during adipocyte differentiation. FFAR4 has also been involved in regulating lipid droplet formation. Reducing FFAR4 effectiveness through small interfering RNA has been shown to arrest both adipocyte differentiation and lipid buildup in 3T3-L1 cells. Conversely, activation of FFAR4 by alpha-linolenic acid has been found to promote the differentiation of 3T3-L1 adipocytes (Iwaski et al. 2014). In addition to its role in adipocyte metabolism, FFAR4 regulates thermogenesis. It is notably expressed in BAT and is significantly upregulated in response to cold exposure in mice. Activation of FFAR4 enhances thermogenesis by upregulating BAT-specific proteins, such as UCP1 (Kalderon et al. 2012). Additionally, FFAR4 activation promotes fatty acid absorption and metabolism, modifies cellular respiration within mitochondria, and decreases adipose tissue mass in BAT. These effects are thought to be mediated through FFAR4-dependent stimulation of Gq/11, leading to increased Ca2+ accumulation (Stone et al. 2014). FFAR4 also plays a critical role in insulin responses and lipolysis regulation. It enhances glucose uptake by facilitating the activation and translocation of GLUT4, a glucose carrier, to the cell membrane in fat cells and 3T3-L1 lipocytes. Disruption of FFAR4 leads to decreased GLUT4 and IRS-1 expression, underscoring its involvement in insulin-stimulated glucose uptake. Research comparing wild-type (WT) mice with FFAR4 knockout (KO) mice shows that FFAR4 activation by omega-3 fatty acids improves glucose uptake stimulated by insulin and enhances insulin specificity in muscle and liver tissues

(Rohwedder et al. 2014). FFAR4 regulates lipolysis, as evidenced by reduced plasma FFAs and glycerol levels in mice treated with the FFAR4 agonist Compound B, without altering plasma insulin concentrations. This effect is further supported by experiments showing that Compound B decreases glycerol release from adipocytes in wild-type mice, but this effect is absent in FFAR4 KO mice. Recent studies indicate that FFAs released during adipocyte generation limit further lipolysis (Husted et al. 2020). Consequently, FFAR4's ability to interact with Gi/o, rather than Gq/11, is essential for regulating lipolysis.

Exploring FFAR4 as a Novel Target for Anti-Diabetic Drug Development

GPCRs have been recognized for their ability to bind with FFAs as ligands, representing the largest family of human proteins, characterized by seven transmembrane helical segments connected by extracellular and intracellular loops (Glukhova et al. 2018). GPCRs activated by FFAs have emerged as a promising focus for drug development. GPR40 and GPR120 are specifically activated by intermediate- and long-chain fatty acids, while GPR41 and GPR43 respond to short-chain fatty acids (Ichimura et al. 2012). GPR40, predominantly found in pancreatic β-cells, has been identified as a key promoter of insulin secretion. Various ligands targeting GPR40 have shown potential not only as antidiabetic agents but also for their wound-healing properties (Milligan et al. 2017). In comparison, GPR41 and GPR43 are less understood, though they have been observed in microglia, neurons, various cancers, and inflammatory conditions. Extensive research on GPR120 since its deorphanization has demonstrated that FFAs can enhance incretin secretion via this receptor. Current studies highlight GPR120's involvement in a range of diseases, including cancer, inflammation, neuroprotection, and notably type 2 diabetes mellitus (T2DM). From a medicinal chemistry perspective, the focus is on the structure-activity correlations of GPR120 agonists and their potential use in T2DM management, with valuable insights drawn from patent literature (Hirasawa et al. 2005).

Investigating GPR120 Agonists for Type 2 Diabetes Mellitus Drug Development

The first identified ligand (Figure 2) was found to boost GLP-1 secretion, underscoring its potential as a target for diabetic care approaches. Research has since demonstrated the intricate pharmacology of GPR120 and its promise for managing metabolic conditions like T2DM. Early research efforts to develop synthetic GPR120 agonists initially concentrated on GPR40 ligands due to their similar amino acid sequences (Abdel et al. 2016). It has since been established that GPR40 agonists can also activate GPR120. Following the identification of selective GPR120 agonist 4 (Figure 2), a variety of new derivatives, mainly including carboxylic acid and sulfonamide compounds, have been developed and assessed for their potential as effective antidiabetic agents (Shimpukade et al. 2012). These advancements highlight the evolving understanding of GPR120's role and the ongoing efforts to find effective treatments for diabetes and related metabolic conditions.

Targeting FFAR4 in Dietary Strategies for Obesity and Type 2 Diabetes Control

FFAR4 interacts with intermediate- to long-chain fatty acids, such as omega-3 fatty acids, and is found in lipocytes, phagocytes, and gustatory receptors. It is essential for insulin signaling, gustatory recognition, and mediating inflammation-reducing responses. Its presence in adipose tissue and macrophages highlights its importance in metabolic regulation. Activation of FFAR4 by omega-3 fatty acids, such as GW-9508, has been shown to activate phosphatidylinositol-4,5-bisphosphate 3-kinase (PI3K) in adipocytes, resulting in the translocation of GLUT4 to the cell membrane, which increases glucose uptake (Oh et al. 2010). In phagocytes, activation of FFAR4 diminishes pro-inflammatory responses triggered by LPS and TNF-α, leading to higher levels of cytokines associated with the M2 macrophage phenotype, while reducing the secretion of M1 cytokines (Oh et al. 2010). Liu et al. demonstrated that activation of FFAR4 by DHA resulted in decreased COX-2 levels and lower levels of prostaglandin E2 (PGE2) in RAW264.7 macrophages. Conversely, Liu et al. (2014) found that DHA could increase PGE2 production in macrophages. Despite these conflicting results, both studies suggest a shift toward an M2 macrophage phenotype, characterized by decreased levels of pro-inflammatory cytokines such as IL-6. FFAR4 is also present in the intestinal tract, where it stimulates GLP-1 release from enteroendocrine cells, similar to FFAR1 (Hirasawa et al. 2005). Additionally, FFAR4 has been linked to anti-diabetic effects, mitigating chronic inflammation associated with diabetes due to its role in macrophages. In adipocytes, FFAR4 activation enhances glucose uptake, whereas in macrophages, it reduces M1-linked cytokines in response to DHA, GW9508, and EPA (Ichimura et al. 2012). Although FFAR4 is expressed at lower levels in the pancreas compared to FFAR1, its activation in pancreatic delta cells triggers somatostatin production (Stone, 2014). FFAR4 also stimulates GLP-1 secretion and is vital for the secretion of gastric inhibitory peptide (GIP) by enteroendocrine K-cells in the gastrointestinal tract. Mice lacking FFAR4 exhibited a 75% decrease in GIP secretion following fat ingestion compared to wild-type mice (Iwasaki et al. 2015).

Conclusion

FFAR4 plays a vital role in enhancing GLP-1 secretion and improving insulin sensitivity through multiple mechanisms. Activation of FFAR4 by long-chain free fatty acids stimulates GLP-1 release from intestinal L-cells, which, in turn, enhances glucose-dependent insulin secretion, inhibits glucagon release, slows gastric emptying, and promotes satiety. Furthermore, FFAR4 activation offers anti-inflammatory effects and enhances insulin signaling in both adipose tissue and pancreatic beta cells. These findings highlight the therapeutic potential of targeting FFAR4 in the pharmacotherapy of type 2 diabetes and other metabolic disorders. Nevertheless, further research is needed to develop effective and safe clinical therapies based on these insights.

References

Abdel-Magid, A. F. (2015). Therapeutic potential of GPR120 agonists for the treatment of type 2 diabetes. *ACS Medicinal Chemistry Letters*, 6(11), 1097-1098.

Alvarez-Curto, E., Inoue, A., Jenkins, L., Raihan, S. Z., Prihandoko, R., Tobin, A. B., & Milligan, G. (2016). Targeted Elimination of G Proteins and Arrestins Defines Their Specific Contributions to Both Intensity and Duration of G Protein-coupled Receptor Signaling. *The Journal of biological chemistry*, 291(53), 27147–27159.

Anbazhagan, A. N., Priyamvada, S., Gujral, T., Bhattacharyya, S., Alrefai, W. A., Dudeja, P. K., & Borthakur, A. (2016). A novel anti-inflammatory role of GPR120 in intestinal epithelial cells. American *Journal of Physiology-Cell Physiology*, 310(7), C612–C621.

Ballatore, C., Huryn, D. M., & Smith III, A. B. (2013). Carboxylic acid (bio) isosteres in drug design. *ChemMedChem*, 8(3), 385-395.

Belete, T. M. (2020). A recent achievement in the discovery and development of novel targets for the treatment of type-2 diabetes mellitus. *Journal of experimental pharmacology*, 12, 1-15.

Briscoe, C. P., Peat, A. J., McKeown, S. C., Corbett, D. F., Goetz, A. S., Littleton, T. R., McCoy, D. C., Kenakin, T. P., Andrews, J. L., Ammala, C., Fornwald, J. A., Ignar, D. M., & Jenkinson, S. (2006). Pharmacological regulation of insulin secretion in MIN6 cells through the fatty acid receptor GPR40: identification of agonist and antagonist small molecules. *British journal of pharmacology*, 148(5), 619–628.

Danforth, E. (2000). Failure of adipocyte differentiation causes type II diabetes mellitus? *Nature Genetics*, 26(1), 13–13.

Drucker, D. J. (2006). The biology of incretin hormones. *Cell Metabolism*, 3(3), 153-165.

Engelstoft, M. S., Park, W. M., Sakata, I., Kristensen, L. V., Husted, A. S., Osborne-Lawrence, S., Piper, P. K., Walker, A. K., Pedersen, M. H., Nøhr, M. K., Pan, J., Sinz, C. J., Carrington, P. E., Akiyama, T. E., Jones, R. M., Tang, C., Ahmed, K., Offermanns, S., Egerod, K. L., Zigman, J. M., Schwartz, T. W. (2013). Seven transmembrane G protein-coupled receptor repertoire of gastric ghrelin cells. *Molecular metabolism*, 2(4), 376–392.

Glukhova, A., Draper-Joyce, C. J., Sunahara, R. K., Christopoulos, A., Wootten, D., & Sexton, P. M. (2018). Rules of engagement : GPCRs and G proteins. *ACS pharmacology & translational science*, 1(2), 73-83

Hirasawa, A., Tsumaya, K., Awaji, T., Katsuma, S., Adachi, T., Yamada, M., Sugimoto, Y., Miyazaki, S., & Tsujimoto, G. (2005). Free fatty acids regulate gut incretin glucagon-like peptide-1secretionthroughGPR120. *Naturemedicine*, 11(1), 90–94,

Holst, J. J. (2007). The physiology of glucagon-like peptide 1. *Physiological Reviews*, 87(4), 1409-1439.

Htike, Z. Z., Zaccardi, F., Papamargaritis, D., Webb, D. R., Khunti, K., & Davies, M. J. (2017). Efficacy and safety of glucagon-like peptide-1 receptor agonists in type 2 diabetes: a systematic review and mixed treatment comparison analysis. *Diabetes, Obesity and Metabolism*, 19(4), 524-536.

Hudson, B. D., Shimpukade, B., Mackenzie, A. E., Butcher, A. J., Pediani, J. D., Christiansen, E., Heathcote, H., Tobin, A. B., Ulven, T., & Milligan, G. (2013). The pharmacology of TUG-891, a potent and selective agonist of the free fatty acid receptor 4 (FFA4/GPR120), demonstrates both potential opportunity and possible challenges to therapeutic agonism. *Molecular pharmacology*, 84(5), 710–725,

Hudson, B. D., Shimpukade, B., Milligan, G., & Ulven, T. (2014). The molecular basis of ligand interaction at free fatty acid receptor 4 (FFA4/GPR120). *The Journal of biological chemistry*, 289(29), 20345–20358.

Husted, A. S., Ekberg, J. H., Tripp, E., Nissen, T. A. D., Meijnikman, S., O'Brien, S. L., Ulven, T., Acherman, Y., Bruin, S. C., Nieuwdorp, M., Gerhart-Hines, Z., Calebiro, D., Dragsted, L. O., & Schwartz, T. W. (2020). Autocrine negative feedback regulation of lipolysis through sensing of NEFAs by FFAR4/GPR120 in WAT. *Molecular Metabolism*, 42, 101103.

Ichimura, A., Hirasawa, A., Hara, T., & Tsujimoto, G. (2009). Free fatty acid receptors act as nutrient sensors to regulate energy homeostasis. *Prostaglandins & other lipid mediators*, 89(3-4), 82–88.

Iwasaki, K., Harada, N., Sasaki, K., Yamane, S., Iida, K., Suzuki, K., Hamasaki, A., Nasteska, D., Shibue, K., Joo, E., Harada, T., Hashimoto, T., Asakawa, Y., Hirasawa, A., & Inagaki, N. (2015). Free Fatty Acid Receptor GPR120 Is Highly Expressed in Enteroendocrine K Cells of the Upper Small Intestine and Has a Critical Role in GIP Secretion After Fat Ingestion. *Endocrinology*, 156(3), 837–846.

Kalderon, B., Azazmeh, N., Azulay, N., Vissler, N., Valitsky, M., & Bar-Tana, J. (2012). Suppression of adipose lipolysis by long-chain fatty acid analogs. *Journal of Lipid Research*, 53(5), 868–878.

Lee, S., Lee, H., Kim, Y., & Kim, E. (2019). Effect of DPP-IV inhibitors on glycemic variability in patients with T2DM: a systematic review and meta-analysis. *Scientific reports*, 9(1), 13296.

Li, X., Yu, Y., & Funk, C. D. (2013). Cyclooxygenase-2 induction in macrophages is modulated by docosahexaenoic acid via interactions with free fatty acid receptor 4 (FFA4). *The FASEB Journal*, 27(12), 4987–4997.

Liu, Y., Chen, L., Sokolowska, M., Eberlein, M., Alsaaty, S., Martinez-Anton, A., Logun, C., Qi, H., & Shelhamer, J. H. (2014). The fish oil ingredient, docosahexaenoic acid, activates cytosolic phospholipase A 2 via GPR120 receptor to produce prostaglandin E 2 and plays an anti-inflammatory role in macrophages. *Immunology*, 143(1), 81–95.

Lombardo, M., Bender, K., London, C., Plotkin, M. A., Kirkland, M., Mane, J., Pachanski, M., Geissler, W., Cummings, J., Habulihaz, B., Akiyama, T. E., Di Salvo, J., Madeira, M., Pols, J., Powles, M. A., Finley, M. F., Johnson, E., Roussel, T., Uebele, V. N., Crespo, A., Leung, D., Alleyne, C., Trusca, D., Lei, Y., Howard, A. D., Ujjainwalla, F., Tata, J. R., & Sinz, C. J. (2016). Discovery of benzofuran propanoic acid GPR120 agonists: From uHTS hit to mechanism-based pharmacodynamic effects. *Bioorganic & Medicinal Chemistry Letters*, 26(23), 5724-5728.

Matsuzaka, T., & Shimano, H. (2011). Molecular mechanisms involved in hepatic steatosis and insulin resistance: Disordered lipid metabolism and diabetes. *Journal of Diabetes Investigation*, 2(3), 170–175.

Milligan, G., Alvarez-Curto, E., Watterson, K. R., Ulven, T., & Hudson, B. D. (2015). Characterizing pharmacological ligands to study the long-chain fatty acid receptors GPR 40/FFA 1 and GPR 120/FFA 4. *British journal of pharmacology*, 172(13), 3254-3265.

Milligan, G., Shimpukade, B., Ulven, T., & Hudson, B. D. (2017). Complex pharmacology of free fatty acid receptors. Chemical Reviews, 117(1), 67.

Moniri, N. H. (2016). Free-fatty acid receptor-4 (GPR120): Cellular and molecular function and its role in metabolic disorders. *Biochemical pharmacology*, 110, 1-15

Moore, K., Zhang, Q., Murgolo, N., Hosted, T., & Duffy, R. (2009). Cloning, expression, and pharmacological characterization of the GPR120 free fatty acid receptor from cynomolgus monkey: comparison with human GPR120 splice variants. *Comparative Biochemistry and Physiology Part B: Biochemistry and Molecular Biology*, 154(4), 419-426.

Oh, D. Y., Talukdar, S., Bae, E. J., Imamura, T., Morinaga, H., Fan, W., Li, P., Lu, W. J., Watkins, S. M., & Olefsky, J. M. (2010). GPR120 is an omega-3 fatty acid receptor mediating potent anti-inflammatory and insulin-sensitizing effects. *Cell metabolism*, 142(5), 687–698.

Roder, P. V., Wu, B., Liu, Y., & Han, W. (2016). Pancreatic regulation of glucose homeostasis. *Experimental and molecular medicine*, 48, 1-19.

Rohwedder, A., Zhang, Q., Rudge, S. A., & Wakelam, M. J. O. (2014). Lipid droplet formation in response to oleic acid in Huh-7 cells is a fatty acid receptor mediated event. *Journal of Cell Science*, 127(Pt 14), 3104-3115.

Schenk, S., Saberi, M., & Olefsky, J. M. (2008). Insulin sensitivity: modulation by nutrients and inflammation. *The Journal of clinical investigation*, 118(9), 2992-3002.

Segerstolpe, Å., Palasantza, A., Eliasson, P., Andersson, E. M., Andréasson, A. C., Sun, X., Picelli, S., Sabirsh, A., Clausen, M., Bjursell, M. K., Smith, D. M., Kasper, M., Ämmälä, C., & Sandberg, R. (2016). Single-Cell Transcriptome Profiling of Human Pancreatic Islets in Health and Type 2Diabetes. *Cell metabolism*, 24(4), 593–607.

Shimpukade, B., Hudson, B. D., Hovgaard, C. K., Milligan, G., & Ulven, T. (2012). Discovery of a potent and selective GPR120 agonist. *Journal of medicinal chemistry*, 55(9), 4511-4515.

Sparks, S. M., Chen, G., Collins, J. L., Danger, D., Dock, S. T., Jayawickreme, C., Jenkinson, S., Laudeman, C., Leesnitzer, M. A., Liang, X., Maloney, P., McCoy, D. C., Moncol, D., Rash, V., Rimele, T., Vulimiri, P., Way, J. M., & Ross, S. (2014). Identification of diarylsulfonamides as agonists of the free fatty acid receptor 4 (FFA4/GPR120). *Bioorganic & medicinal chemistry letters*, 24(14), 3100-3103.

Stone, V. M., Dhayal, S., Brocklehurst, K. J., Lenaghan, C., Sörhede Winzell, M., Hammar, M., Xu, X., Smith, D. M., & Morgan, N. G. (2014). GPR120 (FFAR4) is preferentially expressed in pancreatic delta cells and regulates somatostatin secretion from murine islets of Langerhans. *Diabetologia*, 57(6), 1182–1191.

Suckow, A. T., Polidori, D., Yan, W., Chon, S., Ma, J. Y., Leonard, J., & Briscoe, C. P. (2014). Alteration of the Glucagon Axis in GPR120 (FFAR4) Knockout Mice. *Journal of Biological Chemistry*, 289(22), 15751–15763.

Watson, S. J., Brown, A. J., & Holliday, N. D. (2012). Differential signaling by splice variants of the human free fatty acid receptor GPR120. *Molecular Pharmacology*, 81(5), 631-642.

Winters, M. P., Sui, Z., Wall, M., Wang, Y., Gunnet, J., Leonard, J., Hua, H., Yan, W., Suckow, A., Bell, A., Clapper, W., Jenkinson, C., Haug, P., Koudriakova, T., Huebert, N., & Murray, W. V. (2018). Discovery of N-arylpyrroles as agonists of GPR120 for the treatment of type II diabetes. *Bioorganic & Medicinal Chemistry Letters*, 28(5), 841-846.

Yan, Y., Jiang, W., Spinetti, T., Tardivel, A., Castillo, R., Bourquin, C., Guarda, G., Tian, Z., Tschopp, J., & Zhou, R. (2013). Omega-3 Fatty Acids Prevent Inflammation and Metabolic Disorder through Inhibition of NLRP3 Inflammasome Activation. *Immunity*, 38(6), 1154–1163.

Zhang, X., Cai, C., Winters, M., Wells, M., Wall, M., Lanter, J., Sui, Z., Ma, J., Novack, A., Nashashibi, I., Wang, Y., Yan, W., Suckow, A., Hua, H., Bell, A., Haug, P., Clapper, W., Jenkinson, C., Gunnet, J., Leonard, J., & Murray, W. V. (2017). Design, synthesis, and SAR of a novel series of heterocyclic phenylpropanoic acids as GPR120 agonists. *Bioorganic & Medicinal Chemistry Letters*, 27(15), 3272-3278.

Chapter 5

Insulin Receptors: Central Mediators of Glucose Homeostasis

Megha Tonk[1,2]
Shikha Baghel Chauhan[2]
Rajan Swami[3]
K. S. Gayathri[4]
Elezebeth Mathews[5]
Indu Singh[2]
and Alagu Manickavelu[4,*]

[1]Raj Kumar Goel Institute of Technology (Pharmacy), Ghaziabad, Uttar Pradesh, India
[2]Amity Institute of Pharmacy, Amity University, Noida, Uttar Pradesh, India
[3]Chitkara College of Pharmacy, Chitkara University, Punjab, India
[4]Department of Genomic Science, Central University of Kerala, Tejaswini Hills, Periye, Kasaragod, Kerala, India
[5]Department of Public Health and Community Medicine, Central University of Kerala, Tejaswini Hills, Periye, Kasaragod, Kerala, India

Abstract

Insulin receptors are crucial components in the regulation of glucose homeostasis, serving as central mediators that facilitate the body's ability to maintain optimal blood glucose levels. These receptors, located on the surfaces of various cell types, including liver, muscle, and adipose tissue, are activated by insulin, a hormone produced by pancreatic beta cells in response to elevated blood glucose levels. Upon insulin binding, these receptors initiate a cascade of intracellular signaling pathways that enhance glucose uptake, storage, and utilization. This process is essential for lowering blood glucose levels post-prandially and ensuring energy availability for cellular functions. Dysregulation of insulin receptor function, through mechanisms such as receptor resistance or impaired signaling, is a hallmark of metabolic disorders like type 2 diabetes mellitus, leading to chronic hyperglycemia and associated complications. Understanding the molecular mechanisms governing insulin receptor activity and its interaction with intracellular signaling networks

---

* Corresponding Author's Email: amanicks@cukerala.ac.in

In: Receptor-Targeted Therapies in Diabetes Mellitus
Editors: Ajmer Singh Grewal, Neelam Singh, Swati Verma et al.
ISBN: 979-8-89530-587-4

is critical for developing targeted therapies aimed at restoring proper glucose homeostasis in diabetic patients.

Keywords: insulin receptors, glucose, homeostasis, hyperglycemia, blood glucose, hormone

Abbreviations

AS160	Akt substrate 160 kDa
CR	Cysteine-rich
ECD	Ectodomain
FnIII	Fibronectin type III domains
FOXO	Forkhead box
GS	Glycogen synthase
GSK3	Glycogen synthase kinase 3
ID	Insert domain
IGF-1	Insulin-like growth factor 1
IGF-2	Insulin-like growth factor 2
IR	Insulin receptor
IRR	IR-related receptor
IRS	Insulin responsive substrates
MAPK	Ras-mitogen-activated protein kinase
mTORC1	mammalian target of rapamycin complex 1
PDK1	Phosphoinositide-dependent protein kinase 1
PI3K	Phosphoinositide 3-kinase
PIP3	Phosphatidylinositol 3,4,5-trisphosphate
PKB	AKT/protein kinase B
PKG	cGMP-dependent protein kinase
T2DM	Type 2 diabetes mellitus
TSC	Tumour suppressor complex
WAT	White adipose tissue

Introduction

Insulin is a hormone consisting of 51 amino acids that help control metabolism, support cell growth, and maintain balanced blood sugar levels. Dr. Frederick Banting was the pioneer in Toronto in 1921-1922, isolating and purifying insulin. Since its discovery, scientists have worked extensively to improve the quality of insulin. In 1923, the Nobel Prize in Physiology or Medicine was awarded for this groundbreaking discovery (Tattersall and Matthews, 2024). Other hormones, including glucagon, were also discovered as a result of the discovery of insulin. Individuals with type 2 diabetes or other types of diabetes mellitus rely on insulin as their primary treatment. Insulin has proven to be a lifeline for those with type 1 diabetes (Mathieu, 2021). Initially, it was thought that this hormone could only be produced by pancreatic β cells, but recent research has revealed that some neurons in the central nervous system may also produce small amounts of insulin (Haeusler, 2018). Insulin is an anabolic hormone that has a wide range of cell-mediated responses and effects. Its primary physiological role is to maintain glucose homeostasis. Blood glucose levels are typically maintained in the range of 80–100 mg/dL, or 4–6 mM, under healthy conditions (Ali, 2018). The function of pancreatic β- and α-cells is crucial for preserving blood glucose homeostasis. A higher blood glucose level after meals stimulates pancreatic β-cells to secrete insulin, which enhances cellular glucose absorption and lowers blood glucose levels. Conversely, low glucose levels between meals trigger pancreatic α-cells to release glucagon, activating metabolic pathways to increase systemic glucose concentrations. In muscle cells, insulin promotes glucose uptake and protein synthesis; in adipose tissue, insulin facilitates fatty acid absorption and suppresses lipolysis and glucose production; in the liver, insulin reduces glucose generation; and in the brain, it regulates glucose balance, eating behavior, and nutritional fluxes (Cignarelli, 2019; Boucsein, 2021). Despite these varying effects, the proximal components of insulin signal transduction are very similar in all insulin-responsive cells. Distinct distal effectors play a key role in the variety of physiological insulin responses seen in different cell types. The mechanism of insulin action involves binding to the insulin receptor, a member of the extensive tyrosine kinase family of receptors. This binding increases the quantity of glucose transporter proteins at the cell surface, thereby enhancing glucose uptake through the activation of the phosphoinositide 3-kinase (PI3K) intracellular signaling pathway (Mauvais-Jarvis, 2018). In this chapter, we will cover the current understanding of glucose homeostasis and the processes behind the insulin receptor's role as a central mediator of glucose homeostasis. Additionally, disorders related to insulin receptor dysfunction (insulin resistance) will be addressed, along with a summary of the mechanisms of insulin resistance.

Glucose Homeostasis

Glucose is the primary energy source for most cells in the body and serves as a substrate for various metabolic processes (Sędzikowska and Szablewski, 2021). In plasma, glucose is derived either from dietary intake or through two main metabolic processes: glycogenolysis and gluconeogenesis. To maintain glucose levels within the healthy physiological range of 4–6 mM, the body regulates glucose usage and production based on fed or fasted states, a process known as glucose homeostasis (Rieusset, 2018). Glucose homeostasis involves several mechanisms, including gluconeogenesis in the liver and kidneys, uptake by muscle and adipocytes, absorption in the gastrointestinal tract, and reabsorption and excretion by the liver and kidneys (Matschinsky and Wilson, 2019). The body employs a complex neurohormonal system to carefully monitor and regulate glucose levels within this narrow physiological range (Bizzotto, 2021). Various organs and hormones are essential for glucose regulation at the tissue level, with insulin and glucagon playing key roles in controlling each organ's metabolism, including glucose intake, storage, mobilization, and breakdown. Pancreatic β-cells release insulin in response to elevated blood glucose levels. Insulin, in turn, promotes glucose homeostasis by enhancing glucose uptake by skeletal muscle and white adipose tissue (WAT) while inhibiting hepatic glucose production (Norton, 2022). Maintaining glucose homeostasis is essential to prevent potentially fatal central nervous system damage from prolonged hypoglycemia and to avoid the adverse effects of chronic hyperglycemia, such as nephropathy, retinopathy, and vascular complications (Hamilton, 2021).

Insulin Receptor

In 1972, the IR was initially identified in the membranes of fat and liver cells (Lawrence, 2021). The IR is a dimeric protein essential for maintaining glucose homeostasis, regulating the metabolism of fats, proteins, and carbohydrates, and adjusting the levels of neurotransmitters in the brain (Viola, 2023). It is an $\alpha 2\beta 2$ tetramer that is glycosylated and disulfide-linked and belongs to the receptor tyrosine kinase subfamily, which also includes the insulin receptor-related receptor (IRR) and the insulin-like growth factor 1 (IGF-1) receptor (Saltiel, 2021). There are two isoforms of the IR, A and B. The B isoform has been suggested to mediate most of the metabolic effects of insulin, as it is much more selective for the hormone; it is also the predominant isoform expressed in differentiated liver, muscle, and white adipose tissue (WAT). The A isoform, produced by splicing out exon 11, is widely expressed during fetal development, as its high affinity for insulin-like growth factor 2 (IGF2) is particularly beneficial (Vella, 2018). Insulin and IGF2 are two closely related ligands that can activate insulin receptors (IRs). Insulin and IGF2 bind to the insulin receptor (IR) with different strengths and activate it in distinct ways. This enables them to perform various biological functions through the same receptor, depending on the tissue, metabolic conditions, or developmental stage (An, 2024). The IR has two binding sites for insulin but exhibits "negative cooperativity." This means that when insulin binds to one site, it makes it more difficult for insulin to bind to the second site. Current information suggests that one insulin molecule binds to and activates one IR at physiological concentrations (Shtykova, 2019). Since the 1980s, the receptor's basic structure has been identified as consisting of an intracellular tyrosine kinase domain, a single transmembrane helix, and an extracellular region known as the ectodomain (ECD). The binding of insulin to the dimeric ECD initiates the auto-phosphorylation of the tyrosine kinase domain, which, in turn, activates downstream signaling pathways. The insulin receptor is denoted as $(\alpha\beta)_2$, a dimer of heterodimers composed of two α-chains and two β-chains. The entire insulin receptor ECD consists of the α-chain and about 190 residues from the β-chain's N-terminus, which are located on the extracellular side of the plasma membrane (Figure 1). The remaining β-chain comprises the juxtamembrane domain, the intracellular tyrosine kinase domain, and a transmembrane helix (Xu, 2022, Bershatsky, 2023). McKern et al. described the structural organization of the insulin receptor (IR), showing that each ECD monomer is composed of three fibronectin type III domains (FnIII-1 to FnIII-3), followed by a leucine-rich repeat (L1) domain, a cysteine-rich (CR) region, and a second leucine-rich repeat (L2). The α-β cleavage site is located within the 120-residue insert domain (ID) of FnIII-2. The cysteines C647 and C860 are involved in the disulfide bond that connects the α- and β-chains. Additionally, α-α disulfide bonds exist between the triplets C682, C683, and C685 in the ID, and at position C524 in the FnIII-1 domain (McKern, 2006; Yunn, 2021).

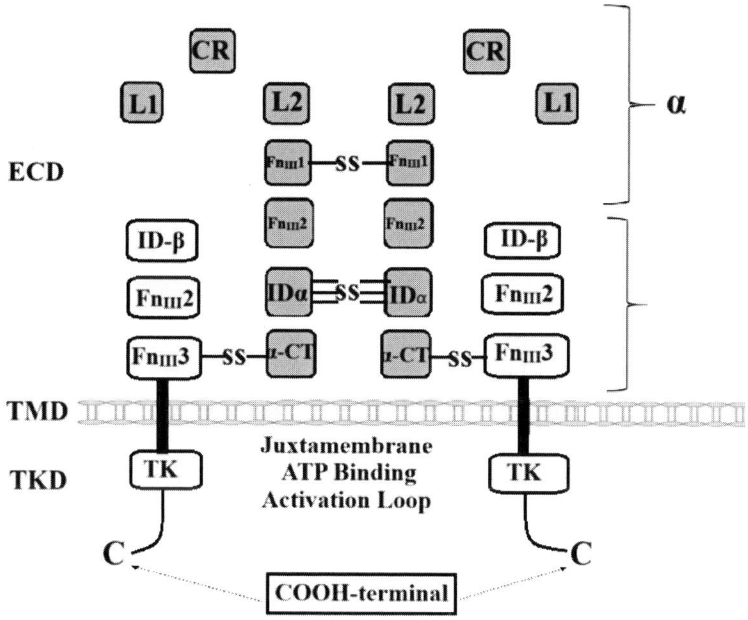

Figure 1. Structure of the mature IR. It is made up of two covalently bonded transmembrane β-subunits and extracellular α-subunits (Scapin, 2018).

Insulin Signaling

The identification and characterization of the IR have significantly advanced our understanding of the molecular mechanisms governing insulin's role in glucose homeostasis. Insulin binds to the cell surface IR, initiating intracellular signaling cascades that lead to specific cellular responses (Martín and Ramos, 2021). Insulin directly binds to the extracellular α-subunits of the IR receptor. This binding induces a conformational change that activates the tyrosine kinase domain of the intracellular β-subunits. The activated β-subunit then undergoes intramolecular transphosphorylation, phosphorylating adjacent subunits on specific tyrosine residues (Akhtar and Sah, 2020). This process facilitates the tyrosine phosphorylation of intracellular substrate proteins known as insulin receptor substrates (IRS). Four IRS proteins with distinct functions are recognized, among which IRS-1 and IRS-2 undergo phosphorylation in response to insulin stimulation. This activation initiates two major signaling pathways: the Ras-mitogen-activated protein kinase (MAPK) pathway and the phosphatidylinositol 3-kinase (PI3K)-AKT/protein kinase B (PKB) pathway (Gupta, 2022). The PI3K/AKT pathway mediates the majority of insulin's metabolic effects (Kwon and Pessin, 2020). Upon phosphorylation of IRS-1, it binds to and activates the lipid kinase PI3K, triggering a cascade of additional kinases, including AKT (White and Kahn, 2021). This pathway promotes glucose uptake by skeletal muscle and adipose tissue by facilitating the translocation of insulin-responsive glucose transporters (GLUTs) to the cell membrane (Czech, 2017). Additionally, activation of the PI3K/AKT pathway enhances glycogen synthesis and suppresses gluconeogenesis in the liver. The MAPK pathway, on the other hand, is primarily involved in insulin's effects on cell growth, including mitogenesis, differentiation, migration, and survival, but does not play a role in insulin's metabolic functions (Wen, 2022).

PI3K-AKT/PKB Signaling Pathway

Insulin stimulates the absorption of glucose through mechanisms that are both dependent and independent of phosphatidylinositol (PI) 3-kinase (PI3K) (Świderska, 2018). Upon tyrosine phosphorylation, IRS proteins bind to the p85 regulatory subunit of PI3K, activating the enzyme and directing it to the plasma membrane. Phosphatidylinositol 3,4,5-trisphosphate (PIP3), a lipid molecule produced by the enzyme, controls the location and function of several proteins (Gabbouj, 2019). These lipids influence the activity or subcellular localization of many signaling molecules by binding to their pleckstrin homology (PH) domains. PIP3 regulates three main groups of signaling molecules: the Tec family of tyrosine kinases, which includes BTK (Bruton's tyrosine kinase) and ITK (Interleukin-2 inducible T cell kinase); the AGC (cyclic AMP [cAMP]-dependent protein kinase 1 [protein kinase A {PKA}], cGMP-dependent protein kinase, and protein kinase C [PKC]) superfamily of serine/threonine protein kinases; and the guanine nucleotide exchange proteins of the Rho family of GTPases (Saltiel, 2016; Ringheim, 2021). A leading kinase, phosphoinositide-dependent protein kinase 1 (PDK1), phosphorylates at least 23 AGC kinases at the activation loop, a critical location for their activity. In signaling, PDK1 is essential for the downstream signaling of growth factors, insulin, and PI3K (Sacerdoti, 2023). Protein kinase B (PKB, also known as Akt) is a crucial component of this family, involved in various forms of cell survival and growth promotion. Due to its PH domain, AKT exhibits affinity for PIP3 in the same way as PDK1 (Powis, 2023).

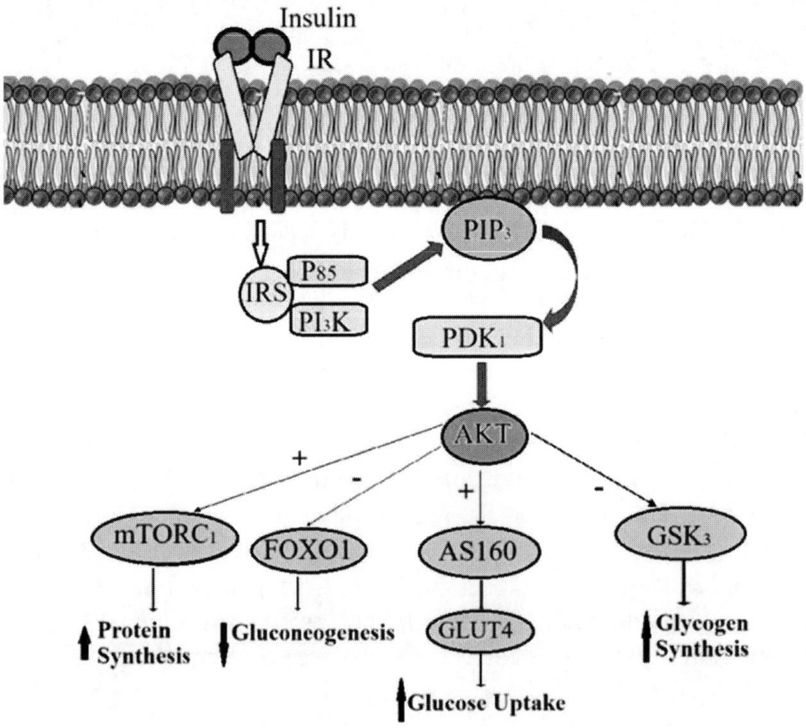

Figure 2. Molecular mechanism of insulin PI3K-AKT/PKB signaling pathway.

Upon binding to PIP3, AKT undergoes conformational changes that expose the phosphorylation site. PDK1 can then phosphorylate AKT on Thr 308 when the two are nearby. This process causes AKT to detach from the plasma membrane, enabling it to activate a range of downstream effectors (Zhang, 2019; Zheng, 2022). More than 100 substrates of Akt have been documented in scholarly publications. The first known substrate of Akt was glycogen synthase kinase 3 (GSK3) (Esteban-Villarrubia, 2020). It was discovered that GSK3 phosphorylates glycogen synthase (GS) to inhibit it, thereby altering glucose metabolism. In response to insulin, GSK3 is phosphorylated and inactivated, which allows GS activation and the deposition of glucose as glycogen (Wang, 2022). The transcription factors of the forkhead box (FOXO) family are another key substrate of Akt (Lee, 2020). These transcription factors are typically located in the nucleus, where Akt signaling causes their translocation, inhibiting their transcriptional activity. This process prevents the activation of programs controlling gluconeogenesis and lipid synthesis through FOXO (Homan, 2021). By directly phosphorylating AS160 (Akt substrate 160 kDa), Akt inhibits the function of the Rab-GTPase-activating protein, which leads to GLUT4 translocation and glucose absorption. Additionally, Akt regulates multiple proteins involved in protein synthesis by activating mTORC1 (mammalian target of rapamycin complex 1) through suppression of the tumor suppressor complex (TSC1/TSC2) (Khalid, 2021; Maines 2021). The whole molecular mechanism of the insulin signaling pathway is diagrammatically represented in Figure 2.

Insulin Resistance

When an organism's body, tissues, or cells are unable to respond efficiently to normal insulin levels, it is said to have developed insulin resistance. As a result, insulin's ability to maintain glucose and lipid homeostasis is impaired (Petersen and Shulman, 2018). When insulin fails to achieve normoglycemia, compensatory hyperinsulinemia occurs, leading to an increased amount of insulin secreted by β-cells. Prolonged insulin release eventually exhausts pancreatic β-cells, causing them to die (Hall, 2020). Furthermore, insulin resistance promotes lipolysis in adipose tissue, disrupts muscle glucose absorption, and enhances gluconeogenesis in the liver. Both genetic and acquired factors contribute to insulin resistance. Common genetic disorders include mutations and polymorphisms in insulin receptors, glucose transporters, and signaling proteins involved in insulin signal transduction. Acquired causes of insulin resistance include obesity, physical inactivity, advanced glycation end products (AGEs), excess free fatty acids (FFAs), psychological stress, smoking, alcohol use, and certain medications (Barber, 2021, Zhao, 2023). Much work has been done to identify the mechanism behind insulin resistance and two major reasons are responsible: (i) Dysregulation of IR binding (ii) Post IR defects.

- *Dysregulation of IR binding*: When insulin binds to its cell-surface receptors, it activates adaptor proteins, including the IRS proteins, which in turn promote downstream insulin signaling that regulates glucose homeostasis. This is how insulin functions biologically. Defective IR binding is primarily characterized by a reduction in the quantity and sensitivity of target receptors on the cell membrane or structural anomalies of the target receptors that impair insulin binding. As a result, many insulin resistance phenotypes can be explained by changes in IR expression, ligand binding, phosphorylation states, and/or kinase activity. Consequently, insulin resistance is influenced by various defects in signal transduction (Sakurai, 2021; Tagi, 2019).

- *Post-IR defects*: It includes irregularities in mitogenic and metabolic signals, as well as impacts on substrates and negative modulators of insulin signaling (Le, 2023). Numerous key elements of the insulin signaling system have previously been discussed. These can be divided into two groups: the proximal part, which comprises the core canonical signaling pathway, including the insulin receptor, insulin receptor substrate (IRS), phosphoinositide 3-kinase (PI3K), and AKT; and the distal part, which consists of various components downstream of AKT, such as FOXO1, GSK3, and AS160. Insulin resistance has been associated with deficiencies in proximal insulin signaling that are linked to cellular stress (Mastrototaro and Roden, 2021). Numerous intracellular stresses trigger various Ser/Thr kinases that phosphorylate the IR or IRS proteins, including mTOR, novel protein kinase C (PKC), mitogen-activated protein kinases (MAPKs), and S6 kinase. This is believed to be a negative-feedback mechanism that inhibits insulin signaling (James, 2021).

Metabolic Disorders Associated with Insulin Resistance

IR is one of the primary features of T2DM. Additionally, it is associated with several metabolic disorders, including polycystic ovarian syndrome, metabolic syndrome, obesity, nonalcoholic fatty liver disease (NAFLD), hypertension, and hyperlipidemia. According to epidemiological research, more than 80% of T2DM patients develop IR. Therefore, here we summarize T2DM and its treatment options (Ormazabal, 2018).

Type 2 Diabetes Mellitus (T2DM)

T2DM is the most prevalent metabolic disorder globally, accounting for over 90% of reported diabetes cases. It is pathologically characterized by insulin resistance, leading to glucolipid metabolism dysfunction. In addition to having a significant hereditary component, T2DM is influenced by lifestyle factors such as age, pregnancy, and obesity (Lu, 2023). Insulin resistance marks the initial stage of T2DM pathogenesis, followed by oxidative stress, which accelerates β-cell insufficiency, increased plasma glucose levels (leading to excessive insulin secretion by β-cells), worsening hyperglycemia, β-cell apoptosis, and ultimately the development of overt T2DM (Gu, 2020). Insulin resistance, a primary indicator of T2DM, is observed as reduced tissue sensitivity to insulin, making it a crucial target for developing effective management therapies (Chao, 2018). In 2021, the world celebrated a century since the groundbreaking discovery of insulin, the first pharmaceutical therapy for diabetes mellitus. Over these 100 years, the FDA has approved ten distinct classes of medications for managing T2DM, with most approvals occurring in the last two decades (Perreault, 2021). Various pharmaceutical drugs have been used to enhance insulin sensitivity and prevent T2DM, primarily including biguanides, thiazolidinediones, and GLP-1 receptor agonists (Table 1) (Li, 2022). Despite the numerous treatment options available, the pipeline for novel T2DM treatments remains robust and highly innovative (Nauck, 2021; Dahlén, 2022). Organizations developing new formulations aim to make them novel, best in class, and either superior to or complementary to existing therapies. These novel treatments focus on maximizing safety, offering non-glycaemic benefits, preventing complications for at-risk patients, and helping individuals achieve personalized glycaemic targets (Blaslov, 2018). In addition to medications, T2DM management involves lifestyle modifications such as regular exercise, a balanced diet, stress management, and disease prevention, along with alternative therapeutic approaches (Magkos, 2020).

Table 1. Medication for management of T2DM (Bellary, 2021)

Category	Drug	Dose (mg)	Mechanism of action
Thiazolidinediones	Pioglitazone	15-45	It stimulates insulin-dependent glucose elimination, improves impaired glucose homeostasis, and increases cellular insulin response.
	Rosiglitazone	2-8	It is a strong and highly specific agonist for the peroxisome proliferator-activated receptor gamma (PPARγ) and increases insulin sensitivity, which helps in glycemic management.
Biguanides	Metformin (IR, SR/XR formulations)	500-3000	Lowers intestinal glucose absorption, decreases hepatic glucose synthesis, and improves insulin sensitivity by increasing peripheral glucose uptake and utilization.
Sulfonylureas	Glimepiride	1-6	It reduces blood sugar levels by inducing endogenous insulin production, which is followed by peripheral insulin receptor sensitivity enhancement and decreased glycogenolysis.
	Glibenclamide	2.5-20	
	Gliclazide	40-320	
	Gliclazide MR	30-100	
	Glipizide	2.5-20	
DPP4 inhibitors	sitagliptin	25-100	It prevents the breakdown of incretins, glucose-dependent insulinotropic peptide (GIP), and glucagon-like peptide-1 (GLP-1). Consequently, prevent the production of glucagon, which raises insulin secretion, reduces stomach emptying, and lowers blood glucose.
	Alogliptin	6.25-25.00	
	Linagliptin	5	
	Saxagliptin	2.5-5.0	
	Vildagliptin	50-100	
GLP-1 receptor agonists	Dulaglutide	0.75–1.50 QW	Activates receptors for GLP-1. Thereby enhances insulin release, reduces glucagon release, slows down stomach emptying, and boosts feelings of satiety.
	Semaglutide	0.5–1.0 QW	
	Liraglutide	0.6–1.8 OD	
	Exenatide	5–10 μg BD	
	Lixisenatide	10–20 μg OD	
Meglitinides	Nateglinide	60-540	It lowers blood sugar by promoting the body's inherent synthesis of insulin.
	Repaglinide	0.5-16.0	
SGLT2 inhibitors	Canagliflozin	100-300	SGLT2 inhibitors work primarily by blocking the sodium-glucose co-transporter 2 (SGLT2) in the proximal renal tubules of the kidneys. This action prevents reabsorption of glucose back into the bloodstream, leading to increased glucose excretion through urine (glycosuria)
	Dapagliflozin	5-10	
	Empagliflozin	10-25	
	Ertugliflozin	5-15	
PPAR full agonists	Chiglitazar Sodium	48	It controls the overexpression of ANGPTL4 and PDK4, which are components of the PPAR signal pathway and it controls insulin resistance-associated PPARγ phosphorylation and implicated in glucose and lipid metabolism.

Conclusion

Insulin receptors play a critical role in regulating glucose levels throughout the body and are essential for maintaining glucose homeostasis. They lower blood glucose levels after meals by facilitating glucose uptake by cells, particularly those in muscle, liver, and adipose tissue. This process is vital for energy metabolism and the storage of glucose as glycogen in the liver and muscles. Two primary signaling pathways are activated by insulin: the MAPK pathway and the PI3K-AKT/PKB pathway. Among these, the PI3K/AKT pathway mediates most of insulin's metabolic effects. Disruption of these downstream signaling pathways leads to insulin resistance, increasing the risk of type 2 diabetes mellitus (T2DM) and associated comorbidities, including glucose intolerance. Thus, insulin receptors play a crucial role in maintaining glucose balance in the bloodstream, which is essential for cellular function and overall health.

A deeper understanding of insulin action and resistance has the potential to transform diabetes management. This knowledge can aid in the development of novel therapeutics and optimize the use of existing antidiabetic medications. Most importantly, it can inform preventative strategies to significantly reduce the growing incidence of T2DM.

References

Akhtar, A., & Sah, S. P. (2020). Insulin signaling pathway and related molecules: Role in neurodegeneration and Alzheimer's disease. *Neurochemistry International*, 135, 104707.

Ali, J. B., Hamdi, T., Fnaiech, N., Di Costanzo, V., Fnaiech, F., & Ginoux, J. M. (2018). Continuous blood glucose level prediction of type 1 diabetes based on artificial neural network. *Biocybernetics and Biomedical Engineering*, 38(4), 828-840.

An, W., Hall, C., Li, J., Hung, A., Wu, J., Park, J., Wang, L., Bai, X. C., & Choi, E. (2024). Activation of the insulin receptor by insulin-like growth factor 2. *Nature Communications*, 15(1), 2609.

Barber, T. M., Kyrou, I., Randeva, H. S., & Weickert, M. O. (2021). Mechanisms of insulin resistance at the crossroad of obesity with associated metabolic abnormalities and cognitive dysfunction. *International Journal of Molecular Sciences*, 22(2), 546.

Bellary, S., Kyrou, I., Brown, J. E., & Bailey, C. J. (2021). Type 2 diabetes mellitus in older adults: Clinical considerations and management. *Nature Reviews Endocrinology*, 17(9), 534-548.

Bershatsky, Y. V., Kuznetsov, A. S., Idiatullina, A. R., Bocharova, O. V., Dolotova, S. M., Gavrilenkova, A. A., Serova, O. V., Deyev, I. E., Rakitina, T. V., Zangieva, O. T., & Pavlov, K. V. (2023). Diversity of structural, dynamic, and environmental effects explain a distinctive functional role of transmembrane domains in the insulin receptor subfamily. *International Journal of Molecular Sciences*, 24(4), 3906.

Bizzotto, R., Tricò, D., Natali, A., Gastaldelli, A., Muscelli, E., De Fronzo, R. A., Arslanian, S., Ferrannini, E., & Mari, A. (2021). New insights on the interactions between insulin clearance and the main glucose homeostasis mechanisms. *Diabetes Care*, 44(9), 2115-2123.

Blaslov, K., Naranđa, F. S., Kruljac, I., & Renar, I. P. (2018). Treatment approach to type 2 diabetes: Past, present, and future. *World Journal of Diabetes*, 9(12), 209.

Boucsein, A., Kamstra, K., & Tups, A. (2021). Central signalling cross-talk between insulin and leptin in glucose and energy homeostasis. *Journal of Neuroendocrinology*, 33(4), e12944.

Chao, P. C., Li, Y., Chang, C. H., Shieh, J. P., Cheng, J. T., & Cheng, K. C. (2018). Investigation of insulin resistance in the popularly used four rat models of type-2 diabetes. *Biomedicine and Pharmacotherapy*, 101, 155-161.

Cignarelli, A., Genchi, V. A., Perrini, S., Natalicchio, A., Laviola, L., & Giorgino, F. (2019). Insulin and insulin receptors in adipose tissue development. International Journal of Molecular Sciences, 20(3), 759.

Czech, M. P. (2017). Insulin action and resistance in obesity and type 2 diabetes. *Nature Medicine*, 23(7), 804-814.

Dahlén, A. D., Dashi, G., Maslov, I., Attwood, M. M., Jonsson, J., Trukhan, V., & Schiöth, H. B. (2022). Trends in antidiabetic drug discovery: FDA-approved drugs, new drugs in clinical trials and global sales. *Frontiers in Pharmacology*, 12, 807548.

Esteban-Villarrubia, J., Soto-Castillo, J. J., Pozas, J., San Román-Gil, M., Orejana-Martín, I., Torres-Jiménez, J., Carrato, A., Alonso-Gordoa, T., & Molina-Cerrillo, J. (2020). Tyrosine kinase receptors in oncology. *International Journal of Molecular Sciences*, 21(22), 8529.

Gabbouj, S., Ryhänen, S., Marttinen, M., Wittrahm, R., Takalo, M., Kemppainen, S., Martiskainen, H., Tanila, H., Haapasalo, A., Hiltunen, M., & Natunen, T. (2019). Altered insulin signaling in Alzheimer's disease brain–special emphasis on PI3K-Akt pathway. *Frontiers in Neuroscience*, 13, 629.

Gu, X., Al Dubayee, M., Alshahrani, A., Masood, A., Benabdelkamel, H., Zahra, M., Li, L., Abdel Rahman, A. M., & Aljada, A. (2020). Distinctive metabolomics patterns associated with insulin resistance and type 2 diabetes mellitus. *Frontiers in Molecular Biosciences*, 7, 609806.

Gupta, A. (2022). Insulin-mediated signaling pathways in healthy state and insulin resistance state. *Journal of Pure and Applied Science and Technology*, 12(2), 1-30.

Haeusler, R. A., McGraw, T. E., & Accili, D. (2018). Biochemical and cellular properties of insulin receptor signalling. *Nature Reviews Molecular Cell Biology*, 19(1), 31-44.

Hall, C., Yu, H., & Choi, E. (2020). Insulin receptor endocytosis in the pathophysiology of insulin resistance. *Experimental and Molecular Medicine*, 52(6), 911-920.

Hamilton, J. S., & Klett, E. L. (2021). Linoleic acid and the regulation of glucose homeostasis: A review of the evidence. *Prostaglandins, Leukotrienes and Essential Fatty Acids*, 175, 102366.

Homan, E. P., Brandão, B. B., Softic, S., El Ouaamari, A., O'Neill, B. T., Kulkarni, R. N., Kim, J. K., & Kahn, C. R. (2021). Differential roles of FOXO transcription factors on insulin action in brown and white adipose tissue. *The Journal of Clinical Investigation*, 131(19), e143328.

James, D. E., Stöckli, J., & Birnbaum, M. J. (2021). The aetiology and molecular landscape of insulin resistance. *Nature Reviews Molecular Cell Biology*, 22(11), 751-771.

Khalid, M., Alkaabi, J., Khan, M. A., & Adem, A. (2021). Insulin signal transduction perturbations in insulin resistance. *International Journal of Molecular Sciences*, 22(16), 8590.

Kwon, H., & Pessin, J. E. (2020). Insulin-mediated PI3K and AKT signaling. *In The Liver: Biology and Pathobiology* (pp. 485-495).

Lawrence, M. C. (2021). Understanding insulin and its receptor from their three-dimensional structures. *Molecular Metabolism*, 52, 101255.

Le, T. K. C., Dao, X. D., Nguyen, D. V., Luu, D. H., Bui, T. M. H., Le, T. H., Nguyen, H. T., Le, T. N., Hosaka, T., & Nguyen, T. T. T. (2023). Insulin signaling and its application. *Frontiers in Endocrinology*, 14, 1226655.

Lee, S., Zhu, C., Yamauchi, J., Zhu, P., Feng, X., Qu, S., & Dong, H. H. (2020). The forkhead box O family in insulin action and lipid metabolism. *In Lipid Signaling and Metabolism* (pp. 247-272). Academic Press.

Li, M., Chi, X., Wang, Y., Setrerrahmane, S., Xie, W., & Xu, H. (2022). Trends in insulin resistance: insights into mechanisms and therapeutic strategy. *Signal Transduction and Targeted Therapy*, 7(1), 216.

Lu, S., Li, Y., Qian, Z., Zhao, T., Feng, Z., Weng, X., & Yu, L. (2023). Role of the inflammasome in insulin resistance and type 2 diabetes mellitus. *Frontiers in Immunology*, 14, 1052756.

Magkos, F., Hjorth, M. F., & Astrup, A. (2020). Diet and exercise in the prevention and treatment of type 2 diabetes mellitus. *Nature Reviews Endocrinology*, 16(10), 545-555.

Maines, E., Franceschi, R., Martinelli, D., Soli, F., Lepri, F. R., Piccoli, G., & Soffiati, M. (2021). Hypoglycemia due to PI3K/AKT/mTOR signaling pathway defects: Two novel cases and review of the literature. *Hormones*, 20, 623-640.

Martín, M. Á., & Ramos, S. (2021). Dietary flavonoids and insulin signaling in diabetes and obesity. *Cells*, 10(6), 1474.

Mastrototaro, L., & Roden, M. (2021). Insulin resistance and insulin-sensitizing agents. *Metabolism*, 125, 154892.

Mathieu, C., Martens, P. J., & Vangoitsenhoven, R. (2021). One hundred years of insulin therapy. *Nature Reviews Endocrinology*, 17(12), 715-725.

Matschinsky, F. M., & Wilson, D. F. (2019). The central role of glucokinase in glucose homeostasis: A perspective 50 years after demonstrating the presence of the enzyme in islets of Langerhans. *Frontiers in Physiology*, 10, 430287.

Mauvais-Jarvis, F. (2018). Gender differences in glucose homeostasis and diabetes. *Physiology and Behavior*, 187, 20-23.

McKern, N. M., Lawrence, M. C., Streltsov, V. A., Lou, M. Z., Adams, T. E., Lovrecz, G. O., Elleman, T. C., Richards, K. M., Bentley, J. D., Pilling, P. A., & Hoyne, P. A. (2006). Structure of the insulin receptor ectodomain reveals a folded-over conformation. *Nature*, 443(7108), 218-221.

Nauck, M. A., Wefers, J., & Meier, J. J. (2021). Treatment of type 2 diabetes: Challenges, hopes, and anticipated successes. *The Lancet Diabetes & Endocrinology*, 9(8), 525-544.

Norton, L., Shannon, C., Gastaldelli, A., & DeFronzo, R. A. (2022). Insulin: The master regulator of glucose metabolism. *Metabolism*, 129, 155142.

Ormazabal, V., Nair, S., Elfeky, O., Aguayo, C., Salomon, C., & Zuñiga, F. A. (2018). Association between insulin resistance and the development of cardiovascular disease. *Cardiovascular Diabetology*, 17, 1-14.

Perreault, L., Skyler, J. S., & Rosenstock, J. (2021). Novel therapies with precision mechanisms for type 2 diabetes mellitus. *Nature Reviews Endocrinology*, 17(6), 364-377.

Petersen, M. C., & Shulman, G. I. (2018). Mechanisms of insulin action and insulin resistance. *Physiological Reviews*, 98(4), 2133-2223.

Powis, G., Meuillet, E. J., Indarte, M., Booher, G., & Kirkpatrick, L. (2023). Pleckstrin Homology (PH) domain, structure, mechanism, and contribution to human disease. *Biomedicine and Pharmacotherapy*, 165, 115024.

Rieusset, J. (2018). The role of endoplasmic reticulum-mitochondria contact sites in the control of glucose homeostasis: An update. *Cell Death and Disease*, 9(3), 388.

Ringheim, G. E., Wampole, M., & Oberoi, K. (2021). Bruton's tyrosine kinase (BTK) inhibitors and autoimmune diseases: Making sense of BTK inhibitor specificity profiles and recent clinical trial successes and failures. *Frontiers in Immunology*, 12, 662223.

Sacerdoti, M., Gross, L. Z., Riley, A. M., Zehnder, K., Ghode, A., Klinke, S., Anand, G. S., Paris, K., Winkel, A., Herbrand, A. K., & Godage, H. Y. (2023). Modulation of the substrate specificity of the kinase PDK1 by distinct conformations of the full-length protein. *Science Signaling*, 16(789), eadd3184.

Sakurai, Y., Kubota, N., Yamauchi, T., & Kadowaki, T. (2021). Role of insulin resistance in MAFLD. *International Journal of Molecular Sciences*, 22(8), 4156.

Saltiel, A. R. (2016). Insulin signaling in the control of glucose and lipid homeostasis. *In Metabolic Control* (pp. 51-71).

Saltiel, A. R. (2021). Insulin signaling in health and disease. The Journal of Clinical Investigation, 131(1).

Scapin, G., Dandey, V. P., Zhang, Z., Prosise, W., Hruza, A., Kelly, T., Mayhood, T., Strickland, C., Potter, C. S., & Carragher, B. (2018). Structure of the insulin receptor–insulin complex by single-particle cryo-EM analysis. *Nature*, 556(7699), 122-125.

Sędzikowska, A., & Szablewski, L. (2021). Human glucose transporters in renal glucose homeostasis. *International Journal of Molecular Sciences*, 22(24), 13522.

Shtykova, E. V., Petoukhov, M. V., Mozhaev, A. A., Deyev, I. E., Dadinova, L. A., Loshkarev, N. A., Goryashchenko, A. S., Bocharov, E. V., Jeffries, C. M., Svergun, D. I., & Batishchev, O. V. (2019). The dimeric ectodomain of the alkali-sensing insulin receptor–related receptor (ectoIRR) has a droplike shape. *Journal of Biological Chemistry*, 294(47), 17790-17798.

Świderska, E., Strycharz, J., Wróblewski, A., Szemraj, J., Drzewoski, J., & Śliwińska, A. (2018). Role of PI3K/AKT pathway in insulin-mediated glucose uptake. *Blood Glucose Levels*, 1, 1-18.

Tagi, V. M., Giannini, C., & Chiarelli, F. (2019). Insulin resistance in children. *Frontiers in Endocrinology*, 10, 342.

Tattersall, R. B., & Matthews, D. R. (2024). The history of diabetes mellitus. *In Textbook of Diabetes* (pp. 1-21).

Vella, V., Milluzzo, A., Scalisi, N. M., Vigneri, P., & Sciacca, L. (2018). Insulin receptor isoforms in cancer. *International Journal of Molecular Sciences*, 19(11), 3615.

Viola, C. M., Frittmann, O., Jenkins, H. T., Shafi, T., De Meyts, P., & Brzozowski, A. M. (2023). Structural conservation of insulin/IGF signalling axis at the insulin receptors level in Drosophila and humans. *Nature Communications*, 14(1), 6271.

Wang, L., Li, J., & Di, L. J. (2022). Glycogen synthesis and beyond, a comprehensive review of GSK3 as a key regulator of metabolic pathways and a therapeutic target for treating metabolic diseases. *Medicinal Research Reviews*, 42(2), 946-982.

Wen, X., Zhang, B., Wu, B., Xiao, H., Li, Z., Li, R., Xu, X., & Li, T. (2022). Signaling pathways in obesity: mechanisms and therapeutic interventions. *Signal Transduction and Targeted Therapy*, 7(1), 298.

White, M. F., & Kahn, C. R. (2021). Insulin action at a molecular level–100 years of progress. *Molecular Metabolism*, 52, 101304.

Xu, Y., Margetts, M. B., Venugopal, H., Menting, J. G., Kirk, N. S., Croll, T. I., Delaine, C., Forbes, B. E., & Lawrence, M. C. (2022). How insulin-like growth factor I binds to a hybrid insulin receptor type 1 insulin-like growth factor receptor. *Structure*, 30(8), 1098-1108.

Yunn, N. O., Park, M., Park, S., Lee, J., Noh, J., Shin, E., & Ryu, S. H. (2021). A hotspot for enhancing insulin receptor activation revealed by a conformation-specific allosteric aptamer. *Nucleic Acids Research*, 49(2), 700-712.

Zhang, Z., Liu, H., & Liu, J. (2019). Akt activation: A potential strategy to ameliorate insulin resistance. *Diabetes Research and Clinical Practice*, 156, 107092.

Zhao, X., An, X., Yang, C., Sun, W., Ji, H., & Lian, F. (2023). The crucial role and mechanism of insulin resistance in metabolic disease. *Frontiers in Endocrinology*, 14, 1149239.

Zheng, S., Chen, N., Kang, X., Hu, Y., & Shi, S. (2022). Irisin alleviates FFA induced β-cell insulin resistance and inflammatory response through activating PI3K/AKT/FOXO1 signaling pathway. *Endocrine*, 75(3), 740-751.

Chapter 6

Insulin Receptors in the Hypothalamus: Key Regulators of Glucose Homeostasis and Diabetes

Prashant Upadhyay[1]
Shipra Sharma[2,3]
Tapasvi Gupta[4]
and Reetika Rawat[3,*]
[1]School of Pharmaceutical Science, IFTM University, Moradabad, Uttar Pradesh, India
[2]Faculty of Pharmacy, IFTM university, Moradabad, Uttar Pradesh, India
[3]Department of Pharmacy, Shri Ram Murti Smarak, College of Engineering and Technology, Bareilly, Uttar Pradesh, India
[4]School of Pharmacy, Suresh Gyan Vihar University, Jaipur, Rajasthan, India

Abstract

Insulin receptors (IR) play a critical role in maintaining glucose homeostasis, particularly through central mechanisms in the hypothalamus. Hypothalamic IR signaling regulates hepatic glucose production (HGP) by modulating enzymatic activity and interacting with neural circuits. Glucose-responsive neurons in the arcuate and ventromedial regions of the hypothalamus detect fluctuations in glucose levels, initiating hormonal and behavioral responses to maintain euglycemia. Insulin's central action on K^+-ATP channels significantly reduces HGP; however, this process can be disrupted by sulfonylureas such as tolbutamide. Additionally, insulin regulates HGP through the vagus nerve and the cytokine interleukin-6 (IL-6), highlighting the roles of the autonomic nervous system and inflammatory pathways in glucose metabolism.

Advanced techniques, including adenoviral delivery and neuron-specific ablation, are used to identify the neuronal populations and mechanisms involved. This chapter explores hypothalamic IR signaling and its therapeutic potential for diabetes, emphasizing the intricate regulatory network of insulin within the central nervous system (CNS).

Keywords: Insulin receptors, hepatic glucose production, diabetes, glucose homeostasis

* Corresponding Author's Email: reetika.rawat@srmscet.edu

In: Receptor-Targeted Therapies in Diabetes Mellitus
Editors: Ajmer Singh Grewal, Neelam Singh, Swati Verma et al.
ISBN: 979-8-89530-587-4

Abbreviations

AgRP	Agouti-related peptide
ANS	Autonomic nervous system
ARC	Arcuate nuclei
CNS	Central nervous system
cryo-EM	Cryogenic electron microscopy
DMN	Dorsomedial nucleus
ERK	Extracellular signal-regulated kinase
FOXO	Forkhead Box O
G6Pase	Glucose-6-phosphatase
GABA	Gamma-aminobutyric acid signals
GE	Glucose-excited neuron cells
G:	Glucose-inhibited neuron cells
GLP-1	Glucagon-like peptide
GLUT	Glucose transporter
GSK3	Glycogen synthase kinase 3
HGP	Hepatic glucose production
ICV	Intracerebroventricular
IL-6	Interleukin-6
IR	Insulin receptors
JNK	c-Jun NH2-terminal kinase
KATP	ATP-sensitive potassium channels
LCFA	Long-chain fatty acids
LH	Lateral hypothalamic
MAPK	Mitogen-activated protein kinase
MC4R	Melanocortin 4 receptor
MCH	Melanin-concentrating hormone
mTOR	Mechanistic target of rapamycin
NP-Y	Neuropeptide Y
NTS	Nucleus tractus solitarius
OCH	Orexin-concentrating hormone
PDK1	Phosphoinositide-dependent protein kinase-1
PEPCK P	hosphoenolpyruvate carboxykinase
PI3K/AKT	Phosphoinositide 3-kinase
PIP3	Phosphatidylinositol-3,4,5-triphosphate
POMC	Pro-opiomelanocortin-related peptide
PTB1B	Protein tyrosine phosphatase 1B
PV	Paraventricular nucleus
RBCs	Red blood cells
SCL2A	Solute carrier family 2 members
SF-1	Steroidogenic factor 1-expressing neurons
SHC	Src homology 2 domain-containing transforming protein
SOCS3	Suppressor of cytokine signaling 3
STAT3	Signal transducer and activator of transcription 3

Tyr	Tyrosine residues
VM	Ventromedial nucleus
α-MSH	α-melanocyte-stimulating hormone

Introduction

Insulin receptors in the hypothalamus play a pivotal role in regulating glucose homeostasis and maintaining overall metabolic balance. The hypothalamus, a critical brain region, integrates various metabolic signals and influences peripheral glucose metabolism through neural and hormonal pathways (Pan et al. 2023). Recent studies have demonstrated that insulin action in the hypothalamus significantly impacts hepatic glucose production (HGP). For example, blocking insulin signaling in the brain impairs the suppression of HGP, while central insulin administration effectively reduces HGP, independent of circulating insulin levels. This effect is mediated through KATP channels in hypothalamic neurons and the vagus nerve, linking central insulin action to liver function. Furthermore, insulin in the hypothalamus increases hepatic IL-6 expression, activating STAT3 signaling to inhibit gluconeogenesis (Petersen and Shulman, 2018). These mechanisms highlight the critical role of hypothalamic insulin signaling pathways in controlling peripheral glucose metabolism and maintaining glucose homeostasis. Dysfunction in hypothalamic insulin signaling has significant implications for metabolic disorders such as diabetes. Impairments in glucose sensing and glucose tolerance have been observed with the deletion of insulin-responsive GLUT4 in the brain, further emphasizing the hypothalamus's role in glucose regulation (Flores-Cortez et al. 2023). These findings suggest that insulin resistance in the hypothalamus can contribute to the pathogenesis of diabetes by disrupting the brain's ability to regulate glucose levels and insulin secretion (Alonge et al. 2020). Understanding the mechanisms by which insulin receptors influence glucose homeostasis could pave the way for novel therapeutic strategies to treat diabetes and other metabolic disorders (Cai et al. 2020).

The Crucial Role of the Insulin Receptor in Glucose Regulation

Insulin, a crucial anabolic peptide hormone produced by pancreatic β-cells, plays a central role in regulating human metabolism. Beyond its well-established function in glucose homeostasis, insulin exerts diverse effects throughout the body (Beaupere et al. 2021). Found in all metazoans, insulin-like signaling controls evolutionarily conserved processes such as reproduction and lifespan. When insulin binds to its receptor (IR), it initiates a series of structural changes and self-phosphorylation events, activating a cascade of kinase signaling pathways (De Meyts, 2004). The PI3K/AKT pathway is pivotal in mediating insulin's metabolic effects, facilitating glucose uptake into muscle and adipose tissues by translocating GLUT4 transporters. In the liver, insulin enhances glycogen and lipid synthesis while suppressing gluconeogenesis (Savova et al. 2023). Additionally, IR signaling supports cellular growth, proliferation, and development. Alongside the PI3K/AKT pathway, the MAPK pathway mediates insulin's mitogenic effects (Rahman et al. 2021). Dysfunction in IR signaling, due to pancreatic β-cell loss or insulin resistance, disrupts these processes, leading to the persistent elevation of blood glucose levels characteristic of diabetes mellitus. Understanding these pathways is crucial for developing therapies that restore proper insulin function and effectively manage metabolic disorders. Patients with diabetes face numerous complications that result in various disease states, underscoring the urgent need to target IR for diabetes treatment (Martín-Timón, 2014). Although the detailed mechanism of insulin-binding-induced IR activation is not fully understood, recent advancements in cryo-EM have expanded our knowledge by revealing various structures of ligand-bound IR, including those with insulin, peptides, and aptamers. Challenges remain, however, in elucidating how insulin accesses and triggers structural changes at apolipoprotein IR binding sites, coordinates extracellular domain conformational changes with cytoplasmic kinase domain autophosphorylation, and determines how agonists bias IR towards specific metabolic effects through functional selectivity (Zakir et al. 2023).

Insulin Receptor Activation: Insight and Challenges

Insulin initiates a cascade of events upon binding to the insulin receptor (IR) in peripheral tissues, crucially activating the receptor and triggering intracellular signaling pathways. The initial steps in IR activation involve the auto-phosphorylation of specific tyrosine residues within the receptor (Le et al. 2023). Notably, three tyrosine residues Tyr1146, Tyr1150, and Tyr1151 located in the kinase activation loop of IR isoform A are sequentially phosphorylated. This process is essential for regulating the kinase activity of IR. In its inactive state, the unphosphorylated activation loop obstructs the catalytic site of the kinase, inhibiting its function by preventing substrate and ATP binding (Yunn et al. 2023). Upon insulin binding, these tyrosine residues undergo phosphorylation, causing the activation loop to move away from the catalytic site. These conformational changes enhance IR kinase activity, enabling interactions with substrates and ATP, thereby initiating downstream signaling events. Insulin also induces phosphorylation of additional tyrosine residues located in the juxtamembrane and C-terminal regions of IR (Kim and Novak, 2007). Among these, phosphorylation of Tyr960 (pY960) in the juxtamembrane creates a docking site for IR substrate proteins and SHC. This interaction facilitates IR-mediated phosphorylation of IR substrate-1 (IRS-1) and SHC, which are crucial for propagating insulin signaling within the cell. The roles of phosphorylated Tyr1316 (pY1316) and Tyr1322 (pY1322) in the C-terminal domain are less clearly understood but are implicated in regulating IR kinase activity and its interaction with adaptor proteins. Insulin receptor activation primarily triggers two major signaling pathways: the PI3K/AKT and MAPK pathways. The PI3K/AKT pathway is responsible for most of the metabolic effects induced by insulin in peripheral tissues (Tennagels et al. 2000). IRS proteins bind to the p85 regulatory subunit of PI3K, activating it to produce PIP3. PIP3 recruits PDK1 and activates AKT, which phosphorylates various downstream targets (Denley et al. 2009). These targets include GLUT4, which promotes glucose uptake; GSK3, which promotes glycogen synthesis; and mTOR, which promotes protein and lipid synthesis (Hahn and Denlinger, 2007). Additionally, AKT phosphorylates FOXO transcription factors, regulating gene expression (Lee et al. 2022). Conversely, the MAPK pathway, initiated by SHC and IR substrate proteins, regulates insulin's mitogenic effects on cell growth, proliferation, and differentiation. This pathway involves the Grb2-Sos-Ras-Raf-ERK signaling cascade. ERK phosphorylates cytoplasmic and nuclear proteins, influencing cellular responses and acting as a transcription factor. Thus, insulin receptor activation orchestrates a complex network of signaling pathways that regulate critical metabolic and growth processes in response to insulin stimulation in peripheral tissues (Borisov et al. 2009).

Role of Hypothalamus in Glucose Homeostasis

The rising global epidemic of obesity and metabolic disorders, particularly type 2 diabetes, poses a significant biomedical challenge. Obesity-related type 2 diabetes is characterized by impaired glucose homeostasis, yet the underlying mechanisms remain poorly understood (Chobot et al. 2018). Maintaining glucose homeostasis is vital for mammalian survival, as glucose is minimally stored in the body and its levels must be tightly regulated through communication with peripheral organs (Perreault et al. 2016). Interestingly, glucose levels in the central nervous system (CNS) are significantly lower than those in circulation, typically ranging between 1 mmol/L and 2.5 mmol/L, and can drop to as low as 0.5 mmol/L. The hypothalamus, a key region for glucose regulation, contains various nuclei with distinct neuronal populations that express neuropeptides and neurotransmitters essential for energy homeostasis (Roh et al. 2016). Its ability to sense and respond to fluctuations in glucose levels underscores its critical role in maintaining glucose balance (Karnani and Burdakov, 2011). These nuclei and neuronal populations are adept at detecting changes in glucose levels and other metabolic cues, integrating this information, and orchestrating appropriate physiological responses. This function is crucial not only for normal metabolic processes but also in the context of metabolic disorders (Alvarsson and Stanley, 2018). Dysregulation of hypothalamic function can contribute to the development and progression of type 2 diabetes and other metabolic conditions. Furthermore, the hypothalamus's role in glucose sensing is significant in the context of type 1 diabetes, particularly concerning the development of hypoglycemia unawareness—a dangerous condition in which patients fail to recognize symptoms of low blood sugar (Lundqvist et al. 2019). Understanding the mechanisms by which the hypothalamus senses glucose and its impact on metabolic health is therefore critical for developing novel therapeutic strategies to manage and treat diabetes and related metabolic disorders (Zhao et al. 2023).

Hypothalmic Glucose-Sensing Neurons: Location and Function

Higher organisms have developed specialized sensor and effector mechanisms to maintain systemic glucose homeostasis. The brain, which consumes 60–70% of total glucose, predominantly utilizes high-affinity transporters such as GLUT-1 and GLUT-3, enabling effective glucose uptake independent of insulin. This highlights the brain's critical role in glucose surveillance. Recent evidence suggests that continuous glucose monitoring occurs through specific cell types across various brain regions, including the brainstem, corticolimbic areas, and hypothalamus. While much focus has been on neuronal glucose sensing, the role of non-neuronal cells is gaining attention. Among these regions, the hypothalamus has been identified as a central hub in the complex and distributed glucose-sensing network (Agrawal et al. 2021). The hypothalamus comprises distinct nuclei, such as the paraventricular (PV), ventromedial (VM), lateral (LH), and arcuate (ARC) nuclei, each containing specific populations of glucose-sensing neurons. The ARC, located adjacent to the third ventricle and median eminence, houses opposing neuronal populations: orexigenic AgRP-producing neurons and anorexigenic POMC-derived neurons. Together with MC4R-expressing neurons, these form the melanocortin system, which is crucial for regulating appetite, energy expenditure, and glucose homeostasis (Bétry et al. 2018). The interaction between α-MSH and AgRP at MC4Rs influences downstream pathway activation. AgRP neurons, which send inhibitory GABAergic signals to POMC neurons, also express the orexigenic neuropeptide Y (NPY). The balance between orexigenic and anorexigenic signals ultimately determines metabolic outcomes. While AgRP neurons are primarily classified as gastrointestinal (GI) neurons, POMC neurons are generally considered glucose-excitatory (GE) neurons (Deem et al. 2022). However, recent findings suggest that glucose modulation of POMC neuron activity may result from presynaptic inputs rather than direct glucose detection. ARC POMC and AgRP neurons project to various hypothalamic and extrahypothalamic regions, including the ventromedial nucleus (VMN), where neurons sense changes in extracellular glucose levels. Notably, SF1-expressing neurons in the VMN express receptors for key metabolic hormones, although only about 10% are responsive to glucose (Bell et al. 2018). The VMN is essential for regulating energy balance and initiating counter-regulatory responses to hypoglycemia. The LH is a heterogeneous structure containing various neuronal populations, including orexin and melanin-concentrating hormone (MCH) neurons. Orexin neurons are generally classified as GI, while some MCH neurons are considered GE. This area plays a vital role in regulating arousal, appetite, and reward (Chan and Sherwin, 2013).

Mechanism of Neuronal Glucose Sensing in the Hypothalamus

The hypothalamus regulates blood glucose levels by sensing, integrating, and responding to fluctuations through its control of the autonomic nervous system (ANS) and the endocrine system. It contains two types of glucose-sensing neurons: GE neurons, which activate when glucose levels rise, and glucose-inhibited (GI) neurons, which activate when glucose levels drop (Routh, 2010). In the ARC, GE neurons, such as POMC neurons, respond to high glucose levels by increasing activity and releasing α-MSH, which reduces appetite and increases energy expenditure. Conversely, GI neurons in the ARC, including those expressing AgRP and NPY, are activated under low glucose conditions, stimulating feeding to restore glucose levels (Jais and Brüning, 2022). The VM hypothalamic nucleus contains steroidogenic factor-1 (SF1)-expressing neurons that respond to low glucose levels by initiating processes that increase blood sugar, such as glucagon secretion and hepatic glucose production. These neurons integrate signals from GE and GI neurons to maintain glucose homeostasis (Hirschberg et al. 2020). Additionally, glucose-sensing neurons in the LH and brainstem regions, such as the nucleus of the solitary tract and the dorsal motor nucleus of the vagus, contribute to glucose regulation by transmitting signals from peripheral organs to the brain. This intricate network ensures stable blood glucose levels, which is vital for preventing metabolic disorders like diabetes (Boychuk et al. 2015).

Role of Hypothalamus in Regulating Hepatic Glucose Production

The hypothalamus regulates food intake and energy expenditure by monitoring blood levels of key hormones and nutrients. The ARC, situated near the median eminence and surrounding the third ventricle, senses these metabolic signals due to its strategic location (Tran et al. 2022). The ARC contains orexigenic neurons that produce NP and AgRP, as well as anorexigenic neurons that produce POMC and cocaine-amphetamine regulated transcript (α-MSH), which activate pathways that reduce food intake and increase energy expenditure via melanocortin receptors. AgRP counteracts α-MSH by binding to these receptors (Bouret, 2022).

The PV nucleus produces catabolic neuropeptides and controls sympathetic output to enhance fatty acid oxidation. The VM hypothalamus senses glucose and leptin, producing brain-derived neurotrophic factor to regulate satiety and glucose homeostasis (Yu and Kim, 2012). The DMN and LH also play roles, with the LH functioning as a feeding center due to its production of MCH and orexin, which regulate appetite and energy balance (Lee et al. 2021).

Brain-Based Mechanism for Managing Glucose Levels

A specialized group of neurons in the brain detects metabolic signals, including hormones like insulin and leptin, as well as nutrients such as glucose and fatty acids, primarily in the hypothalamus and brainstem. These brain regions contain neurons that adjust their excitability in response to changes in extracellular glucose levels. Two main types of glucose-sensing neurons exist: glucose-excited neurons, which activate when extracellular glucose levels rise, and glucose-inhibited neurons, which become active when glucose levels drop (Jordan et al. 2010). Glucose-excited neurons are predominantly found in the ventromedial (VM) ARC, and paraventricular nucleus (PVN). In contrast, glucose-inhibited neurons are located in the lateral hypothalamus (LH), ARC, and PVN (De Backer et al. 2016). Both types are also present in the dorsal vagal complex of the brainstem, which includes the nucleus of the solitary tract (NTS), the area postrema, and the dorsal motor nucleus of the vagus (Khodai et al. 2018).

Detection and Response to Glucose Change

Maintaining stable blood glucose levels requires a rapid response to fluctuations in plasma glucose. When glucose-sensing neurons in the hypothalamus and other regions detect a potential drop in blood sugar, they initiate a core response. This detection activates a series of neural and hormonal mechanisms designed to prevent further declines in glucose levels and restore normal blood sugar levels (euglycemia) (Stanley et al. 2019).

Mechanism of Glucose Level Detection by Hypothalamic Neurons

Proper management of glucose metabolism is crucial for brain physiological processes, which are monitored by glucose-detecting neurons. These neurons modify their electrical activity in response to changing glucose levels. Importantly, these neurons can directly sense glucose level changes without relying on indirect presynaptic modulation. These specialized neurons are concentrated in the hypothalamic region and outside the hypothalamus (Yoon and Diano, 2021). The hypothalamus plays a crucial role in blood glucose regulation, as it can detect, process, and respond to changes in circulating signals. This intricate function is achieved through its influence on the ANS and the endocrine system (Fioramonti, 2023). The hypothalamus contains two types of glucose-responsive neurons: those excited by glucose and those inhibited by it. Rising glucose levels activate GE neurons, while low glucose conditions stimulate GI neurons. The ARC and VMH nuclei play important roles in understanding their glucose-detecting mechanisms and their role in glucose metabolism, particularly in hypothalamic regions (Jordan et al. 2010). The GE neurons and pancreatic β-cells both increase their activity when glucose levels rise. In β-cells, this process involves glucose uptake via GLUT2, glucose phosphorylation by glucokinase, and glucose metabolism leading to increased ATP production. This increase in ATP closes KATP channels, depolarizes the membrane, and allows calcium entry, triggering insulin release. Given these similarities, researchers have investigated the involvement of GLUT2, glucokinase, and KATP channel components (SUR1, SUR2, and Kir6.2) in central glucose sensing (Jordan et al. 2010; Thorens, 2015). GLUT2 is found in brain regions containing glucose-responsive neurons. Studies involving genetically modified mice have shown that GLUT2 in the CNS plays a role in counteracting low blood sugar (Sun et al. 2023). In pancreatic β-cells, glucokinase controls ATP production through glycolysis and regulates KATP channel activity. The pancreatic variant of glucokinase is also present in glucose-sensing brain areas and is involved in approximately 70% of GE neurons. Furthermore, when glucokinase was selectively reduced in cultured neurons from the VM hypothalamus, these neurons lost their ability to sense glucose (De Backer et al. 2016). In the brain, KATP channels (composed of subunits SUR1 and Kir6.2) play a crucial role in linking glucose metabolism to changes in electrical activity, particularly in the glucose-sensing regions of the hypothalamus. Electrophysiological studies have shown that inhibiting or activating KATP channels can alter how GE neurons respond to changes in glucose levels in laboratory settings and living organisms (Mc Traggart et al. 2010). Extensive research suggests that GE neurons respond to elevated extracellular glucose like pancreatic β-cells. This process involves increased ATP levels, which lead to the closure of KATP channels. This closure results in membrane depolarization, followed by calcium influx through voltage-gated channels, ultimately enhancing neuronal activity and neurotransmitter release (Fridyland et al. 2011). However, some evidence also suggests the presence of alternative glucose-sensing mechanisms in neurons that may not rely on KATP channels or GLUT2.

Hormonal, Physiological and Behavioural Responses to Restore Euglycemia

The brain relies heavily on glucose for fuel, necessitating precise regulation of blood sugar levels (glucose homeostasis) through hormonal and physiological responses to prevent hypoglycemia, which is rare in healthy individuals (Mergenthaler et al. 2013). However, diabetes mellitus, particularly in patients treated with insulin, can lead to frequent hypoglycemic episodes, which may result in confusion, seizures, and even coma or death (Spargue et al. 2011). In healthy individuals, blood sugar levels are maintained through predictable responses activated by the sympathetic nervous system, with physiological and behavioral reactions occurring at specific glucose thresholds (Stanley et al. 2019). Three primary protective mechanisms are initiated: insulin production decreases as pancreatic β-cells reduce output, glucagon production increases from pancreatic α-cells, and the adrenal medulla releases more epinephrine into the bloodstream (Sprague and Arbeláez, 2011; Senthilkumaran et al. 2024). As glucose levels fall within the normal range (4.4-4.7 mmol/L or 80-85 mg/dL), the pancreas reduces insulin production, promoting glucose production while decreasing its use by non-brain tissues. If levels drop below normal (3.6-3.9 mmol/L or 65-70 mg/dL), counterregulatory hormones, such as glucagon and epinephrine, stimulate glucose production in the liver and limit glucose use in insulin-sensitive tissues. At even lower levels (2.8-3.0 mmol/L or 50-55 mg/dL), symptoms of hypoglycemia appear, and brain function becomes impaired below 2.8 mmol/L or 50 mg/dL. In poorly controlled diabetics, these thresholds shift higher, while individuals with frequent low blood sugar or excessive insulin production may develop lower thresholds. These mechanisms prompt individuals to consume carbohydrates to restore normal blood sugar levels (euglycemia) (Verhulst et al. 2022). Unlike glucagon and epinephrine, which act quickly, growth hormone and cortisol have a delayed impact during hypoglycemia. Research using controlled hormone suppression and replacement techniques has revealed time-dependent effects; for instance, when cortisol levels were kept low, glucose production decreased, and utilization increased after 6 hours, resulting in lower blood glucose levels after 9.5 hours, despite unchanged glucagon, insulin, and growth hormone levels (Stanley et al. 2019). A study comparing healthy adults with patients lacking growth hormone and cortisol due to hypopituitarism found that the hormone-deficient group had lower blood glucose levels starting 2.5 hours after insulin infusion began, becoming statistically significant by 12 hours. However, both groups recovered quickly from hypoglycemia once insulin infusion stopped, indicating that growth hormone and cortisol do not play a crucial role in the immediate correction of low blood sugar (Stanley et al. 2019; Defeo et al. 1989).

Involvement of the Autonomous Nervous System and Inflammatory Pathways

The CNS plays a crucial role in the development of diabetes, which is primarily a disorder of peripheral tissues. The hypothalamus, a key structure within the CNS, is central to regulating glucose levels due to its position at the intersection of neuroendocrine and autonomic systems. Emerging evidence suggests that hypothalamic inflammation significantly disrupts glucose homeostasis. Although the exact cause of this inflammation remains unclear, it is closely linked to various forms of cellular stress, including endoplasmic reticulum stress, RNA stress, oxidative damage, and autophagy defects. These stress factors can trigger or enhance the activation of pro-inflammatory NF-κB pathways. The effectiveness of anti-inflammatory treatments and therapies targeting these pathways in alleviating diabetic symptoms indicates their potential for managing the widespread disease and its complications. The underlying mechanisms of hypothalamic inflammation involve multiple dynamic processes (Inoue, 2016).

Influence of Insulin on HGP via Vagal Nerve

The liver plays a crucial role in maintaining overall glucose balance by regulating glucose production based on energy needs. Insulin, present in high concentrations in portal blood, is the primary regulator of HGP. In diabetes, increased HGP is correlated with elevated fasting blood glucose levels. Insulin directly influences liver cells to control HGP (Sharabi et al. 2018). When insulin binds to its receptors, it activates a signaling cascade involving PI3K, IRS, PDK1, and Akt, which suppresses HGP. Consequently, mice lacking liver-specific insulin receptors or having impaired PI3K signaling exhibit high insulin levels and glucose intolerance, along with reduced insulin-mediated suppression of HGP. Meanwhile, insulin regulates HGP through both direct and indirect pathways (Petersen and Shulman, 2018). While direct control occurs via insulin receptors in the liver, indirect regulation involves insulin's effect on other organs. Studies have shown that insulin can still partially suppress HGP even when PI3K signaling is inhibited in the liver. Moreover, research comparing I.V. and I.P. insulin administration revealed that the magnitude of insulin levels reflects direct insulin action on liver cells. These findings suggest that the relationship between insulin and HGP regulation is more complex. Insulin indirectly inhibits HGP through two main mechanisms. First, it decreases the release of glycerol and free fatty acids from adipose tissue, which are essential materials and energy sources for gluconeogenesis. Second, it reduces the expression of key genes involved in gluconeogenesis in the liver, especially those encoding PEPCK and G6Pase (Inoue et al. 2016; Egerton et al. 2017). The vagus nerve plays a crucial role in how central insulin action regulates HGP. Cutting the hepatic branch of the vagus nerve reduces the HGP-suppressing effect of ICV insulin administration. The vagus nerve typically maintains steady activity, but studies in anesthetized rats show that blood glucose increases enhance this activity, while insulin increases inhibit it. HGP is also lowered by ICV α-MSH administration. Furthermore, administering diazoxide (a KATP channel activator that hyperpolarizes neurons) to the dorsal motor nucleus of the vagus suppresses HGP. These findings suggest that HGP suppression may result from vagus nerve activation (Matsuhisa et al. 2000). The vagus nerve's influence extends beyond HGP regulation to broader hepatic glucose metabolism. This is evidenced by insulin resistance in vagotomized rats, increased hepatic glycogen synthase activity following vagal stimulation in rabbits, and enhanced glucose utilization in perfused rat livers when the vagus is stimulated in the presence of insulin. Notably, the insulin resistance induced by vagotomy in rats can be mitigated by intraportal administration of acetylcholine. However, this suggests that the control of HGP by central insulin action cannot be explained solely by the direct effect of acetylcholine released by the vagus on liver cells (Matsuhisa et al. 2000; Kistner et al. 2022; Ellingsgaard et al. 2020; Nieto-Vazquez et al. 2008; Erta et al. 2012; Febbraio et al. 2004; De Melo Madureira et al. 2022).

Conclusion

This chapter explores the intricate mechanisms underlying glucose homeostasis, emphasizing the critical role of the insulin receptor (IR) and its activation in regulating blood glucose levels. The insulin receptor is essential for glucose uptake and metabolism, and its proper activation is crucial for maintaining euglycemia. Despite advancements in understanding IR function, challenges remain in optimizing therapeutic targeting, necessitating further research to enhance diabetes management strategies. The hypothalamus's role in glucose regulation is also examined, highlighting its function through glucose-sensing neurons that monitor glucose levels and adjust hepatic glucose production accordingly. This central control illustrates the hypothalamus's significant influence on metabolic processes. Additionally, mechanisms involved in detecting glucose changes and initiating appropriate physiological responses to stabilize glucose levels are discussed. The interplay between hormonal, physiological, and behavioral responses, along with contributions from the autonomic nervous system and inflammatory pathways, is essential for restoring euglycemia. Lastly, the cytokine IL-6's role in modulating insulin's effects sheds light on the regulatory network affecting insulin sensitivity and glucose metabolism, paving the way for future research on glucose-related disorders.

References

Agrawal, R., Reno, C. M., Sharma, S., Christensen, C., Huang, Y., & Fisher, S. J. (2021). Insulin action in the brain regulates both central and peripheral functions. *American Journal of Physiology-Endocrinology and Metabolism*, 321(1), E156–E163.

Alonge, K. M., D'Alessio, D. A., & Schwartz, M. W. (2021). Brain control of blood glucose levels: Implications for the pathogenesis of type 2 diabetes. *Diabetologia*, 64(1), 5–14.

Alvarsson, A., & Stanley, S. A. (2018). Remote control of glucose-sensing neurons to analyze glucose metabolism. *American Journal of Physiology-Endocrinology and Metabolism*, 315(3), E327–E339.

Beaupere, C., Liboz, A., Fève, B., Blondeau, B., & Guillemain, G. (2021). Molecular mechanisms of glucocorticoid-induced insulin resistance. *International Journal of Molecular Sciences*, 22(2), 623.

Bell, B. B., Harlan, S. M., Morgan, D. A., Guo, D. F., & Rahmouni, K. (2018). Differential contribution of POMC and AgRP neurons to the regulation of regional autonomic nerve activity by leptin. *Molecular Metabolism*, 8, 1–12.

Bétry, C., Thobois, S., Laville, M., & Disse, E. (2018). Deep brain stimulation as a therapeutic option for obesity: A critical review. *Obesity Research & Clinical Practice*, 12(3), 260–269.

Borisov, N., Aksamitiene, E., Kiyatkin, A., Legewie, S., Berkhout, J., Maiwald, T., Kaimachnikov, N. P., Timmer, J., Hoek, J. B., & Kholodenko, B. N. (2009). Systems-level interactions between insulin–EGF networks amplify mitogenic signaling. *Molecular Systems Biology*, 5(1), 256.

Bouret, S. G. (2022). Developmental programming of hypothalamic melanocortin circuits. *Experimental & Molecular Medicine*, 54(4), 403–413.

Boychuk, C. R., Gyarmati, P., Xu, H., & Smith, B. N. (2015). Glucose sensing by GABAergic neurons in the mouse nucleus tractus solitarii. *Journal of Neurophysiology*, 114(2), 999–1007.

Cai, M., Liao, Z., Zou, X., Xu, Z., Wang, Y., Li, T., Li, Y., Ou, X., Deng, Y., Guo, Y., Peng, T., & Li, M. (2020). Herpes Simplex Virus 1 UL2 inhibits the TNF-α–mediated NF-κB activity by interacting with p65/p50. *Frontiers in Immunology*, 11, 549.

Chan, O., & Sherwin, R. (2013). Influence of VMH fuel sensing on hypoglycemic responses. *Trends in Endocrinology & Metabolism*, 24(12), 616–624.

Chobot, A., Górowska-Kowolik, K., Sokołowska, M., & Jarosz-Chobot, P. (2018). Obesity and diabetes—Not only a simple link between two epidemics. *Diabetes/Metabolism Research and Reviews*, 34(7), e3042.

D'souza, A. M., Neumann, U. H., Glavas, M. M., & Kieffer, T. J. (2017). The glucoregulatory actions of leptin. *Molecular Metabolism*, 6(9), 1052–1065.

De Backer, I., Hussain, S. S., Bloom, S. R., & Gardiner, J. V. (2016). Insights into the role of neuronal glucokinase. *American Journal of Physiology-Endocrinology and Metabolism*, 311(1), E42–E55.

De Melo Madureira, Á. N., de Oliveira, J. R. S., & de Menezes Lima, V. L. (2022). The role of IL-6 released during exercise to insulin sensitivity and muscle hypertrophy. *Mini Review in Medicinal Chemistry*, 22(18), 2419–2428.

De Meyts, P. (2004). Insulin and its receptor: Structure, function and evolution. *BioEssays*, 26(12), 1351–1362.

Deem, J. D., Faber, C. L., & Morton, G. J. (2022). AgRP neurons: Regulators of feeding, energy expenditure, and behavior. *The FEBS Journal*, 289(8), 2362–2381.

Defeo, P., Perriello, G., Torlone, E., Ventura, M. M., Santeusanio, F., Brunetti, P., Gerich, J. E., & Bolli, G. B. (1989). Demonstration of a role for growth hormone in glucose counter-regulation. *American Journal of Physiology*, 256, E835–E843.

Denley, A., Gymnopoulos, M., Kang, S., Mitchell, C., & Vogt, P. K. (2009). Requirement of phosphatidylinositol (3,4,5) trisphosphate in phosphatidylinositol 3-kinase-induced oncogenic transformation. *Molecular Cancer Research*, 7(7), 1132–1138.

Dilworth, L., Facey, A., & Omoruyi, F. (2021). Diabetes mellitus and its metabolic complications: The role of adipose tissues. *International Journal of Molecular Sciences*, 22(14), 7644.

Edgerton, D. S., Kraft, G., Smith, M., Farmer, B., Williams, P. E., Coate, K. C., Printz, R. L., O'Brien, R. M., & Cherrington, A. D. (2017). Insulin's direct hepatic effect explains the inhibition of glucose production caused by insulin secretion. *JCI Insight*, 2(6), e91863.

Ellingsgaard, H., Seelig, E., & Timper, K. (2020). GLP-1 secretion is regulated by IL-6 signalling: A randomised, placebo-controlled study. *Diabetologia*, 63, 362–373.

Erta, M., Quintana, A., & Hidalgo, J. (2012). Interleukin-6, a major cytokine in the central nervous system. *International Journal of Biological Sciences*, 8(9), 1254–1266.

Febbraio, M. A., Hiscock, N., Sacchetti, M., Fischer, C. P., & Pedersen, B. K. (2004). Interleukin-6 is a novel factor mediating glucose homeostasis during skeletal muscle contraction. *Diabetes*, 53(7), 1643–1648.

Fioramonti, X. (2023). A new role for hypothalamic glucose-sensing neurons in hypoglycemia unawareness. *Diabetes*, 72(8), 1055–1056.

Flores-Cortez, Y. A., Barragán-Bonilla, M. I., Mendoza-Bello, J. M., & Espinoza-Rojo, M. (2023). Insulin: A connection between pancreatic β cells and the hypothalamus. *World Journal of Diabetes*, 14(2), 76–91.

Hahn, D. A., & Denlinger, D. L. (2007). Meeting the energetic demands of insect diapause: Nutrient storage and utilization. *Journal of Insect Physiology*, 53(8), 760–773.

Hirschberg, P. R., Sarkar, P., Teegala, S. B., & Routh, V. H. (2020). Ventromedial hypothalamus glucose-inhibited neurones: A role in glucose and energy homeostasis? *Journal of Neuroendocrinology*, 32(1), e12773.

Inoue, H. (2016). Central insulin-mediated regulation of hepatic glucose production [Review]. *Endocrine Journal*, 63(1), 1–7.

Jais, A., & Brüning, J. C. (2022). Arcuate nucleus-dependent regulation of metabolism—Pathways to obesity and diabetes mellitus. *Endocrine Reviews*, 43(2), 314–328.

Jordan, S. D., Könner, A. C., & Brüning, J. C. (2010). Sensing the fuels: Glucose and lipid signaling in the CNS controlling energy homeostasis. *Cellular and Molecular Life Sciences*, 67(19), 3255–3273.

Karnani, M., & Burdakov, D. (2011). Multiple hypothalamic circuits sense and regulate glucose levels. *American Journal of Physiology-Regulatory, Integrative and Comparative Physiology*, 300(1), R47–R55.

Khodai, T., Nunn, N., Worth, A. A., Feetham, C. H., Belle, M. D. C., Piggins, H. D., & Luckman, S. M. (2018). PACAP neurons in the ventromedial hypothalamic nucleus are glucose inhibited and their selective activation induces hyperglycaemia. *Frontiers in Endocrinology*, 9, 632.

Kim, S. K., & Novak, R. F. (2007). The role of intracellular signaling in insulin-mediated regulation of drug metabolizing enzyme gene and protein expression. *Pharmacology & Therapeutics*, 113(1), 88–120.

Kistner, T. M., Pedersen, B. K., & Lieberman, D. E. (2022). Interleukin 6 as an energy allocator in muscle tissue. *Nature Metabolism*, 4(2), 170–179.

Le, T. K. C., Dao, X. D., Nguyen, D. V., Luu, D. H., Bui, T. M. H., Le, T. H., Nguyen, H. T., Le, T. N., Hosaka, T., & Nguyen, T. T. T. (2023). Insulin signaling and its application. *Frontiers in Endocrinology*, 14, 1226655.

Lee, J., Raycraft, L., & Johnson, A. W. (2021). The dynamic regulation of appetitive behavior through lateral hypothalamic orexin and melanin concentrating hormone expressing cells. *Physiology & Behavior*, 229, 113234.

Lee, S. H., Park, S. Y., & Choi, C. S. (2022). Insulin resistance: From mechanisms to therapeutic strategies. *Diabetes & Metabolism Journal*, 46(1), 15–37.

Li, R. J. W., Zhang, S.-Y., & Lam, T. K. T. (2020). Interaction of glucose sensing and leptin action in the brain. *Molecular Metabolism*, 39, 101011.

Lundqvist, M. H., Almby, K., Abrahamsson, N., & Eriksson, J. W. (2019). Is the brain a key player in glucose regulation and development of type 2 diabetes? *Frontiers in Physiology*, 10, 457.

Martín-Timón, I. (2014). Type 2 diabetes and cardiovascular disease: Have all risk factors the same strength? *World Journal of Diabetes*, 5(4), 444.

Matsuhisa, M., Yamasaki, Y., Shiba, Y., Nakahara, I., Kuroda, A., Tomita, T., Iida, M., Ikeda, M., Kajimoto, Y., Kubota, M., & Hori, M. (2000). Important role of the hepatic vagus nerve in glucose uptake and production by the liver. *Metabolism*, 49(1), 11–16.

McTaggart, J. S., Clark, R. H., & Ashcroft, F. M. (2010). The role of the KATP channel in glucose homeostasis in health and disease: More than meets the islet. *The Journal of Physiology*, 588(17), 3201–3209.

Mergenthaler, P., Lindauer, U., Dienel, G. A., & Meisel, A. (2013). Sugar for the brain: The role of glucose in physiological and pathological brain function. *Trends in Neuroscience*, 36(10), 587–597.

Nieto-Vazquez, I., Fernández-Veledo, S., & Lorenzo, M. (2008). Dual role of interleukin-6 in regulating insulin sensitivity in murine skeletal muscle. *Diabetes*, 57(12), 3211–3221.

Obici, S., Feng, Z., Morgan, K., Stein, D., Karkanias, G., & Rossetti, L. (2002). Central administration of oleic acid inhibits glucose production and food intake. *Diabetes*, 51(2), 271–275.

Pan, S., Worker, C. J., & Feng Earley, Y. (2023). The hypothalamus as a key regulator of glucose homeostasis: Emerging roles of the brain renin-angiotensin system. *American Journal of Physiology-Cell Physiology*, 325(1), C141–C154.

Perreault, K., Lagacé, J. C., Brochu, M., & Dionne, I. J. (2016). Association between fat-free mass and glucose homeostasis: Common knowledge revisited. *Ageing Research Reviews*, 28, 46–61.

Petersen, M. C., & Shulman, G. I. (2018). Mechanisms of insulin action and insulin resistance. *Physiological Reviews*, 98(4), 2133–2223.

Rahman, M. S., Hossain, K. S., Das, S., Kundu, S., Adegoke, E. O., Rahman, M. A., Hannan, M. A., Uddin, M. J., & Pang, M.-G. (2021). Role of insulin in health and disease: An update. *International Journal of Molecular Sciences*, 22(12), 6403.

Roh, E., Song, D. K., & Kim, M. S. (2016). Emerging role of the brain in the homeostatic regulation of energy and glucose metabolism. *Experimental & Molecular Medicine*, 48(3), e216.

Routh, V. H. (2010). Glucose sensing neurons in the ventromedial hypothalamus. *Sensors*, 10(10), 9002–9025.

Savova, M. S., Mihaylova, L. V., Tews, D., Wabitsch, M., & Georgiev, M. I. (2023). Targeting PI3K/AKT signaling pathway in obesity. *Biomedicine & Pharmacotherapy*, 159, 114244.

Senthilkumaran, M., Koch, C., Herselman, M. F., & Bobrovskaya, L. (2024). Role of the adrenal medulla in hypoglycaemia-associated autonomic failure: A diabetic perspective. *Metabolites*, 14(2), 100.

Sharabi, K., Tavares, C. D., Rines, A. K., & Puigserver, P. (2015). Molecular pathophysiology of hepatic glucose production. *Molecular Aspects of Medicine*, 46, 21–33.

Sohn, J. W., & Ho, W. K. (2020). Cellular and systemic mechanisms for glucose sensing and homeostasis. *Pflügers Archiv - European Journal of Physiology*, 472(11), 1547–1561.

Sprague, J. E., & Arbeláez, A. M. (2011). Glucose counterregulatory responses to hypoglycemia. *Pediatric Endocrinology Review*, 9(1), 463–473.

Stanley, S., Moheet, A., & Seaquist, E. R. (2019). Central mechanisms of glucose sensing and counterregulation in defense of hypoglycemia. *Endocrine Reviews*, 40(3), 768–788.

Sun, B., Chen, H., Xue, J., Li, P., & Fu, X. (2023). The role of GLUT2 in glucose metabolism in multiple organs and tissues. *Molecular Biology Reports*, 50(8), 6963–6974.

Tennagels, N., Bergschneider, E., Al-Hasani, H., & Klein, H. W. (2000). Autophosphorylation of the two C-terminal tyrosine residues Tyr 1316 and Tyr 1322 modulates the activity of the insulin receptor kinase *in vitro*. *FEBS Letters*, 479(1–2), 67–71.

Thorens, B. (2015). GLUT2, glucose sensing and glucose homeostasis. *Diabetologia*, 58, 221–232.

Tran, L. T., Park, S., Kim, S. K., Lee, J. S., Kim, K. W., & Kwon, O. (2022). Hypothalamic control of energy expenditure and thermogenesis. *Experimental & Molecular Medicine*, 54(4), 358–369.

Verhulst, C. E. M., Fabricius, T. W., Teerenstra, S., Kristensen, P. L., Tack, C. J., McCrimmon, R. J., Heller, S., Evans, M. L., Amiel, S. A., Pedersen-Bjergaard, U., & de Galan, B. E. (2022). Glycaemic thresholds for counterregulatory hormone and symptom responses to hypoglycaemia in people with and without type 1 diabetes: A systematic review. *Diabetologia*, 65(10), 1601–1612.

Yoon, N. A., & Diano, S. (2021). Hypothalamic glucose-sensing mechanisms. *Diabetologia*, 64(5), 985–993.

Yu, J. H., & Kim, M.-S. (2012). Molecular mechanisms of appetite regulation. *Diabetes & Metabolism Journal*, 36(6), 391.

Yunn, N. O., Kim, J., Ryu, S. H., & Cho, Y. (2023). A stepwise activation model for the insulin receptor. *Experimental & Molecular Medicine*, 55(10), 2147–2161.

Zakir, M., Ahuja, N., Surksha, M. A., Sachdev, R., Kalariya, Y., Nasir, M., Kashif, M., Shahzeen, F., Tayyab, A., Khan, M. S. M., Junejo, M., Manoj Kumar, F., Varrassi, G., Kumar, S., Khatri, M., & Mohamad, T. (2023). Cardiovascular complications of diabetes: From microvascular to macrovascular pathways. *Cureus*, 15(9), e45835.

Zhao, X., An, X., Yang, C., Sun, W., Ji, H., & Lian, F. (2023). The crucial role and mechanism of insulin resistance in metabolic disease. *Frontiers in Endocrinology*, 14, 1149239.

Chapter 7

Glucagon-Like Peptide-1 Receptors (GLP-1R): Enhancing Insulin Secretion

Priyanka Singh*
Manu Sharma
and Namita Badoniya
Department of Pharmacy, Banasthali Vidhyapith, Banasthali, Rajasthan, India

Abstract

Glucagon-like peptide-1 receptors (GLP-1R) are essential modulators of glucose homeostasis, primarily by enhancing insulin secretion. GLP-1, an incretin hormone released from intestinal L-cells in response to meal consumption, binds to GLP-1R on pancreatic β-cells, activating glucose-dependent insulin secretion and improving glycemic control. This mechanism has been utilized to develop GLP-1R agonist drugs that mimic the incretin effect, providing significant benefits for patients with type 2 diabetes mellitus (T2DM).

Activation of GLP-1R not only enhances insulin secretion but also reduces glucagon release, slows gastric emptying, and increases satiety, addressing hyperglycemia and obesity in T2DM patients. Clinical trials have demonstrated that GLP-1R agonists effectively decrease hemoglobin A1c (HbA1c) levels, promote weight loss, and reduce cardiovascular risks, making them a cornerstone in diabetes treatment. This chapter explores the physiological mechanisms of GLP-1R-mediated insulin secretion, the pharmacodynamics of GLP-1R agonists, and their clinical implications. Additionally, it discusses emerging trends and future directions in GLP-1R research aimed at advancing diabetes treatment and improving patient outcomes.

Keywords: GLP-1 receptors agonists, insulin secretion, incretin effect, type 2 DM, glucose homeostasis

* Corresponding Author's Email: spriyaa35@gmail.com

In: Receptor-Targeted Therapies in Diabetes Mellitus
Editors: Ajmer Singh Grewal, Neelam Singh, Swati Verma et al.
ISBN: 979-8-89530-587-4

Abbreviation

ADP	Adenosine diphosphate
ATP	Adenosine triphosphate
cAMP	Cyclic AMP
DPP-IV	Dipeptidyl peptidase-IV
Epac-2	Exchange Protein directly activated by cAMP 2
$FADH_2$	Flavin adenine dinucleotide
GIP	Glucose-dependent insulinotropic polypeptide
GLP-1R	Glucagon-like peptide-1 receptor
GLUT	Glucose transporter
GPC-R	G protein-coupled receptor
GSIS	Glucose-stimulated insulin secretion
GTPase	Guanosine triphosphatase
Gαs	Stimulatory G protein alpha subunit
HbA1c	Hemoglobin A1c
K^+ATP	ATP-sensitive potassium channel
Kv	Voltage-dependent K^+ channels
mRNA	Messenger ribonucleic acid
NADH	Nicotinamide-adenine dinucleotide
PKA	Protein kinase A
RAP-1	Ras-associated protein-1
T2DM	Type 2 diabetes mellitus
$VDCa^{2+}$	Voltage-dependent calcium channels

Introduction

The regulation of insulin release and blood glucose levels is vital for maintaining metabolic balance. Insulin, a crucial metabolic hormone, is secreted by pancreatic β-cells in response to rising blood glucose levels, typically following the consumption of a carbohydrate-rich meal. These β-cells are highly sensitive to nutrient levels and adjust insulin secretion accordingly to ensure that glucose is effectively utilized and stored. Conversely, during periods of nutrient deprivation, the pancreas releases glucagon to raise blood sugar levels. In individuals with type 2 diabetes mellitus (T2DM), insulin secretion is impaired, resulting in chronic hyperglycemia. In this context, glucagon-like peptide-1 receptor (GLP-1R) agonists, an endogenous incretin, represent a promising treatment alternative for maintaining glucose homeostasis (Müllere et al. 2019). GLP-1 is a peptide released by intestinal L-cells in response to meal ingestion and consists of thirty amino acids. It is derived from the post-translational processing of preproglucagon, which serves as a precursor for various glucagon-related peptides. To demonstrate its regulatory effects, glucagon-like peptide-1 (GLP-1) binds to and activates the GLP-1R, a member of the class B family of G-protein coupled receptors (GPCRs). This receptor is expressed in multiple organs, including the brain, pancreas, kidneys, heart, and gastrointestinal tract (Rorsman and Ashcroft, 2018). Recent studies have shown that GLP-1R is predominantly expressed in pancreatic β-cells, with less frequent presence in α- and δ-cells.

This was demonstrated through experiments involving GLP-1R mRNA and protein co-localization with islet cell hormones in rats, mice, and humans. Upon activation of the β-cell receptor, there is a rapid increase in cyclic AMP (cAMP) levels and intracellular Ca^{2+}, leading to the exocytosis of insulin in a glucose-dependent manner. However, research has also indicated that GLP-1 influences certain extra-pancreatic tissues even in the absence of GLP-1R, suggesting that this hormone may operate through currently unidentified receptors or mechanisms (Gandasi et al. 2024). Given these findings, GLP-1-based therapies could provide new treatment strategies for diseases unrelated to T2DM in tissues responsive to GLP-1. Due to its therapeutic potential, several GLP-1R agonists and dipeptidyl peptidase IV (DPP-IV) inhibitors have been developed to prevent the degradation of endogenous GLP-1 (Chichura et al. 2023). This chapter explores the mechanisms of insulin secretion, glucose regulation, the role of incretin hormones like GLP-1, and the latest advancements in therapies for T2DM.

Glucose Regulation by Insulin Secretion

The secretion of insulin is essential for regulating fuel homeostasis in animals. It is released into the circulation by beta cells located in the islets of Langerhans in the pancreas. These "fuel-sensing" β-cells are activated to secrete insulin when blood glucose levels rise, typically after consuming a carbohydrate-rich diet. The primary function of insulin is to interact with and activate specific membrane-bound receptors on cells, promoting the storage of excess carbohydrates as glycogen in the muscles and liver, or as fatty acids in adipose tissue. Conversely, during nutrient deprivation or starvation, the pancreas increases blood glucose levels by secreting glucagon. Furthermore, the release of insulin by pancreatic beta cells is precisely regulated and influenced by various physiological and biochemical factors, with glucose being the main trigger. This regulation involves multiple steps and signaling pathways, ensuring that insulin release aligns with the body's metabolic demands (Yang et al. 2023).

Mechanism of Glucose-Stimulated Insulin Release (GSIR)

- *Uptake and metabolism of glucose:* Glucose is transported into β-cells through glucose transporters, such as GLUT1 in humans and GLUT2 in rats, as blood glucose levels rise. Once inside the β-cells, glucose undergoes metabolism, generating ATP through glycolysis and the tricarboxylic acid cycle. This process also produces reducing equivalents like NADH and FADH2. These reducing equivalents further contribute to ATP production when oxidized by the electron transport chain in the mitochondria. As a result of this high-energy environment, the ATP-to-ADP ratio in beta cells increases, leading to the inhibition of ATP-sensitive potassium channels (K+ATP), which causes plasma membrane depolarization (Fridlyand and Philipson, 2010).
- *K+ATP Channels:* The closure of K+ATP channels, induced by the rising ATP-to-ADP ratio, is a crucial initial step in initiating insulin secretion. This membrane depolarization plays a significant role in the subsequent signaling pathways (Ashcroft, 2023).

- *Voltage-dependent calcium channels ($VDCa^{2+}$ Channels):* The depolarization of the membrane opens $VDCa^{2+}$, allowing the influx of Ca^{2+}. This increase in intracellular Ca^{2+} concentration serves as the primary catalyst for insulin granule exocytosis (Lim et al. 2009).
- *Insulin granule exocytosis:* The influx of Ca^{2+} triggers a cascade of downstream signaling events, including the activation of protein kinases and the translocation of insulin-containing granules toward the plasma membrane. These granules then merge with the plasma membrane, leading to the release of insulin into the bloodstream (Rutter et al. 2006).

Blood Glucose Regulation by the Incretin Hormone GLP-1

The intestinal mucosa secretes incretin hormones in response to oral nutrient consumption, which enhance glucose-stimulated insulin production and lower blood glucose levels. Notably, within the normal glucose range, incretins can also reduce insulin release (Nauck et al. 2023). The two main forms of incretin hormones identified are GLP-1 and glucose-dependent insulinotropic polypeptide (GIP). Among these, GLP-1 is particularly significant as it not only lowers glucose levels but also delays gastric emptying and inhibits glucagon secretion. The term "incretin effect" refers to the ability of the intestinally produced GIP and GLP-1 to stimulate pancreatic insulin production through their glucoregulatory effects following oral glucose intake. The insulin-secreting effects of GLP-1 and GIP lead to a more significant reduction in blood glucose levels compared to insulin secretion stimulated by intravenous glucose administration without the involvement of intestinally released GLP-1 or GIP (Nauck et al. 2016). This incretin effect is more pronounced in healthy individuals than in those with T2DM. However, administering pharmacological doses of GLP-1 intravenously can acutely increase plasma insulin levels, resulting in lowered blood glucose levels in T2DM patients. A critical clinical feature of GLP-1's action is that insulin secretion from beta cells depends on glucose levels; GLP-1 effectively stimulates insulin secretion only when blood glucose levels are elevated. Consequently, GLP-1's effects on insulin secretion and blood glucose reduction are self-limiting, which reduces the risk of hypoglycemia in T2DM patients. In contrast, sulfonylureas like tolbutamide stimulate insulin secretion regardless of glucose levels and lack a self-limiting effect, increasing the likelihood of hypoglycemia (Boer and Holst, 2020). Research in mice has shown that, beyond stimulating insulin secretion, GLP-1 also acts as a growth factor for β-cells, enhancing insulin biosynthesis and promoting insulin gene expression (Leech et al. 2011). Additionally, GLP-1 has been shown to stimulate beta cell division (mitosis) and prevent beta cell death (apoptosis). While the effects of GLP-1 on humans remain to be confirmed, these findings suggest that long-term treatment with GLP-1 receptor (GLP-1R) agonists may lead to an increase in beta cell mass and islet insulin content. This beneficial antidiabetic effect is not observed with sulfonylureas. It is also essential to recognize that GLP-1's regulation of glucose involves more than its direct effects on pancreatic beta cells; GLP-1R analogs also act on pancreatic alpha cells to decrease glucagon secretion, which helps inhibit glucose synthesis in the liver (Alsalim et al. 2023). Moreover, GLP-1 has effects outside the pancreas, including slowing gastric emptying, reducing appetite, and enhancing cardiovascular performance (De Mesquita et al. 2016). GLP-1 actions may be modulated by both its class B

G-protein-coupled receptor and a conventional pathway triggered by GLP-1 metabolites, specifically (9-36) GLP-1 amide and (28-36) GLP-1 amide (Tomas and Habener, 2010). There is ongoing speculation about whether this unidentified non-conventional mechanism allows GLP-1 to exert 'insulin mimetic' effects on the liver. However, it remains unclear which GLP-1R analogs used to treat type-2 DM might activate this non-traditional pathway. Furthermore, the potential adverse effects of GLP-1 metabolism inhibitors, which could prevent the production of (9-36) GLP-1 amide and (28-36) GLP-1 amide, are also not well understood. This presents an opportunity to deepen our understanding of the pharmacology and physiology of GLP-1.

β-Cell Depolarization and Improved K^{+}_{ATP} Channel Closure Through GLP-1R Activation

GLP-1 acutely enhances GSIS primarily by activating GLP-1R, which interacts with the stimulatory Gαs subunit. This interaction leads to an increase in intracellular cAMP levels by activating adenylate cyclase. The acute GSIS in pancreatic β-cells is largely influenced by changes in the cell's energy balance, specifically the ATP/ADP ratio, which is directly linked to glucose metabolism. In pancreatic β-cells, glucose metabolism is not limited by glucose transporters; instead, glucokinase acts as the rate-limiting enzyme. Glucokinase functions as a glucose sensor with an enzymatic threshold of approximately 4 mM and demonstrates strong cooperation for glucose binding. When plasma glucose levels exceed this threshold, the rates of glucose metabolism increase through glycolysis and oxidative phosphorylation in the cytoplasm and mitochondria, respectively. As the ATP/ADP ratio rises, it affects K+ATP channels. ATP binds to the pore-forming subunits (Kir 6.2), promoting the release of ADP from the regulatory subunits (SUR1) and causing the channels to close. This closure leads to membrane depolarization, which opens voltage-dependent Ca^{2+} channels and triggers insulin exocytosis (Mayendraraj et al. 2022; Meloni et al. 2013). Moreover, *in vitro* studies using human and mouse pancreatic islets have shown that GLP-1R activation raises intracellular cAMP levels, which subsequently enhances glucose-induced insulin release. The elevated cAMP levels also increase the ATP sensitivity of K+ATP channels, effectively shifting the ATP sensitivity curve to the left. This mechanism is mediated by two key intermediaries: protein kinase A (PKA) and guanine nucleotide exchange factor (GEF). Both SUR1 and Kir 6.2 subunits of the K+ATP channel possess PKA phosphorylation sites. The activation of PKA through GLP-1R leads to the phosphorylation of SUR1 subunits, which reduces their affinity for ADP. Additionally, PKA activation influences exocytosis dynamics by phosphorylating snapin, which regulates Epac-2 and synaptosomal proteins (Pabreja et al. 2014; Light et al. 2022). Similarly, the cAMP-dependent activation of Epac-2 enhances the K+ATP channel's sensitivity to ATP, affecting vesicle priming and fusion, thereby increasing GSIS. Activation of Epac-2 likely works alongside PKA-dependent snapin activation, potentially involving GTPase RAP-1 and its target, phospholipase C, which may further enhance vesicle priming (Dzhura et al. 2011). While the enhancement of GSIS through GLP-1R is primarily dependent on the Gαs/cAMP pathway, some studies using supra physiological GLP-1 levels have suggested that β-arrestin 1 may also play a role in mediating part of the cAMP/GSIS response. Understanding the β-arrestin 1-dependent pathway could be significant for the development of low molecular weight drugs (Sonoda et al. 2008). In insulinoma cell lines, GLP-1R activation also promotes insulin expression by stabilizing insulin mRNA and increasing insulin transcription. This effect is mediated through the stimulation of cAMP-responsive element-binding protein (CREB) and T-cell-activated nuclear factor, operating via both PKA-dependent and PKA-independent pathways (Lawrence et al. 2002).

GLP-1's Inhibiting Effects on β-cell of Voltage-Dependent K^+ Channels (Kv)

Pancreatic β-cell electrical activity is significantly regulated by Kv channels. When glucose induces membrane depolarization, these channels allow potassium ions to exit the cell, promoting membrane repolarization. Recent research has highlighted the Kv1.0 and Kv2.0 family of channels, particularly the Kv2.1 channel, as crucial regulators of insulin secretion (Lubberding et al. 2022). Functional knockout studies of these channels have shown that their absence leads to increased insulin secretion in response to glucose stimulation. Specifically, in rat β-cells, stimulation of the GLP-1 receptor (GLP-1R) has been found to reduce Kv currents by approximately 40%. This inhibition of Kv currents by GLP-1 is attributed to increased voltage-dependent steady-state inactivation of the channels. Both the cAMP/PKA (protein kinase A) and phosphatidylinositol-3 kinase (PI3K) signaling pathways are implicated in GLP-1's modulation of Kv currents. Consequently, the insulin-stimulating effect of GLP-1 may, in part, result from its ability to inhibit Kv channels, leading to increased amplitude and prolonged action potential duration (Doyle and Egan, 2007). This action enhances the overall electrical activity of β-cells, facilitating greater insulin secretion in response to elevated glucose levels.

Voltage Gated Calcium Channel Activity Increased by GLP-1

GLP-1 plays a crucial role in regulating β-cell membrane potential by inhibiting K+ATP and Kv channels. This inhibition results in membrane depolarization, which activates voltage-gated Ca^{2+} channels, leading to an influx of Ca^{2+} ions and triggering calcium-dependent insulin exocytosis. Research indicates that GLP-1 enhances the overall Ca^{2+} current in both human and mouse β-cells. This enhancement is primarily attributed to delayed inactivation of the Ca^{2+} channels, which allows for prolonged calcium influx. Furthermore, GLP-1 appears to shift the gating of Ca^{2+} channels towards more negative voltages, facilitating regenerative electrical activity at voltages where action potentials would not typically occur. The enhancement of Ca^{2+} channel activity mediated by GLP-1 is linked to PKA-dependent phosphorylation of the channels. This is supported by findings that the specific PKA inhibitor, cAMPS, can block the increase in Ca^{2+} current induced by GLP-1 (Smith et al. 2019).

T2DM Treatment Using GLP-1 Based Medicine

GLP-1 agonists, or incretin mimetics, are a class of medications used primarily to manage DM and, in some cases, obesity (Berman et al. 2023). Following the FDA's approval of exenatide in 2005 for type 2 DM treatment, there has been a surge in the development of new GLP-1R stimulators that offer enhanced efficacy and longer-lasting effects. Exenatide requires administration at least twice daily to maintain therapeutic concentrations between meals, leading to reduced levels between doses. In contrast, liraglutide, approved in 2009, features a free fatty acid side chain that binds to albumin in plasma and interstitial fluid. This modification allows liraglutide to remain predominantly albumin-bound (around 98%), creating a reservoir for prolonged action and enabling once-daily injections, with an elimination half-life of approximately 13 hours. Subsequent advancements aimed to extend the duration between injections to once weekly. A novel formulation of exenatide is gradually released from a matrix after subcutaneous injection, achieving steady-state concentrations over 8 to 10 weeks, though it has a delayed onset of action (Kim et al. 2007; Drucker et al. 2008). Other strategies include linking modified GLP-1 to larger proteins, such as albumin (albiglutide) or the immunoglobulin Fc fragment (efpeglenatide and dulaglutide). These modifications typically result in slower degradation, with half-lives around one week, allowing for effective circulating levels shortly after subcutaneous injection, which helps in lowering plasma glucose levels quickly. Semaglutide, a GLP-1 analog structurally similar to liraglutide but with tighter albumin binding, also allows for weekly subcutaneous injections. For oral administration, semaglutide requires daily dosing due to decreased bioavailability through the gastrointestinal tract, making it the first GLP-1R stimulant approved for oral use. Both subcutaneous and oral formulations of semaglutide show similar effects on HbA1c, body weight, and side effects at equivalent doses (Aroda et al. 2023; Davies et al. 2017). Combining a GLP-1R agonist with basal insulin achieves HbA1c control comparable to intensified basal-bolus insulin regimens but with a significantly lower risk of weight gain and hypoglycemia. Furthermore, integrating insulin into a GLP-1R agonist regimen effectively manages fasting plasma glucose levels. GLP-1R agonists also influence postprandial glucose through mechanisms such as slowing gastric emptying, enhancing insulin secretion, and reducing glucagon secretion. Research comparing basal insulin, GLP-1R agonists, and their combination demonstrates that combination therapy leads to the most significant HbA1c reduction, with changes in body weight falling between the extremes of GLP-1R agonist (least weight gain) and insulin (most weight gain) (Diamant et al. 2014). Recent drug design advancements have resulted in combination therapies featuring GLP-1R agonists alongside innovative bioactive peptides. An example is tirzepatide, which combines sequences from both GLP-1 and GIP into a single co-agonist molecule. While both GLP-1 and GIP enhance insulin secretion, GLP-1 also aids in appetite suppression, whereas GIP has an immediate impact on fat cells. Therefore, tirzepatide offers the metabolic advantages of both hormones, making it a highly effective medication for lowering glucose levels and promoting weight loss (Boer et al. 2023). Other combination therapies currently under investigation include novel molecules that integrate GLP-1, GIP, and glucagon, leveraging glucagon's metabolic effects to enhance energy expenditure and potentially leading to greater weight loss (Knerr et al. 2022). Additionally, combining GLP-1 with amylin, known for its ability to delay gastric emptying and reduce appetite, has shown superior outcomes in glucose control and weight loss compared to each hormone used individually (Melson et al. 2024). Another approach involves the use of DPP-IV inhibitors, which increase circulating levels of GLP-1 without directly stimulating its secretion from L-cells. Medications such as vildagliptin (Galvus) and sitagliptin (Januvia) are currently employed in the treatment of type 2 diabetes mellitus (T2DM). While DPP-IV inhibitors may operate through unconventional mechanisms that could limit their efficacy, they remain promising alternatives due to their availability in oral dosage forms (Kalra et al. 2024; Saini et al. 2023).

Conclusion

GLP-1-based therapies, including DPP-IV inhibitors and GLP-1R agonists, have revolutionized the management of type 2 diabetes mellitus (T2DM) by enhancing insulin secretion, reducing glucagon release, delaying gastric emptying, and stimulating β-cell proliferation. Compared to traditional medications such as sulfonylureas, these therapies offer distinct advantages, including a lower risk of hypoglycemia and minimal weight gain. Clinical trials have demonstrated the efficacy of various GLP-1R agonists, such as exenatide, liraglutide, and semaglutide, in achieving significant weight loss, improving glycemic control, and enhancing cardiovascular health. Recent advancements have introduced combination therapies, such as tirzepatide, which integrates GLP-1 and GIP sequences, resulting in superior metabolic outcomes.

The ongoing development of GLP-1-based therapies has led to numerous patents focusing on novel compounds, dual agonists, advanced medication formulations, and innovative delivery systems, highlighting the continuous progress in diabetes management.

References

Alsalim, W., Lindgren, O., & Ahrén, B. (2023). Glucose-dependent insulinotropic polypeptide and glucagon-like peptide-1 secretion in humans: Characteristics and regulation. *Journal of Diabetes Investigation*, 14(3), 354–361.

Aroda, V. R., Frias, J. P., Ji, L., Niemoeller, E., Nguyên-Pascal, M. L., Denkel, K., Espinasse, M., Guo, H., Baek, S., Choi, J., & Lingvay, I. (2023). Efficacy and safety of once-weekly efpeglenatide in people with suboptimally controlled type 2 diabetes: The Amplitude-D, Amplitude-L and Amplitude-S randomized controlled trials. *Diabetes, Obesity & Metabolism*, 25(8), 2084–2095.

Ashcroft, F. M. (2023). KATP Channels and the Metabolic Regulation of Insulin Secretion in Health and Disease: The 2022 Banting Medal for Scientific Achievement Award Lecture. *Diabetes*, 72(6), 693–702.

Berman, C., Vidmar, A. P., & Chao, L. C. (2023). Glucagon-like Peptide-1 Receptor Agonists for the Treatment of Type 2 Diabetes in Youth. *Touch Reviews in endocrinology*, 19(1), 38–45.

Boer, G. A., & Holst, J. J. (2020). Incretin Hormones and Type 2 Diabetes-Mechanistic Insights and Therapeutic Approaches. *Biology*, 9(12), 473.

Boer, G. A., Hay, D. L., & Tups, A. (2023). Obesity pharmacotherapy: incretin action in the central nervous system. *Trends in Pharmacological Sciences*, 44(1), 50–63.

Chichura, K. S., Elfers, C. T., Salameh, T. S., Kamat, V., Chepurny, O. G., McGivney, A., Milliken, B. T., Holz, G. G., Applebey, S. V., Hayes, M. R., Sweet, I. R., Roth, C. L., & Doyle, R. P. (2023). A peptide triple agonist of GLP-1, neuropeptide Y1, and neuropeptide Y2 receptors promotes glycemic control and weight loss. *Scientific Reports*, 13(1), 9554.

Davies, M., Pieber, T. R., Hartoft-Nielsen, M. L., Hansen, O. K. H., Jabbour, S., & Rosenstock, J. (2017). Effect of Oral Semaglutide Compared with Placebo and Subcutaneous Semaglutide on Glycemic Control in Patients with Type 2 Diabetes: A Randomized Clinical Trial. *JAMA*, 318(15), 1460–1470.

De Mesquita Araújo, L., Feguri, S., de Oliveira, T., Pedrosa, F., Guimarães, R., de Sá, L., Rocha, D. and Arbex, A. (2016) Extra Glycemic Impacts of GLP-1 Receptor Agonists: Benefits of a Class Effect? *Open Journal of Endocrine and Metabolic Diseases*, 6, 43-57.

Diamant, M., Nauck, M. A., Shaginian, R., Malone, J. K., Cleall, S., Reaney, M., de Vries, D., Hoogwerf, B. J., MacConell, L., Wolffenbuttel, B. H., & 4B Study Group (2014). Glucagon-like peptide 1 receptor agonist or bolus insulin with optimized basal insulin in type 2 diabetes. *Diabetes Care*, 37(10), 2763–2773.

Doyle, M. E., & Egan, J. M. (2007). Mechanisms of action of glucagon-like peptide 1 in the pancreas. *Pharmacology & Therapeutics*, 113(3), 546–593.

Drucker, D. J., Buse, J. B., Taylor, K., Kendall, D. M., Trautmann, M., Zhuang, D., Porter, L., & DURATION-1 Study Group (2008). Exenatide once weekly versus twice daily for the treatment of type 2 diabetes: a randomised, open-label, non-inferiority study. *Lancet*, 372(9645), 1240–1250.

Dzhura, I., Chepurny, O. G., Leech, C. A., Roe, M. W., Dzhura, E., Xu, X., Lu, Y., Schwede, F., Genieser, H. G., Smrcka, A. V., & Holz, G. G. (2011). Phospholipase C-ε links Epac2 activation to the potentiation of glucose-stimulated insulin secretion from mouse islets of Langerhans. *Islets*, 3(3), 121–128.

Fridlyand, L. E., & Philipson, L. H. (2010). Glucose sensing in the pancreatic beta cell: a computational systems analysis. *Theoretical Biology & Medical Modelling*, 7, 15.

Gandasi, N. R., Gao, R., Kothegala, L., Pearce, A., Santos, C., Acreman, S., Basco, D., Benrick, A., Chibalina, M. V., Clark, A., Guida, C., Harris, M., Johnson, P. R. V., Knudsen, J. G., Ma, J., Miranda, C., Shigeto, M., Tarasov, A. I., Yeung, H. Y., Thorens, B. Rorsman, P. (2024). GLP-1 metabolite GLP-1(9-36) is a systemic inhibitor of mouse and human pancreatic islet glucagon secretion. *Diabetologia*, 67(3), 528–546.

Kalra, S., Zargar, A. H., Sridhar, G. R., Das, A. K., Ahmed, J., Mohan, J. C., Vijayakumar, G., Kumar, A., Sahay, R. K., Ayer, V., Pandit, K., Bantwal, G., Srinivas, A., Unnikrishnan, A. G., Jindal, S., Ray, S., Baruah, M. P., Ganguly, K., Mittal, S., Joshi, A., Sharma, B. (2024). Expert eValuation of Efficacy and Rationality of Vildagliptin "EVER-Vilda": An Indian Perspective. Clinical medicine insights. *Endocrinology and diabetes*, 17, 11795514231203911.

Kim, D., MacConell, L., Zhuang, D., Kothare, P. A., Trautmann, M., Fineman, M., & Taylor, K. (2007). Effects of once-weekly dosing of a long-acting release formulation of exenatide on glucose control and body weight in subjects with type 2 diabetes. *Diabetes Care*, 30(6), 1487–1493.

Knerr, P. J., Mowery, S. A., Douros, J. D., Premdjee, B., Hjøllund, K. R., He, Y., Kruse Hansen, A. M., Olsen, A. K., Perez-Tilve, D., DiMarchi, R. D., & Finan, B. (2022). Next generation GLP-1/GIP/glucagon triple agonists normalize body weight in obese mice. *Molecular Metabolism*, 63, 101533.

Lawrence, M. C., Bhatt, H. S., & Easom, R. A. (2002). NFAT regulates insulin gene promoter activity in response to synergistic pathways induced by glucose and glucagon-like peptide-1. *Diabetes*, 51(3), 691–698.

Leech, C. A., Dzhura, I., Chepurny, O. G., Kang, G., Schwede, F., Genieser, H. G., Holz, G. G. (2011). Molecular physiology of glucagon-like peptide-1 insulin secretagogue action in pancreatic β cells. *Progress in Biophysics and Molecular Biology*, 107(2), 236–247.

Li, A., Su, X., Hu, S., & Wang, Y. (2023). Efficacy and safety of oral semaglutide in type 2 diabetes mellitus: A systematic review and meta-analysis. *Diabetes Research and Clinical Practice*, 198, 110605.

Light, P. E., Manning Fox, J. E., Riedel, M. J., & Wheeler, M. B. (2002). Glucagon-like peptide-1 inhibits pancreatic ATP-sensitive potassium channels via a protein kinase A- and ADP-dependent mechanism. *Molecular Endocrinology*, 16(9), 2135–2144.

Lim, A., Park, S. H., Sohn, J. W., Jeon, J. H., Park, J. H., Song, D. K., Lee, S. H., & Ho, W. K. (2009). Glucose deprivation regulates KATP channel trafficking via AMP-activated protein kinase in pancreatic beta-cells. *Diabetes*, 58(12), 2813–2819.

Lubberding, A. F., Juhl, C. R., Skovhøj, E. Z., Kanters, J. K., Mandrup-Poulsen, T., & Torekov, S. S. (2022). Celebrities in the heart, strangers in the pancreatic beta cell: Voltage-gated potassium channels Kv 7.1 and Kv 11.1 bridge long QT syndrome with hyperinsulinaemia as well as type 2 diabetes. *Acta Physiologica*, 234(3), e13781.

Mayendraraj, A., Rosenkilde, M. M., & Gasbjerg, L. S. (2022). GLP-1 and GIP receptor signaling in beta cells - A review of receptor interactions and co-stimulation. *Peptides*, 151, 170749.

Meloni, A. R., DeYoung, M. B., Lowe, C., & Parkes, D. G. (2013). GLP-1 receptor activated insulin secretion from pancreatic β-cells: mechanism and glucose dependence. *Diabetes, Obesity & Metabolism*, 15(1), 15–27.

Melson, E., Ashraf, U., Papamargaritis, D., & Davies, M. J. (2024). What is the pipeline for future medications for obesity? *International journal of obesity* (2005), 10.1038/s41366-024-01473-y. Advance online publication.

Müller, T. D., Finan, B., Bloom, S. R., D'Alessio, D., Drucker, D. J., Flatt, P. R., Fritsche, A., Gribble, F., Grill, H. J., Habener, J. F., Holst, J. J., Langhans, W., Meier, J. J., Nauck, M. A., Perez-Tilve, D., Pocai, A., Reimann, F., Sandoval, D. A., Schwartz, T. W., Seeley, R. J., Stemmer, K., Tang-Christensen, M.,

Woods, S. C., DiMarchi, R. D., & Tschöp, M. H. (2019). Glucagon-like peptide 1 (GLP-1). *Molecular Metabolism*, 30, 72–130.

Nauck, M. A., & Müller, T. D. (2023). Incretin hormones and type 2 diabetes. *Diabetologia*, 66(10), 1780–1795.

Nauck, M. A., Petrie, J. R., Sesti, G., Mannucci, E., Courrèges, J. P., Lindegaard, M. L., Jensen, C. B., Atkin, S. L., & Study 1821 Investigators. (2016). A phase 2, randomized, dose-finding study of the novel once-weekly human GLP-1 analog, semaglutide, compared with placebo and open-label liraglutide in patients with type 2 diabetes. *Diabetes Care*, 39(2), 231–241.

Pabreja, K., Mohd, M. A., Koole, C., Wootten, D., & Furness, S. G. (2014). Molecular mechanisms underlying physiological and receptor pleiotropic effects mediated by GLP-1R activation. *British Journal of Pharmacology*, 171(5), 1114–1128.

Reed, J., Bain, S., & Kanamarlapudi, V. (2020). Recent advances in understanding the role of glucagon-like peptide 1. *F1000 Research*, 9, F1000 Rev-239.

Rorsman, P., & Ashcroft, F. M. (2018). Pancreatic β-cell electrical activity and insulin secretion: Of mice and men. *Physiological Reviews*, 98(1), 117–214.

Rosenstock, J., Kahn, S. E., Johansen, O. E., Zinman, B., Espeland, M. A., Woerle, H. J., Pfarr, E., Keller, A., Mattheus, M., Baanstra, D., Meinicke, T., George, J. T., von Eynatten, M., McGuire, D. K., Marx, N., & for the CAROLINA Investigators. (2019). Effect of linagliptin vs glimepiride on major adverse cardiovascular outcomes in patients with type 2 diabetes: The CAROLINA randomized clinical trial. *JAMA*, 322(12), 1155–1166.

Rutter, G. A., Pullen, T. J., Hodson, D. J., & Martinez-Sanchez, A. (2006). Pancreatic β-cell identity, glucose sensing, and the control of insulin secretion. *Biochemical Journal*, 464(1), 1–12.

Saini, K., Sharma, S., & Khan, Y. (2023). DPP-4 inhibitors for treating T2DM - hype or hope? an analysis based on the current literature. *Frontiers in Molecular Biosciences*, 10, 1130625.

Smith, N. K., Hackett, T. A., Galli, A., & Flynn, C. R. (2019). GLP-1: Molecular mechanisms and outcomes of a complex signaling system. *Neurochemistry International*, 128, 94–105.

Sonoda, N., Imamura, T., Yoshizaki, T., Babendure, J. L., Lu, J. C., & Olefsky, J. M. (2008). Beta-Arrestin-1 mediates glucagon-like peptide-1 signaling to insulin secretion in cultured pancreatic beta cells. *Proceedings of the National Academy of Sciences*, 105(18), 6614–6619.

Tomas, E., & Habener, J. F. (2010). Insulin-like actions of glucagon-like peptide-1: A dual receptor hypothesis. *Trends in Endocrinology and Metabolism*, 21(2), 59–67.

Tornehave, D., Kristensen, P., Rømer, J., Knudsen, L. B., & Heller, R. S. (2008). Expression of the GLP-1 receptor in mouse, rat, and human pancreas. *The Journal of Histochemistry and Cytochemistry*, 56(9), 841–851.

Yang, C., Wei, M., Zhao, Y., Yang, Z., Song, M., Mi, J., Yang, X., & Tian, G. (2023). Regulation of insulin secretion by the post-translational modifications. *Frontiers in Cell and Developmental Biology*, 11, 1217189.

Chapter 8

Sodium-Glucose Cotransporter-2 (SGLT2): A Key Player in Glucose Homeostasis

Ajmal Tariq Hussain
Suman Baishnab*
Vishwjeet Singh
and Sarah Saeed
Amity Institute of Pharmacy, Amity University Uttar Pradesh, Lucknow Campus, Uttar Pradesh, India

Abstract

Glucose homeostasis is critical for maintaining metabolic balance, ensuring blood glucose levels remain within strict limits through complex cellular and hormonal interactions. Sodium-glucose cotransporter 2 (SGLT2) plays a pivotal role in this process. Primarily located in the renal proximal tubules, SGLT2 facilitates glucose reabsorption from the glomerular filtrate back into circulation by coupling glucose transport with sodium ions. This mechanism not only prevents glucose loss in the urine but also contributes to overall energy balance. SGLT2 is also involved in various metabolic pathways, including insulin signaling, gluconeogenesis, and glycogenolysis. The advent of SGLT2 inhibitors has revolutionized the management of type 2 diabetes by offering an insulin-independent method for lowering blood sugar levels. These inhibitors effectively prevent blood sugar spikes and may also reduce cardiovascular risk while promoting weight loss. However, they are not without drawbacks, as their use can lead to side effects such as urinary tract infections and raise concerns about long-term safety.

Keywords: Sodium-glucose cotransporter 2 (SGLT2), metabolic pathways, renal glucose reabsorption, SGLT2 inhibitors

---

* Corresponding Author's Email: sumanbaishnab51@gmail.com

In: Receptor-Targeted Therapies in Diabetes Mellitus
Editors: Ajmer Singh Grewal, Neelam Singh, Swati Verma et al.
ISBN: 979-8-89530-587-4

Abbreviations

13BPG	1,3-Bisphosphoglycerate
ACE	Angiotensin-converting enzyme
ACTH	Adrenocorticotropic hormone
AMPK	AMP-activated protein kinase
ARBs	Angiotensin II receptor blockers
AT:	Adenosine triphosphate
CKD	Chronic kidney disease
CNS	Central nervous system
DHAP	Dihydroxyacetone phosphate
DKA	Diabetic ketoacidosis
eGFR	Estimated glomerular filtration rate
F16BP	Fructose-1,6-bisphosphate
F6P	Fructose-6-phosphate
FoxO-1	Forkhead box O-1
G3P	Glyceraldehyde-3-phosphate
G6P	Glucose-6-phosphate
GIP	Gastric inhibitory polypeptide
GLP-1	Glucagon-like peptide-1
GLUT	Glucose transporter
GNG	Gluconeogenesis
GSD	Glycogen storage disease
HbA1c	Hemoglobin A1c
MACE	Major adverse cardiovascular events
NADH	Nicotinamide adenine dinucleotide
NASH	Non-alcoholic steatohepatitis
PEP	Phosphoenolpyruvate
SGLT2	Sodium-glucose cotransporter 2
SNP	Single nucleotide polymorphism
SREBP-1c	Sterol regulatory element-binding protein 1c
T2DM	Type 2 diabetes mellitus
UGT	Uridine diphosphate glucuronosyltransferase
VDCC	Voltage-dependent calcium channel

Introduction

Glucose homeostasis is a vital physiological process that maintains blood glucose levels within a narrow range of 4-6 mmol/L, ensuring a consistent energy supply to critical organs, particularly the brain and muscles. Disruptions in this delicate balance can result in severe health complications, with diabetes mellitus being one of the leading causes of morbidity and mortality worldwide (Röder et al. 2016). Key hormones, such as insulin and glucagon, secreted by pancreatic β-cells and α-cells respectively, play pivotal roles in regulating blood glucose levels. Insulin lowers blood glucose by promoting its uptake and storage in adipose and muscle tissues, while glucagon raises blood glucose levels through glycogen breakdown and gluconeogenesis. The pancreas continuously monitors blood glucose levels, dynamically adjusting hormone secretion to maintain homeostasis. This intricate regulation includes the intra-islet insulin axis, where insulin released by β-cells suppresses glucagon secretion from α-cells, thereby preventing excessive glucose production and ensuring metabolic stability (Röder et al. 2016). Furthermore, hepatic glucose metabolism plays a central role in maintaining homeostasis. During fasting, glucagon stimulates glycogenolysis and gluconeogenesis to restore normal glucose levels, while hyperglycemia triggers insulin release, promoting glycogenesis. The liver regulates carbohydrate homeostasis through various pathways, including glycogenesis, glycolysis, and gluconeogenesis. These processes are controlled by key transcription factors such as Sterol Regulatory Element-Binding Protein 1 (SREBP-1c), Carbohydrate Response Element Binding Protein (ChREBP), and Forkhead Box O (FoxO-1) (Han et al. 2016). In addition to pancreatic and hepatic regulation, the central nervous system (CNS) plays a vital role in glucose homeostasis. The hypothalamus detects low blood glucose levels and stimulates the release of Adrenocorticotropic Hormone (ACTH), which increases hepatic glucose production via corticosterone. Concurrently, glucagon is released to enhance glycogenolysis. The CNS also exerts neuronal control, increasing glucose uptake in peripheral tissues and adjusting insulin sensitivity during hypoglycemia (Choi & Kim, 2022). Overall, the CNS coordinates hormonal responses and regulates glucose metabolism, ensuring a system that effectively responds to fluctuations in blood glucose levels. Incretins, such as Gastric Inhibitory Polypeptide (GIP) and Glucagon-Like Peptide-1 (GLP-1), further enhance insulin secretion and inhibit glucagon release after meals, contributing to the postprandial regulation of glucose levels (Röder et al. 2016; Häusl et al. 2019). The liver's capacity to manage glucose homeostasis is crucial, as it synthesizes glucose from non-carbohydrate sources during fasting, primarily utilizing amino acids, lactate, and glycerol (Han et al. 2016). The interconnectedness of metabolic pathways across various organs underscores the complexity of glucose homeostasis regulation. In the fed state, excess glucose is stored as glycogen in the liver through glycogenesis and utilized for energy via glycolysis. During fasting, glycogenolysis and gluconeogenesis increase to maintain blood glucose levels. Hormones like insulin and glucagon regulate these metabolic pathways by targeting critical enzymes and transcription factors. Any disruptions in these processes can lead to common disorders such as diabetes mellitus or rare inborn errors of metabolism. These conditions often manifest in childhood, and poor regulation can result in severe outcomes, including hyperglycemia or hypoglycemia. Understanding these regulatory mechanisms is essential for developing effective therapies and improving long-term outcomes and quality of life for individuals with metabolic disorders (Röder et al. 2016; Han et al. 2016). Overall, glucose metabolism is crucial for energy homeostasis, ensuring an adequate fuel supply to key organs. Disruptions in this delicate balance are associated with increased morbidity and mortality, underscoring the importance of maintaining glucose homeostasis (Zhao et al. 2009).

Sodium-Glucose Cotransporter 2 (SGLT2)

Structure and Function of SGLT2

SGLT2, a member of the SLC5 gene family, encodes a protein consisting of approximately 670 amino acids with 14 transmembrane helices. A central 10-helix bundle within this structure contains the glucose- and sodium-binding sites. Located on the luminal membrane of the S1 and S2 segments of the proximal renal tubule, SGLT2 functions efficiently both in heterologous expression systems and on the apical surface of epithelial cells. It demonstrates a moderate affinity for glucose (KM ~5 mM) and a high turnover number (30-60 cm^3/s) (Ghezzi et al. 2018; Wright, 2021). SGLT2 utilizes a 1:1 sodium-to-glucose transport ratio, powered by the Na+/K+ ATPase pump, to reabsorb glucose from the glomerular filtrate into the bloodstream, contributing to approximately 90% of glucose reabsorption in the proximal tubule of the kidney. This process is crucial for preventing glucosuria and maintaining normal blood glucose levels. After glucose is transported across the luminal membrane by SGLT2, it is further transferred across the basolateral membrane and back into circulation via GLUT2 (Ghezzi et al. 2018; Wright, 2021). The significance of SGLT2 in maintaining whole-body euglycemia has led to the development of antidiabetic drugs targeting this transporter. By inhibiting SGLT2-mediated glucose reabsorption, these drugs effectively lower blood glucose levels, providing a therapeutic approach for managing hyperglycemia in diabetes patients (Ghezzi et al. 2018; Wright, 2021; Packer et al. 2023).

Mechanism of Sodium-Glucose Cotransport

Cotransport Mechanism

Sodium-glucose cotransport via SGLT2 is essential for reclaiming filtered glucose from the urine and returning it to circulation. This process is driven by the electrochemical gradient of Na+, which is maintained by the Na+/K+ ATPase pump located on the basolateral membrane of proximal renal tubule cells. The pump actively maintains a low concentration of Na+ within the cytosol and a high concentration outside the cell, creating a gradient that facilitates glucose reabsorption. When glucose or Na+ binds to SGLT2 on the apical membrane, a conformational change in the transporter allows the co-transport of one glucose molecule with two Na+ ions. This secondary active transport mechanism derives its energy from the Na+ gradient rather than ATP, enabling efficient glucose reabsorption (Ghezzi et al. 2018; Wright et al. 2011).

Stoichiometry of Transport

The SGLT2-mediated sodium-to-glucose coupling ratio is 1:2, meaning that one glucose molecule is transported with two Na+ ions. This process is powered by the Na+ gradient, where Na+ moves from outside to inside the cell along its electrochemical gradient, driving glucose transport against its chemical gradient. SGLT2 sequentially binds Na+ and glucose, causing conformational changes that enable their co-transport across the membrane as a glucose-Na+ complex. Inside the cell, Na+ is extruded by the Na+/K+-ATPase pump, while glucose exits into general circulation through the basolateral membrane. This coupling mechanism efficiently reabsorbs glucose from the tubular fluid into the blood, utilizing the Na+ gradient maintained by the Na+/K+-ATPase pump (Hummel et al. 2011; Vallon, 2011).

SGLT2 Expression in the Body

Tissue Distribution

SGLT2 is primarily expressed in the luminal membrane of epithelial cells in the S1 and S2 segments of the proximal renal tubules, where it facilitates the reabsorption of approximately 90% of filtered glucose from the glomerular filtrate. Although predominantly localized in the kidneys, SGLT2 is also expressed at low levels in extra-renal tissues, including the brain, pancreas, and intestine. However, the physiological or pathological significance of SGLT2 in these non-renal tissues remains largely unexplored (Packer et al. 2023; Ghezzi et al. 2018).

Regulation of Expression

SGLT2 expression is modulated by hormonal regulation and nutritional status. Insulin upregulates SGLT2 expression in the kidneys, which may contribute to increased glucosuria in type 2 diabetes mellitus (T2DM). In contrast, glucagon decreases SGLT2 expression, likely enhancing urinary glucose excretion during fasting or hypoglycemia. Additionally, a high-carbohydrate diet increases SGLT2 expression and may contribute to insulin resistance, while a low-carbohydrate diet or fasting reduces its expression, reflecting an adaptive mechanism to maintain glucose homeostasis in response to changes in nutritional status (Vallon, 2020).

Pathological Conditions

Under pathological conditions such as diabetes mellitus, SGLT2 expression can be upregulated, leading to increased glucose reabsorption and contributing to hyperglycemia. Notably, different levels of SGLT2 expression are observed depending on the glycemic state. In diabetic nephropathy, particularly in type 1 diabetes or insulin-dependent diabetes mellitus (IDDM), SGLT2 expression may eventually decrease as a compensatory mechanism, reducing glucosuria and limiting glucose reabsorption by tubular cells (Nakano et al. 2022). SGLT2 is predominantly expressed in the proximal renal tubules, where it plays a key role in glucose reabsorption. Although its expression in non-renal tissues is minimal, the regulation of SGLT2 by hormonal, nutritional, and pathological factors underscores its critical role in glucose homeostasis and highlights its potential as a therapeutic target for metabolic disorders.

SGLT2 in Glucose Homeostasis

Renal Glucose Reabsorption

SGLT2 plays a crucial role in blood glucose homeostasis by reabsorbing filtered glucose from the renal proximal tubules back into circulation. It is predominantly expressed on the apical membrane of the S1 and S2 segments of the proximal tubule, where it is responsible for reabsorbing 70-90% of the filtered glucose load (Valentine, 2012). The glucose reuptake process relies on the sodium gradient maintained by the Na+/K+ ATPase pump on the basolateral membrane of proximal tubular cells, which drives glucose transport against its concentration gradient. Initially, glucose and Na+ ions bind to SGLT2 on the apical membrane, causing conformational changes that facilitate the co-transport of one glucose molecule with two sodium ions into the cell. This secondary active transport process is driven by the sodium gradient, rather than direct ATP consumption. Once inside the cell, sodium ions are actively pumped out via the Na+/K+ ATPase pump, and glucose exits across the basolateral membrane into circulation through the facilitative glucose transporter GLUT2 (Wilding, 2014; Novikov & Vallon, 2016).

Role in Glucose Homeostasis

SGLT2 in the renal proximal tubules plays a critical role in glucose homeostasis by reabsorbing the majority of filtered glucose, preventing its loss in urine (glucosuria), and ensuring glucose availability for metabolism and energy production. In healthy individuals, approximately 180 grams of glucose are filtered daily by the kidneys, with SGLT2 reabsorbing nearly all of it, while SGLT1 in the distal proximal tubule reabsorbs a smaller portion. When plasma glucose levels exceed the renal threshold of 180-200 mg/dL, the transporters become saturated, leading to glucosuria. In diabetes mellitus, increased expression of SGLT2 and SGLT1 raises this renal threshold, contributing to sustained hyperglycemia. SGLT2 inhibitors, a novel drug class for T2DM, lower blood glucose by enhancing urinary glucose excretion; these drugs block SGLT2, preventing glucose reabsorption in the kidneys (Wilding, 2014; Valentine, 2012). Understanding the role of SGLT2 in glucose reabsorption has therefore been instrumental in the development of these therapies.

Interaction with Other Glucose Transporters

SGLT1 and SGLT2 work in a coordinated but complementary manner to reabsorb filtered glucose in the kidneys. SGLT2, the primary isoform in the glomerular filtrate, reabsorbs approximately 90% of filtered glucose in the early proximal tubule, while SGLT1, located in the late proximal tubule and small intestine, absorbs the remaining 10%. SGLT1 has a lower Km for glucose, allowing it to maintain glucose reabsorption even when SGLT2 function is impaired or glucose levels are low (Ghezzi et al. 2018). Facilitative GLUTs also play a crucial role in glucose handling: GLUT2 on the basolateral membrane of proximal tubular cells allows glucose to exit cells and enter circulation, while GLUT1 in distal tubular segments reabsorbs about 5% of glucose for cellular energy. SGLT2 acts as the primary glucose reabsorber in the early proximal tubule, with SGLT1 providing backup capacity in the late proximal tubule. Several factors influence these glucose reabsorption processes. For instance, fasting upregulates SGLT1 to prevent hypoglycemia, while diabetes mellitus leads to increased SGLT2 expression, exacerbating hyperglycemia. Additionally, hormonal, dietary, and pharmacological factors regulate SGLT2 activity. Understanding these regulatory mechanisms is essential for developing targeted therapies, such as SGLT2 inhibitors, for metabolic diseases like diabetes (Szablewski, 2017; Vallon, 2020).

Pathophysiology Involving SGLT2

SGLT2 plays a critical role in glucose homeostasis by reabsorbing more than 90% of filtered glucose in the early proximal tubule, preventing glycosuria under normal conditions (Novikov & Vallon, 2016). In T2DM, the expression and activity of SGLT2 are often increased, leading to greater glucose reabsorption by the kidneys and preventing glucose depletion in the blood. This upregulation serves as a compensatory mechanism in response to insulin resistance and impaired glucose metabolism, which occur during the disease (Valentine, 2012). In animal models, both genetic and diet-induced rodent models of T2DM show enhanced SGLT2 activity, helping maintain glucose homeostasis despite insulin resistance and beta-cell dysfunction. Similarly, in humans with T2DM, renal glucose reabsorption is increased by 20-30% compared to healthy controls, due to elevated SGLT2 expression and function in the proximal tubules (Novikov & Vallon, 2016). Several factors influence SGLT2 expression, including transcriptional and post-translational modifications in response to hyperglycemia, as well as hormonal regulation by insulin and glucagon signaling (Ghezzi et al. 2018). Increased SGLT2 activity in T2DM contributes to diabetic complications such as nephropathy, retinopathy, and cardiovascular disease. This understanding has led to the development of SGLT2 inhibitors, a class of medications that help control blood sugar levels and reduce the risk of complications in diabetes.

Genetic Variations and Their Implications

Genetic differences in the SGLT2 gene (SLC5A2), which encodes the glucose transporter responsible for reabsorbing glucose from kidney cells, have been linked to abnormal glucose homeostasis and increased susceptibility to T2DM. Specific single nucleotide polymorphisms (SNPs) in the SGLT2 gene, such as rs9934336 and rs6813195, contribute to variations in SGLT2 expression and function. The rs9934336 SNP, in particular, results in reduced SGLT2 activity and expression, where the C allele leads to lower glucose reabsorption without affecting urinary glucose excretion (UGE), potentially increasing UGE and offering protection against T2DM (Prasad & Groop, 2015). Individuals carrying the C allele may also exhibit greater sensitivity to SGLT2 inhibitor treatment. Conversely, the rs6813195 SNP has been associated with higher SGLT2 expression and activity, which likely increases renal glucose reabsorption and contributes to hyperglycemia, thereby raising the risk of T2DM (Scott et al. 2014). These polymorphisms not only influence susceptibility to T2DM but also affect the response to SGLT2 inhibitors. Individuals with the C allele of rs9934336, who have lower SGLT2 activity, may experience a better glycemic response to SGLT2 inhibitors, as their renal glucose reabsorption is reduced. On the other hand, individuals with genetic variants linked to higher SGLT2 expression may show fewer effective responses to these inhibitors due to greater baseline glucose reabsorption. These genetic variations highlight the importance of precision medicine in T2DM management, as they provide insights into both diabetes susceptibility and individual responses to pharmacological treatments, particularly SGLT2 inhibitors (Prasad & Groop, 2015; Scott et al. 2014).

Impact on Insulin Sensitivity and Secretion

The inhibition of SGLT2 and the subsequent reduction in renal glucose reabsorption indirectly influence insulin sensitivity and secretion. The decrease in blood glucose levels due to SGLT2 inhibition is believed to improve insulin sensitivity in peripheral tissues. Insulin resistance, which leads to chronic hyperglycemia and suppression of insulin signaling, reduces glucose uptake in skeletal muscle and adipose tissue. SGLT2 inhibitors may interrupt this process by lowering blood glucose, thus improving whole-body insulin sensitivity and attenuating insulin resistance. Furthermore, SGLT2 inhibitors contribute to weight loss and a reduction in central fat mass, both of which are well-recognized risk factors for developing insulin resistance. The increase in erythropoiesis, along with the reduction in abdominal fat, further contributes to enhanced insulin sensitivity as a result of SGLT2 inhibitor therapy (Novikov & Vallon, 2016; Vallon & Thomson, 2017). SGLT2 inhibition may also influence pancreatic beta-cell function and insulin secretion. SGLT2 is expressed in pancreatic alpha cells, and its inhibition can lead to increased glucagon secretion. Elevated glucagon levels, in turn, stimulate beta cells to release insulin, thereby aiding in maintaining glucose homeostasis. The impact of SGLT2 inhibitors on insulin secretion may vary depending on individual factors and other circumstances. By reducing glucotoxicity, SGLT2 inhibitors can enhance beta-cell function and improve glucose control. These inhibitors primarily lower hemoglobin A1c (HbA1c) by reducing blood glucose levels, which subsequently improves insulin sensitivity and secretion. This effect results in decreased glucotoxicity, reduced insulin resistance, and mitigation of beta-cell failure. Additionally, the weight loss associated with SGLT2 inhibition further enhances insulin sensitivity in peripheral tissues. Collectively, the evidence suggests that SGLT2 inhibition reduces renal glucose reabsorption, leading to improvements in both insulin sensitivity and secretion. This contributes to better glycemic control, including diminished glucotoxicity and reduced body weight (Hiraizumi et al. 2024; Vallon & Thomson, 2017).

Therapeutic Targeting of SGLT2

The identification and development of selective SGLT2 inhibitors as an antidiabetic strategy for T2DM marked a significant breakthrough in disease management. Research into SGLTs began in the 1970s, emphasizing their critical role in renal glucose reabsorption. This research ultimately led to the discovery of SGLT2, which is responsible for reabsorbing approximately 90% of glucose in the proximal renal tubules, paving the way for targeted drug development. Advances in the 1980s and 1990s in understanding the structure, function, and regulation of SGLT2 set the foundation for selective inhibition, resulting in the creation of a new class of oral hypoglycemic agents. The first SGLT2 inhibitor, phlorizin, was developed by Bristol-Myers Squibb in 2000. However, its lack of selectivity and poor pharmacokinetics limited its clinical utility (Bebernitz, 2017). This development was followed by the introduction of more potent and selective SGLT2 inhibitors, including dapagliflozin (AstraZeneca), canagliflozin (Janssen Research & Development), and empagliflozin (Boehringer Ingelheim) in the late 2000s and early 2010s. These inhibitors exhibited enhanced selectivity for SGLT2 over SGLT1 and improved pharmacokinetic profiles, demonstrating robust antihyperglycemic efficacy. The FDA's approval of dapagliflozin in 2014 marked a pivotal milestone, paving the way for the global approval of other SGLT2 inhibitors, such as canagliflozin and empagliflozin. Today, these medications are integral to diabetes management, offering benefits such as reducing blood glucose without increasing the risk of hypoglycemia, lowering HbA1c levels, promoting weight loss, and providing cardiovascular protection (Yau et al. 2022). SGLT2 inhibitors function by blocking glucose reabsorption in the proximal renal tubules, thereby increasing glucose excretion in the urine without elevating blood sugar levels. This insulin-independent mechanism lowers blood glucose, promotes caloric loss through glucose excretion, and aids in weight reduction. Because glucose excretion is capacity-limited by SGLT1 activity in the later proximal tubules, the risk of hypoglycemia is minimized, maintaining stable glycemic levels. Additionally, SGLT2 inhibition mimics the effects of calorie restriction, enhancing glycemia elimination and activating physiological defence mechanisms such as increased plasma glucagon, hepatic glucose production, and lipolysis. These adaptations help prevent hypoglycemic episodes and preserve energy reserves. As a result, SGLT2 inhibitors offer a favorable metabolic profile, encompassing improved glycemic control, weight reduction, and a minimal risk of hypoglycemia (Vallon & Thomson, 2017; Upadhyay, 2024). Pivotal clinical trials have demonstrated the efficacy of SGLT2 inhibitors in treating T2DM. The EMPA-REG OUTCOME trial showed that empagliflozin reduced cardiovascular death and heart failure hospitalizations, while also lowering HbA1c by 0.6%-1% and inducing modest weight loss (Yau et al. 2022). The CANVAS program highlighted the benefits of canagliflozin in reducing cardiovascular events and slowing kidney disease progression, with the CREDENCE trial further confirming its positive effects on renal outcomes and cardiovascular events (Mavrakanas et al. 2023a). Similarly, the DECLARE-TIMI 58 trial demonstrated that dapagliflozin reduced heart failure hospitalizations and slowed kidney disease progression (Chan & Chan, 2023). Overall, SGLT2 inhibitors not only improve glycemic control and induce clinically significant weight loss, but also provide additional benefits such as lowering blood pressure, reducing albuminuria, and decreasing the incidence of cardiovascular events.

Clinical Implications of $SGLT_2$ Inhibitors

Glycaemic Control

SGLT2 inhibitors provide significant benefits in lowering blood glucose levels for individuals with T2DM. These drugs work by inhibiting the SGLT2 transporter in the early proximal tubule of the renal cortex, reducing the reuptake of filtered glucose and increasing glucose excretion via urine (Wilding et al. 2018). Clinical trials have shown that SGLT2 inhibitors can lower HbA1c levels by 0.6% to 1.2% when used as monotherapy and by 0.5% to 0.9% when added to an existing metformin regimen. This improvement in glycemic control occurs through an insulin-independent mechanism, which is particularly beneficial for T2DM patients who do not respond adequately to other antidiabetic treatments (Tsushima et al. 2021).

Weight Loss and Blood Pressure Reduction

In addition to their glycemic benefits, SGLT2 inhibitors have demonstrated other favorable metabolic effects, such as weight loss and reductions in blood pressure. Clinical trials have reported weight loss ranging from 2.5 kg to 3.5 kg with the use of SGLT2 inhibitors, primarily due to increased urinary glucose excretion and caloric loss, rather than a direct reduction in blood sugar levels. These inhibitors also exhibit blood pressure-lowering effects, reducing both systolic and diastolic blood pressure. The mechanism behind this blood pressure-lowering effect is multifactorial, involving osmotic diuresis, decreased arterial stiffness, and improved endothelial function. The improvement in glycemic control, along with weight loss and blood pressure reductions, makes SGLT2 inhibitors an ideal adjunct to current therapies for treating T2DM, particularly in patients with obesity, hypertension, or coexisting cardiovascular disease (Tsushima et al. 2021; Wilding et al. 2018).

Cardiovascular and Renal Benefits

SGLT2 inhibitors have shown significant cardiovascular benefits, particularly in reducing the risk of heart failure and major adverse cardiovascular events (MACE). These benefits have been consistently demonstrated in clinical trials. For instance, the CREDENCE trial found that canagliflozin reduced hospital admissions for heart failure among participants with type 2 diabetes and chronic kidney disease (van der Aart-van der Beek et al. 2022). This finding aligns with results from the EMPA-REG OUTCOME trial, which examined empagliflozin in individuals with established cardiovascular disease and found a significantly reduced risk of heart failure hospitalization (Mavrakanas et al. 2023b). Furthermore, the CANVAS program and the DECLARE-TIMI 58 trial demonstrated that both canagliflozin (Invokana) and dapagliflozin reduced the risk of MACE, including cardiovascular death, myocardial infarction, and non-fatal stroke (Chan & Chan, 2023; Makawi et al. 2024). SGLT2 inhibitors reduce cardiovascular risk through several mechanisms. These drugs lower blood pressure and positively influence cardiovascular risk factors, such as glycosuria and natriuresis. Additionally, they enhance vascular health by improving endothelial function and increasing arterial compliance. SGLT2 inhibitors also provide direct cardiovascular protection by enhancing myocardial energetics. Their renal protective effects are particularly significant, as they slow the progression of CKD, a major cardiovascular risk factor. Furthermore, these inhibitors exert anti-inflammatory and antioxidant effects by reducing oxidative stress and inflammation, both of which play crucial roles in the pathophysiology of cardiovascular changes. In summary, SGLT2 inhibitors improve heart failure outcomes and reduce major adverse cardiovascular events (MACE) through their glycosuric and natriuretic actions, as well as their beneficial effects on cardiac and renal function, ultimately lowering the risk of MACE (van der Aart-van der Beek et al. 2022; Mavrakanas et al. 2023b).

Renal Protection

SGLT2 inhibitors significantly benefit kidney health, particularly by reducing the onset of albuminuria, a key marker of kidney disease. These inhibitors mitigate hyperfiltration by lowering intraglomerular pressure through afferent arteriolar vasoconstriction, a mechanism central to the development of DKD. In addition to decreasing albuminuria, SGLT2 inhibitors exert anti-inflammatory and anti-fibrotic effects, reducing glomerulosclerosis and tubulointerstitial fibrosis. By lowering blood glucose levels, these drugs also decrease glucotoxicity and oxidative stress, both of which contribute to the progression of diabetic nephropathy, thereby enhancing overall glycemic control. The CREDENCE trial demonstrated that SGLT2 inhibitor treatment was associated with a 34% reduction in the risk of progression to end-stage kidney disease compared to placebo, underscoring their potential to improve kidney outcomes in patients with diabetes (Makawi et al. 2024; Bailey et al. 2022; Mavrakanas et al. 2023a).

Future Directions in SGLT2 Research

Emerging Therapies and Innovations

Several new SGLT2 inhibitors are under development, reflecting the growing interest in this class of medications. Sotagliflozin, a dual SGLT1 and SGLT2 inhibitor, has been approved in Europe for treating type 1 diabetes, with ongoing Phase III trials investigating its potential for managing heart failure and chronic kidney disease (Posch et al. 2022). Licogliflozin, an investigational compound, is currently being studied in clinical trials for T2DM, non-alcoholic fatty liver disease, and other metabolic disorders (Harrison et al. 2022). Ipragliflozin, an SGLT2 inhibitor developed in Japan, is seeking approval in the United States for T2DM and may also offer benefits in treating heart failure and chronic kidney disease. Another promising SGLT2 inhibitor, remogliflozin, is under development for T2DM and shows potential for managing non-alcoholic steatohepatitis (NASH) (Shao et al. 2020).

Emerging Therapeutic Approaches

A new therapeutic approach for SGLT2 inhibitors involves several innovative strategies aimed at enhancing their efficacy and expanding their clinical applications. One key development is the use of combination therapies, such as pairing SGLT2 inhibitors with GLP-1 receptor agonists or novel mineralocorticoid receptor antagonists. These combinations seek to improve glycemic control and provide additional cardiorenal benefits through complementary mechanisms of action. Another emerging strategy focuses on tissue-targeting approaches to enhance therapeutic efficacy and minimize off-target effects by modifying SGLT2 inhibitors for better organ specificity, such as targeting the kidney or heart. Advances in drug delivery systems, including oral sustained-release formulations and transdermal patches, are also being explored to increase bioavailability and improve patient compliance. Furthermore, research into genetic and epigenetic factors influencing SGLT2 expression is paving the way for precision medicine approaches, which could optimize therapeutic interventions for individual patients (Di Costanzo et al. 2023).

Potential for Combination Therapies

Future research will help refine the most effective therapeutic strategies, but it is already evident that combining SGLT2 inhibitors with other antidiabetic medications offers synergistic benefits for glycemic control, cardiovascular protection, and renal health. SGLT2 inhibitors lower blood glucose levels by inhibiting glucose reabsorption in the kidneys, while other antidiabetic agents, such as metformin or GLP-1 receptor agonists, improve insulin sensitivity and secretion, enhancing overall glycemic control. Combining these agents results in more effective blood sugar management. Regarding cardiovascular protection, SGLT2 inhibitors have demonstrated the ability to reduce hospitalizations for heart failure and MACE. Their cardioprotective effects can be further enhanced when used in conjunction with other cardiovascular protectors, such as GLP-1 receptor agonists or mineralocorticoid receptor antagonists (Elrakaybi et al. 2022).

SGLT2 inhibitors also provide renal protection by slowing the progression of kidney disease and reducing albuminuria, benefits that can be further enhanced when combined with other renal protective agents, such as ACE inhibitors or ARBs (Bailey et al. 2022). For instance, the combination of metformin and SGLT2 inhibitors has shown synergistic effects on glycemic control and cardiovascular outcomes. This was evidenced in the EMPA-REG OUTCOME trial, which demonstrated superior cardiovascular benefits with empagliflozin plus metformin compared to metformin alone (van der Aart-van der Beek et al. 2022). Similarly, combining SGLT2 inhibitors with GLP-1 receptor agonists has been shown to improve glycemic control and reduce cardiovascular risks, as evidenced by the LEADER trial, which found that liraglutide plus metformin significantly reduced cardiovascular outcomes in patients with type 2 diabetes (Chan & Chan, 2023). Furthermore, the combination of SGLT2 inhibitors and mineralocorticoid receptor antagonists, as demonstrated in the EMPA-KIDNEY trial, results in clinically meaningful reductions in glomerular filtration rate (GFR) loss and improves renal outcomes (Mavrakanas et al. 2023b).

Future Directions

Ongoing clinical trials are exploring the benefits of combining SGLT2 inhibitors with other antidiabetic agents to enhance treatment for T2DM, cardiovascular disease, and kidney disease (Elrakaybi et al. 2022). These combinations are promising because they offer complementary actions that improve glycemic control, cardiovascular protection, and renal outcomes. Current research is increasingly focused on understanding the tissue-specific effects of SGLT2 inhibitors, particularly their direct impact on the heart and kidneys, as well as their role in reducing inflammation and oxidative stress (Bailey et al. 2022; Tsai et al. 2021). Future studies aim to determine the optimal timing for initiating SGLT2 inhibitors, especially in populations with chronic kidney disease and heart failure, and to assess novel drug combinations, such as pairing SGLT2 inhibitors with GLP-1 receptor agonists or mineralocorticoid receptor antagonists or exploring dapagliflozin-statin co-packaged tablets. Additionally, research is investigating the genetic and epigenetic determinants of response to SGLT2 inhibitors, seeking biomarkers that may allow for more personalized care (Nair et al. 2018). Long-term safety and efficacy are being scrutinized through post-marketing surveillance and observational studies. Key trials, such as EMPA-KIDNEY, DAPA-HF, EMPEROR-Reduced, DELIVER, and SOLOIST-WHF, continue to assess the impact of SGLT2 inhibitors on cardiovascular and renal outcomes. Ongoing research into frequent responders (FR) and non-frequent responders (NFR) may further refine how these agents can be optimally used to improve patient-centered metabolic and cardio-renal disease outcomes.

Conclusion

The introduction of SGLT2 inhibitors has marked a significant advancement in the management of T2DM and related metabolic disorders by targeting the reabsorption of glucose in the kidneys. These drugs offer a transformative, insulin-independent mechanism to improve glucose homeostasis, with multiple benefits such as enhanced glycemic control, weight loss, blood pressure reduction, and a decreased risk of cardiovascular and renal complications. Beyond their glucose-lowering effects, SGLT2 inhibitors also provide renal benefits that are independent of their ability to reduce blood sugar, solidifying their role in the diabetes treatment armamentarium. Future research is focused on tissue-specific targeting to minimize off-target effects and exploring the potential of combining SGLT2 inhibitors with other therapeutic agents to achieve synergistic effects. Additionally, genetic and epigenetic studies hold promise for advancing personalized medicine, which may lead to better therapeutic strategies for conditions like heart failure, CKD, and non-alcoholic fatty liver disease. These developments may also uncover novel therapeutic targets and glucose regulatory pathways, further improving glycemic control and overall metabolic health. With these advancements, the future application of SGLT2 inhibitors is poised to expand beyond diabetes care, offering promising treatments for a range of metabolic diseases.

References

Bailey, C. J., Day, C., & Bellary, S. (2022). Renal Protection with SGLT2 Inhibitors: Effects in Acute and Chronic Kidney Disease. *Current Diabetes Reports*, 22(1), 39–52.

Bebernitz, G. (2017). Sodium–Glucose Cotransporters. Comprehensive Medicinal Chemistry III, 491–511.

Chan, J. C. H., & Chan, M. C. Y. (2023). SGLT2 Inhibitors: The Next Blockbuster Multifaceted Drug? *Medicina (Lithuania)*, 59(2), 1–13.

Choi, J. H., & Kim, M. S. (2022). Homeostatic Regulation of Glucose Metabolism by the Central Nervous System. *In Endocrinology and Metabolism* (Vol. 37, Issue 1, pp. 9–25). Korean Endocrine Society.

Di Costanzo, A., Esposito, G., Indolfi, C., & Spaccarotella, C. A. M. (2023). SGLT2 inhibitors: a new therapeutical strategy to improve clinical outcomes in patients with chronic kidney diseases. *International Journal of Molecular Sciences*, 24(10), 8732.

Elrakaybi, A., Laubner, K., Zhou, Q., Hug, M. J., & Seufert, J. (2022). Cardiovascular protection by SGLT2 inhibitors – Do anti-inflammatory mechanisms play a role? *Molecular Metabolism*, 64, 101549.

Ghezzi, C., Loo, D. D. F., & Wright, E. M. (2018). Physiology of renal glucose handling via SGLT1, SGLT2 and GLUT2 Online Mendelian Inheritance in Man. *Diabetologia*, 61, 2087–2097.

Han, H. S., Kang, G., Kim, J. S., Choi, B. H., & Koo, S. H. (2016). Regulation of glucose metabolism from a liver-centric perspective. *Experimental and Molecular Medicine*, 48(3), e218-10.

Harrison, S. A., Manghi, F. P., Smith, W. B., Alpenidze, D., Aizenberg, D., Klarenbeek, N., Chen, C. Y., Zuckerman, E., Ravussin, E., Charatcharoenwitthaya, P., Cheng, P. N., Katchman, H., Klein, S., Ben-Ari, Z., Mendonza, A. E., Zhang, Y., Martic, M., Ma, S., Kao, S., Tanner, S., Pachori, A., Badman, M. K., He, Y., Ukomadu, C., & Sicard, E. (2022). Licogliflozin for nonalcoholic steatohepatitis: A randomized, double-blind, placebo-controlled, phase 2a study. *Nature Medicine*, 28(7), 1432-1438.

Häusl, A. S., Balsevich, G., Gassen, N. C., & Schmidt, M. V. (2019). Focus on FKBP51: A molecular link between stress and metabolic disorders. *Molecular Metabolism*, 29(September), 170–181.

Hiraizumi, M., Akashi, T., Murasaki, K., Kishida, H., Kumanomidou, T., Torimoto, N., Nureki, O., & Miyaguchi, I. (2024). Transport and inhibition mechanism of the human SGLT2–MAP17 glucose transporter. *Nature Structural and Molecular Biology*, 31(1), 159–169.

Hummel, C. S., Lu, C., Loo, D. D. F., Hirayama, B. A., Voss, A. A., & Wright, E. M. (2011). Glucose transport by human renal Na+/D-glucose cotransporters SGLT1 and SGLT2. American Journal of Physiology. *Cell Physiology*, 300(1), C721.

Iyer, G., Dyawanapelly, S., Jain, R., & Dandekar, P. (2022). An overview of oral insulin delivery strategies (OIDS). *International Journal of Biological Macromolecules*, 208(March), 565–585.

Makawi, A. T., Tawfik, Y. M. K., Dixon, D. L., McMahon, G. M., & Buckley, L. F. (2024). Expanding the Impact of SGLT2 Inhibitors in Chronic Kidney Disease. *American Journal of Nephrology*, 55(4), 417-420.

Mavrakanas, T. A., Tsoukas, M. A., Brophy, J. M., Sharma, A., & Gariani, K. (2023a). SGLT-2 inhibitors improve cardiovascular and renal outcomes in patients with CKD: a systematic review and meta-analysis. *Scientific Reports*, 13(1), 1–12.

Nair, A. S., Bagchi, D., Lehmann, T. E., & Nair, S. (2018). Renal Sodium-Glucose Transporter-2 Inhibitors as Antidiabetic Agents. *In Nutritional and Therapeutic Interventions for Diabetes and Metabolic Syndrome* (Second Edi). Elsevier Inc.

Nakano, D., Akiba, J., Tsutsumi, T., Kawaguchi, M., Yoshida, T., Koga, H., & Kawaguchi, T. (2022). Hepatic expression of sodium-glucose cotransporter 2 (SGLT2) in patients with chronic liver disease. *Medical Molecular Morphology*, 55(4), 304–315.

Novikov, A., & Vallon, V. (2016). SGLT2 inhibition in the diabetic kidney – an update. *Current Opinion in Nephrology and Hypertension*, 25(1), 50.

Packer, M., Wilcox, C. S., & Testani, J. M. (2023). Critical Analysis of the Effects of SGLT2 Inhibitors on Renal Tubular Sodium, Water and Chloride Homeostasis and Their Role in Influencing Heart Failure Outcomes. *Circulation*, 148(4), 354–372.

Posch, M. G., Walther, N., Ferrannini, E., Powell, D. R., Banks, P., Wason, S., & Dahmen, R. (2022). Metabolic, intestinal, and cardiovascular effects of sotagliflozin compared with empagliflozin in patients with type 2 diabetes: a randomised, double-blind study. *Diabetes Care*, 45(9), 2118.

Prasad, R. B., & Groop, L. (2015). Genetics of Type 2 Diabetes—Pitfalls and Possibilities. *Genes 2015*, Vol. 6, Pages 87-123, 6(1), 87–123.

Röder, P. V., Wu, B., Liu, Y., & Han, W. (2016). Pancreatic regulation of glucose homeostasis. *Experimental & Molecular Medicine*, 48(December 2015), e219.

Scott, R. A., Fall, T., Pasko, D., Barker, A., Sharp, S. J., Arriola, L., Balkau, B., Barricarte, A., Barroso, I., Boeing, H., Clavel-Chapelon, F., Crowe, F. L., Dekker, J. M., Fagherazzi, G., Ferrannini, E., Forouhi, N. G., Franks, P. W., Gavrila, D., Giedraitis, V., Grioni, S., Groop, L. C., Kaaks, R., Key, T. J., Kühn, T., Lotta, L. A., Nilsson, P. M., Overvad, K., Palli, D., Panico, S., Quirós, J. R., Rolandsson, O., Roswall, N., Sacerdote, C., Sala, N., Sánchez, M. J., Schulze, M. B., Siddiq, A., Slimani, N., Sluijs, I., Spijkerman, A. M., Tjonneland, A., Tumino, R., van der A, D. L., Yaghootkar, H., RISC Study Group, EPIC-InterAct Consortium, McCarthy, M. I., Semple, R. K., Riboli, E., Walker, M., Ingelsson, E., Frayling, T. M., Savage, D. B., Langenberg, C., & Wareham, N. J. (2014). Common genetic variants highlight the role of insulin resistance and body fat distribution in type 2 diabetes, independent of obesity. *Diabetes*, 63(12), 4378-4387.

Shao, S. C., Kuo, L. T., Chien, R. N., Hung, M. J., & Lai, E. C. C. (2020). SGLT2 inhibitors in patients with type 2 diabetes with non-alcoholic fatty liver diseases: an umbrella review of systematic reviews. *BMJ Open Diabetes Research & Care*, 8(2), 1956.

Szablewski, L. (2017). Distribution of glucose transporters in renal diseases. *Journal of Biomedical Science*, 24(1), 1–12.

Tsai, K. F., Chen, Y. L., Chiou, T. T. Y., Chu, T. H., Li, L. C., Ng, H. Y., Lee, W. C., & Lee, C. Te. (2021). Emergence of sglt2 inhibitors as powerful antioxidants in human diseases. *Antioxidants*, 10(8), 1–26.

Tsushima, Y., Lansang, M. C., & Makin, V. (2021a). The role of SGLT-2 inhibitors in managing type 2 diabetes. *Cleveland Clinic Journal of Medicine*, 88(1), 47–58.

Upadhyay, A. (2024). SGLT2 Inhibitors and Kidney Protection: Mechanisms beyond Tubuloglomerular Feedback. *Kidney360*, 5(5), 771–782.

Valentine, V. (2012). The role of the kidney and sodium-glucose cotransporter-2 inhibition in diabetes management. *Clinical Diabetes*, 30(4), 151–155.

Vallon, V. (2011). Molecular determinants of renal glucose reabsorption. Focus on "Glucose transport by human renal Na+/D-glucose cotransporters SGLT1 and SGLT2." *American Journal of Physiology-Cell Physiology*, 300(1), C6-C8.

Vallon, V. (2020). Glucose transporters in the kidney in health and disease. *Pflugers Archiv European Journal of Physiology*, 472(9), 1345–1370.

Vallon, V., & Thomson, S. C. (2017). Targeting renal glucose reabsorption to treat hyperglycaemia: the pleiotropic effects of SGLT2 inhibition. *Diabetologia*, 60(2), 215–225.

van der Aart-van der Beek, A. B., de Boer, R. A., & Heerspink, H. J. L. (2022). Kidney and heart failure outcomes associated with SGLT2 inhibitor use. *Nature Reviews Nephrology*, 18(5), 294–306.

Wilding, J. P. H. (2014). The role of the kidneys in glucose homeostasis in type 2 diabetes: Clinical implications and therapeutic significance through sodium glucose co-transporter 2 inhibitors. *Metabolism: Clinical and Experimental*, 63(10), 1228–1237.

Wilding, J., Fernando, K., Milne, N., Evans, M., Ali, A., Bain, S., Hicks, D., James, J., Newland-Jones, P., Patel, D., & Viljoen, A. (2018). SGLT2 Inhibitors in Type 2 Diabetes Management: Key Evidence and Implications for Clinical Practice. *Diabetes Therapy*, 9(5), 1757–1773.

Wright, E. M. (2021). SGLT2 Inhibitors: Physiology and Pharmacology. Kidney360, 2(12), 2027–2037.

Wright, E. M., LOO, D. D. F. L., & Hirayama, B. A. (2011). Biology of human sodium glucose transporters. *Physiological Reviews*, 91(2), 733–794.

Yau, K., Dharia, A., Alrowiyti, I., & Cherney, D. Z. I. (2022). Prescribing SGLT2 Inhibitors in Patients With CKD: Expanding Indications and Practical Considerations. *Kidney International Reports*, 7(7), 1463–1476.

Zhao, Y., Wieman, H. L., Jacobs, S. R., & Rathmell, J. C. (2009). *NIH Public Access*. 6879(08), 1–16.

Chapter 9

SGLT2 Inhibitors: A Novel Approach to Glycaemic Control

Sweta Kamboj[1]
Rohit Kamboj[1]
Monia Sharma[2]
and Shikha Kamboj[1,*]
[1]Guru Gobind Singh College of Pharmacy, Yamuna Nagar, Haryana, India
[2]Department of Periodontology, J.N. Kapoor D.A.V. (C) Dental College, Yamuna Nagar, Haryana, India

Abstract

Sodium-glucose cotransporter-2 (SGLT2) inhibitors represent a promising class of medications for managing type 2 diabetes mellitus (T2DM). These agents enhance urinary glucose excretion by selectively inhibiting SGLT2 in the renal proximal tubule, effectively lowering blood sugar levels, promoting weight loss, and minimizing the risk of hypoglycemia offering distinct advantages over traditional therapies. SGLT2 inhibitors significantly improve glycemic control in T2DM patients, particularly those struggling with weight management, and have demonstrated substantial cardiovascular and renal benefits. Notably, clinical trials such as CANVAS and DECLARE-TIMI 58 have highlighted the cardiovascular benefits of specific SGLT2 inhibitors, including canagliflozin and dapagliflozin, in reducing cardiovascular complications, a common comorbidity in T2DM. Meta-analyses further validate these findings, showing reduced heart failure-related hospitalizations and overall cardiovascular risk. In addition to their cardiovascular advantages, SGLT2 inhibitors have proven effective in lowering HbA1c levels and improving glycemic control with minimal hypoglycemia risk. They also slow the progression of diabetic kidney disease, addressing another critical comorbidity in T2DM. Overall, SGLT2 inhibitors provide a multifaceted therapeutic approach, making them a valuable addition to diabetes management. Ongoing research continues to explore their full potential and long-term benefits for T2DM patients.

Keywords: SGLT2 inhibitors, type 2 diabetes, glycemic control, hypoglycemia, weight management, cardiovascular disease, kidney disease

---

* Corresponding Author's Email: shikhakamboj21@gmail.com

In: Receptor-Targeted Therapies in Diabetes Mellitus
Editors: Ajmer Singh Grewal, Neelam Singh, Swati Verma et al.
ISBN: 979-8-89530-587-4

Abbreviations

AChE	Acetylcholinesterase
BBB	Blood-brain barrier
CNS	Central nervous system
COPD	Chronic obstructive pulmonary disease
CVOTs	Cardiovascular outcomes trials
DKA	Diabetic ketoacidosis
DPP-4	Dipeptidyl peptidase-4
FENa	fractional excretion of sodium
GFR	Glomerular filtration rate
GLP-1	Glucagon-like peptide-1
GSH	Glutathione
HbA1c	Hemoglobin A1c
HF	Heart failure
MCP-1	Monocyte chemoattractant protein-1
MDA	Malondialdehyde
MI	Myocardial infarction
NAFLD	Non-alcoholic fatty liver disease
RCTs	Randomized controlled trials
ROS	Reactive oxygen species
SGLT2	Sodium-glucose cotransporter-2
T2DM	Type 2 diabetes mellitus
TNF	tumor necrosis factor
UTIs	Urinary tract infections

Introduction

Initially developed for their anti-diabetic effects, sodium-glucose cotransporter-2 (SGLT2) inhibitors are now included in both diabetes and heart failure management guidelines, resulting in their widespread adoption among patients. Numerous post-hoc analyses, meta-analyses, and presentations at various scientific congresses have consistently demonstrated that this class of drugs significantly reduces mortality, lowers cardiovascular event rates, and helps prevent heart failure and renal disease (Jasleen et al. 2023). The eight cardiovascular outcome trials (CVOTs) involving SGLT2 inhibitors in patients with diabetes have consistently demonstrated these benefits. These drugs, commonly recognized by the suffix "flozins," have shown significant advantages for cardiovascular health, including reducing blood pressure, managing heart failure, and controlling heart rate. Additionally, SGLT2 inhibitors have shown potential in respiratory health, aiding in the management of conditions such as acute pulmonary edema, asthma, bronchitis, and chronic obstructive pulmonary disease (COPD). SGLT2 inhibitors, which are also expressed in the blood-brain barrier (BBB), may influence the central nervous system (CNS) by reducing oxidative stress, decreasing BBB permeability, lowering microglial activity, and inhibiting acetylcholinesterase (AChE). Furthermore, these inhibitors provide liver support by addressing non-alcoholic fatty liver disease (NAFLD) and liver toxicity while promoting weight loss. In the pancreas, SGLT2 inhibitors effectively manage hyperglycemia, reduce nephrotoxicity, and slow the decline of the glomerular filtration rate (GFR), making them promising for patients undergoing kidney transplantation (Ernesto et al. 2023). Despite their benefits, SGLT2 inhibitors are associated with adverse effects, including urinary tract infections (UTIs), dehydration, hypotension, dizziness, postural fainting, hyperkalemia-induced cardiac arrest, and pancreatitis. Other medications for type 2 diabetes mellitus (T2DM) also have notable side effects. For example, subcutaneous insulin use has been linked to a more than sixfold increased risk of proliferative retinopathy (Chan et al. 2023). Thiazolidinediones are associated with edema and an increased risk of heart failure (HF) hospitalization and cardiovascular (CV) death. Similarly, oral sulfonylureas are linked to hypoglycemia, myocardial infarction (MI), stroke, and CV death, with more frequent CV events compared to newer antidiabetic medications. Initial studies associated glucagon-like peptide-1 (GLP-1) agonists with pancreatitis and dipeptidyl peptidase-4 (DPP-4) inhibitors with heart failure; however, recent analyses have questioned these associations. Emerging research highlights the potential impact of SGLT2 inhibitors on Alzheimer's disease progression and brain injury in ischemic conditions. Studies have demonstrated that empagliflozin reduces amyloid-beta plaque density and levels of both soluble and insoluble amyloid beta in APP/PS1xdb model mice (Correa et al. 2021). Additionally, SGLT2 inhibitors promote angiogenesis and neurogenesis, thereby reducing central nervous system (CNS) damage caused by ischemia. Empagliflozin has been shown to increase levels of HIF-1α and VEGF-A while significantly decreasing caspase-3, with one study reporting an 85% reduction in caspase-3 levels in mice with ischemia/reperfusion injury. This neuroprotective effect may be attributed to its ability to cross a compromised BBB. Furthermore, research indicates that empagliflozin reduces atherosclerotic plaque formation in the aortic arch and valve in ApoE-/- mice, as well as inflammatory markers such as tumor necrosis factor-alpha (TNF-α), interleukin-6 (IL-6), and monocyte chemoattractant protein-1 (MCP-1) (Hiraizumi et al. 2024). Empagliflozin also decreases infarct size by mitigating oxidative stress, inflammation, and apoptotic markers in the brain. This is achieved through the reduction of malondialdehyde (MDA) levels and the enhancement of catalase and glutathione (GSH) activity, which help preserve the microvascular integrity of brain cells. Beyond SGLT2 inhibition, these drugs exhibit a wide range of kidney and heart benefits, even in the absence of SGLT2 channels in cardiac tissue. Their effects on cardiorenal health include improving risk factors, enhancing myocardial energy utilization, and optimizing ventricular loading conditions through diuretic, natriuretic, and vascular mechanisms (Salvatore et al. 2022). Clinically, SGLT2 inhibitors also demonstrate antifibrotic properties by reducing inflammation and oxidative stress, as well as modulating mitochondrial function and autophagy. This chapter will comprehensively examine the benefits and risks of SGLT2 inhibitors across various organ systems and their implications for clinical practice.

SGLT2 Inhibitors

Mechanism of Action of SGLT2 Inhibitors

The primary mechanism by which SGLT2 inhibitors regulate blood glucose is by reducing glucose reabsorption in the renal proximal tubule, leading to glycosuria. However, the precise mechanisms underlying their cardiovascular and renal protective effects remain under investigation (Abdelrahman et al. 2024). For cardiovascular benefits, proposed mechanisms include enhancing cardiac energy efficiency, lowering blood pressure, reducing inflammation, promoting natriuresis and diuresis, inhibiting sympathetic nervous system activity, and preventing cardiac remodeling. Regarding renal protection, SGLT2 inhibitors reduce intraglomerular pressure by increasing sodium flow through the nephron, which triggers adenosine-mediated constriction of the afferent glomerular arterioles. Additional renal benefits include improved oxygen supply to the tubules and reduced kidney inflammation (Pabel et al. 2023). Other proposed mechanisms involve decreasing inflammatory markers such as IL-6, TNF, IFNγ, NF-κβ, TLR-4, and TGF-β, as well as enhancing mitochondrial function. Ongoing research continues to investigate and clarify these protective mechanisms.

Mechanism of Action of GLP-1 Receptor Agonists

GLP-1 receptor agonists enhance insulin secretion and suppress abnormal glucagon release by leveraging the incretin effect. They are believed to support weight loss by slowing gastric emptying and reducing appetite. The cardiovascular benefits of GLP-1 receptor agonists are likely attributed to their anti-inflammatory properties, as well as their ability to inhibit platelet aggregation and reduce thrombus formation (Tang et al. 2023). Additionally, their renal benefits include reducing renal inflammation and preserving renal structure and function.

Combination Therapy of SGLT2 Inhibitors and GLP-1 Receptor Agonists

Given their complementary yet distinct mechanisms, combining SGLT2 inhibitors with GLP-1 receptor agonists may offer a synergistic effect, resulting in greater reductions in HbA1c and enhanced cardiovascular protection (Young et al. 2023). This discussion examines the benefits of this combination therapy. A meta-analysis revealed that the combined use of these agents led to more substantial reductions in HbA1c, body weight, and systolic blood pressure compared to monotherapy. However, combination therapy was associated with a higher risk of hypoglycemia and other adverse effects specific to each drug class. The analysis confirmed that the combination is both safe and effective. The choice of therapy depends on factors such as patient comorbidities, individual preferences, known mechanisms of action, and findings from recent clinical trials (Sayour et al. 2023).

Short-Term Impact of SGLT2 Inhibitors on HbA1c Levels

SGLT2 inhibitors have emerged as a valuable addition to the treatment options for managing T2DM. These drugs, including canagliflozin, dapagliflozin, and empagliflozin, act by inhibiting the SGLT2 transporter in the renal proximal tubules. This inhibition reduces glucose reabsorption and increases urinary glucose excretion, thereby lowering blood glucose levels and improving glycemic control, as evidenced by reductions in HbA1c levels. Short-term studies demonstrate that SGLT2 inhibitors can reduce HbA1c by approximately 0.5% to 1.0%

within 12 to 24 weeks of initiating therapy. This effect is particularly pronounced when these drugs are added to the treatment regimens of patients who have not achieved adequate glycemic control with other medications, such as metformin, sulfonylureas, or insulin (Davies et al. 2018). The reduction in HbA1c achieved with SGLT2 inhibitors varies depending on baseline levels, with greater reductions typically observed in patients with higher initial HbA1c values. Studies indicate that the HbA1c-lowering effect of SGLT2 inhibitors is comparable to, and in some cases slightly superior to, that of DPP-4 inhibitors, another class of glucose-lowering medications. This sustained reduction in HbA1c is vital for managing T2DM, as it is associated with a decreased risk of both microvascular and macrovascular complications. A significant advantage of SGLT2 inhibitors is their insulin-independent mechanism of action. Unlike many other diabetes therapies, these agents do not depend on endogenous insulin or functioning beta cells to reduce blood glucose levels, making them effective even in patients with beta-cell dysfunction or insulin resistance (Rosenstock et al. 2013). This feature makes SGLT2 inhibitors especially valuable for patients with advanced T2DM, where beta-cell function is often severely compromised. Additionally, their insulin-independent mechanism of action lowers the risk of hypoglycemia, a common adverse effect associated with other antidiabetic medications like insulin and sulfonylureas. While the risk of hypoglycemia is minimal when SGLT2 inhibitors are used as monotherapy or in combination with metformin, it may increase when they are combined with insulin or insulin secretagogues. Beyond HbA1c reduction, SGLT2 inhibitors offer additional metabolic benefits that enhance overall diabetes management. These drugs are associated with modest weight loss, a particularly advantageous effect for patients with T2DM who often struggle with obesity. This weight reduction primarily results from caloric loss due to increased glucose excretion. Furthermore, SGLT2 inhibitors have been shown to lower systolic blood pressure, likely due to their mild diuretic effect, which is beneficial for patients with hypertension a common comorbidity in T2DM. The short-term safety profile of SGLT2 inhibitors is generally favorable, though certain adverse effects require monitoring (Fitchett et al. 2018). The most frequently reported side effects include genital mycotic infections and urinary tract infections, likely caused by increased urinary glucose levels, which create a conducive environment for microbial growth. These infections are typically mild to moderate and can be managed with standard treatments. Educating patients about maintaining good genital hygiene can help mitigate these risks. A less common but potentially serious concern is euglycemic diabetic ketoacidosis (DKA), particularly in cases where insulin doses are reduced or in patients with type 1 diabetes mellitus, for whom SGLT2 inhibitors are not generally recommended. In summary, SGLT2 inhibitors contribute to significant HbA1c reductions in patients with T2DM, typically ranging from 0.5% to 1.0% within the first 12 to 24 weeks of therapy. Their insulin-independent mechanism of action, combined with additional benefits such as weight loss and blood pressure reduction, makes them valuable options for diabetes management. Although generally well-tolerated, clinicians should remain vigilant about potential adverse effects, particularly infections and the rare occurrence of euglycemic DKA. Overall, SGLT2 inhibitors provide an effective, multifaceted approach to achieving short-term glycemic control and managing T2DM (Mahaffey et al. 2018).

Cardiorenal Outcomes in the CANVAS, and DECLARE-TIMI 58

The CANVAS and DECLARE-TIMI 58 trials are landmark studies that have significantly advanced our understanding of the cardiovascular and renal outcomes associated with SGLT2 inhibitors, specifically canagliflozin and dapagliflozin. The CANVAS (Canagliflozin Cardiovascular Assessment Study) program, which included two sub-studies (CANVAS and CANVAS-R), evaluated the cardiovascular safety and efficacy of canagliflozin in patients with T2DM and high cardiovascular risk (Wanner et al. 2016). Enrolling over 10,000 participants and following them for a median of 188 weeks, the CANVAS trial demonstrated that canagliflozin not only lowered HbA1c levels but also provided significant cardiovascular benefits, including a 14% reduction in major adverse cardiovascular events (MACE). This reduction was primarily driven by decreases in cardiovascular death and heart failure hospitalizations. Additionally, the study highlighted notable renal benefits, including a 40% reduction in the risk of doubling serum creatinine, progression to end-stage renal disease (ESRD), or renal-related death. However, safety concerns, such as an increased risk of lower limb amputations and genital infections, were also reported (Mosenzon et al. 2024). Similarly, the DECLARE-TIMI 58 trial investigated the impact of dapagliflozin on cardiovascular and renal outcomes in over 17,000 patients with T2DM at high cardiovascular risk, with a median follow-up of 4.2 years. The study demonstrated a 17% reduction in the risk of hospitalization for heart failure and showed a favorable trend in reducing major adverse cardiovascular events (MACE). However, the reduction in MACE did not reach statistical significance for the primary endpoint (Zelniker and Braunwald, 2024). Importantly, the DECLARE-TIMI 58 trial confirmed the renal protective effects of dapagliflozin, demonstrating a 47% reduction in the risk of the composite renal endpoint, which included a sustained decline in eGFR, end-stage renal disease (ESRD), or renal death. The safety profile of dapagliflozin was consistent with previous studies, showing an increased risk of genital infections but no significant increase in the risk of lower limb amputations or diabetic ketoacidosis (DKA). Together, these trials highlight the cardiovascular and renal benefits of SGLT2 inhibitors, emphasizing that both canagliflozin and dapagliflozin not only improve glycemic control but also provide substantial protective effects against cardiovascular and renal complications in high-risk T2DM populations (Bhatt et al. 2023).

Synergism Between SGLT2 Inhibitors and Loop Diuretics

Diuretics are frequently prescribed for patients with heart failure (HF), with the DAPA-HF study indicating that 93% of participants were on diuretics at baseline. Conducted by McMurray et al. in 2019, this study demonstrated that dapagliflozin significantly reduced the risk of cardiovascular death in patients with heart failure with reduced ejection fraction (HFrEF), regardless of their diabetes status. Consequently, SGLT2 inhibitors are often used with loop diuretics in HF management. The combination of SGLT2 inhibitors and loop diuretics may produce synergistic effects. Research by Heise et al. (2016), Wilcox et al. (2018), and Griffin et al. (2020a) supports this notion, with one double-blind, placebo-controlled trial revealing that the enhancement of fractional excretion of sodium (FENa) was more than four times greater when SGLT2 inhibitors were combined with loop diuretics compared to either agent used alone. However, another study indicated that the initial sodium excretion from combining bumetanide and dapagliflozin was not significantly greater than with bumetanide alone, suggesting a lack of first-dose synergy between the SGLT2 inhibitor and the loop diuretic (Cannon et al. 2023). In patients exhibiting diuretic resistance, a retrospective study found that the combination of SGLT2 inhibitors with loop diuretics resulted in weight loss and enhanced diuretic effectiveness for most individuals experiencing diuretic-resistant acute decompensated heart failure. However, this study involved high initial doses of loop diuretics and lacked a randomized control group. Additionally, the EMPEROR-Reduced trial, conducted by Packer et al. (2021), demonstrated that empagliflozin reduces the risk of cardiovascular death or hospitalization for heart failure, regardless of whether patients were experiencing volume overload. Notably, the benefits of empagliflozin were not more pronounced in patients with recent volume overload, despite their increased susceptibility to fluid retention. Currently, there is limited data regarding the use of SGLT2 inhibitors in conjunction with loop diuretics, necessitating further research to ascertain whether SGLT2 inhibitors could serve as alternatives to thiazide diuretics. Nevertheless, patients with heart failure do appear to benefit from treatment with SGLT2 inhibitors (Zinman et al. 2023).

Safety Profile of SGLT2 Inhibitors

Initial clinical trials of SGLT2 inhibitors revealed several adverse events. Notably, hypoglycemia, a common concern with glucose-lowering agents, did not increase when SGLT2 inhibitors were used alone, as confirmed by a recent meta-analysis (Alahmadb et al. 2024). This finding aligns with the drugs' mechanism, which does not stimulate insulin release or alter glucose synthesis. However, the risk of hypoglycemia can rise when SGLT2 inhibitors are combined with other glucose-lowering medications, such as insulin. Not all initially noted adverse events have been validated in later clinical trials. For instance, a meta-analysis found no significant association between SGLT2 inhibitors and UTIs, with a risk ratio (RR) of 0.97 (95% CI: 0.81 to 1.16). It is worth noting that diabetes itself increases susceptibility to UTIs due to elevated urinary glucose levels, which can promote microbial growth. Although SGLT2 inhibitors do not increase UTI risk, they have been associated with a higher incidence of genital infections. The EMPA-REG trial, for example, reported a greater incidence of genital infections with empagliflozin compared to placebo (Katherine and Clark, 2023). Euglycemic diabetic ketoacidosis (DKA) is another significant concern with SGLT2 inhibitors in patients with diabetes. This condition typically presents with abdominal pain, nausea, vomiting, an increased anion gap, and normal serum glucose levels (Lee and Riella, 2024). The suppression of insulin by SGLT2 inhibitors is thought to raise free fatty acid production, leading to ketone formation. Factors that can elevate the risk of euglycemic DKA include discontinuing insulin therapy, following starvation or low-carbohydrate diets, excessive physical activity, acute illnesses like infections, and heavy alcohol consumption. Patients should be informed of this risk and provided with a "sick-day" plan to mitigate it. For individuals without diabetes, the risk of euglycemic DKA is extremely low, with only one documented case in a large meta-analysis spanning 30,000 participant-years (Li et al. 2022). Finally, while clinicians have expressed concerns about a heightened risk of hypoglycemia, major hypoglycemic events were not observed in large randomized controlled trials involving patients without diabetes. SGLT2 inhibitors lower plasma glucose by inhibiting glucose reabsorption, a mechanism that becomes less effective as plasma glucose levels fall (Khawaja et al. 2023).

Conclusion

In conclusion, integrating SGLT2 inhibitors into HF management represents a promising advancement in treatment. When combined with loop diuretics, SGLT2 inhibitors demonstrate synergistic effects that enhance diuretic efficacy, as evidenced by increased fractional excretion of sodium (FENa), improved weight loss, and better fluid management in patients experiencing diuretic resistance. Although initial studies have reported mixed findings regarding the dose-response relationship between SGLT2 inhibitors and loop diuretics, the overall evidence supports the beneficial role of SGLT2 inhibitors in HF therapy. Landmark trials such as CANVAS and DECLARE-TIMI 58 confirm the cardiovascular and renal benefits of these agents, and further studies, including the EMPEROR-Reduced trial, highlight their effectiveness in reducing cardiovascular death and hospitalization due to heart failure, regardless of volume overload status. While data on the combined use of SGLT2 inhibitors and loop diuretics remain limited, particularly regarding whether SGLT2 inhibitors could replace thiazide diuretics, their positive impact on fluid management and overall HF outcomes is notable. By potentially reducing the need for intensified diuretic therapy, SGLT2 inhibitors could enhance patient outcomes and add value to existing heart failure treatment regimens.

References

Abdelrahman, A. M., Awad, A. S., & Abdel-Rahman, E. M. (2024). Sodium-glucose co-transporter 2 inhibitors: Mechanism of action and efficacy in non-diabetic kidney disease from bench to bedside. *Journal of Clinical Medicine*, 13(956).

Alahmad, A., Farhad, M. A., Thangavel, J. A., Thanaraj, A., Alic, H., Mullac, F. A., & Qaddoumi, M. (2024). Long-term mortality and SGLT2 inhibitors in type 2 diabetes with and without renal impairment: An observational cohort study. *Medical Principles and Practice*, 33, 251-259.

Bhatt, D. L., Szarek, M., Steg, P. G., Cannon, C. P., Leiter, L. A., McGuire, D. K., Wilding, J. P. H., Kosiborod, M. N., Katona, B. G., Pineda, A. L., Al-Shurbaji, A., Saver, J. L., & Ruff, C. T. (2023). Sotagliflozin in patients with diabetes and chronic kidney disease. *New England Journal of Medicine*, 388(4), 405-415.

Cannon, C. P., Pratley, R., Dagogo-Jack, S., Mancuso, J., Huyck, S., Masiukiewicz, U., Charbonnel, B., Frederich, R., Gantz, I., & Inagaki, N. (2023). Cardiovascular outcomes with ertugliflozin in type 2 diabetes: A post hoc analysis of the VERTIS CV trial. *Diabetes, Obesity and Metabolism*, 25(1), 57-65.

Chan, J. C. H., & Chan, M. C. Y. (2023). SGLT2 inhibitors: The next blockbuster multifaceted drug? *Medicina*, 59(2), 388.

Correa, F., & Rotter, C. (2021). Sodium-glucose cotransporter 2 inhibitors mechanisms of action: A review. *Frontiers in Medicine*, 8, 777861.

Davies, M. J., D'Alessio, D. A., Fradkin, J., Kernan, W. N., Mathieu, C., Mingrone, G., Rossing, P., Tsapas, A., Wexler, D. J., & Buse, J. B. (2018). Management of hyperglycemia in type 2 diabetes, 2018: A consensus report by the American Diabetes Association (ADA) and the European Association for the Study of Diabetes (EASD). *Diabetes Care*, 41(12), 2669-2701.

Ernesto, C., & Chung, L. (2023). Comprehensive review of SGLT2 inhibitors efficacy through their diuretic mode of action in diabetic patients. *Frontiers in Endocrinology*, 14, 1174692.

Fitchett, D., Inzucchi, S. E., Zinman, B., Wanner, C., Mattheus, M., George, J. T., & Johansen, O. E. (2018). Empagliflozin reduces mortality and hospitalization for heart failure in patients with type 2 diabetes and a history of myocardial infarction. *Circulation*, 137(5), 405-407.

Hiraizumi, M., Akashi, T., Murasaki, K., Kishida, H., Kumanomidou, T., Torimoto, N., Nureki, O., & Miyaguch, I. (2024). Transport and inhibition mechanism of the human SGLT2–MAP17 glucose transporter. *Nature Structural & Molecular Biology*, 159-169.

Jasleen, B., Vishal, J. K., Sameera, M., Fahad, M., Brendan, O., Deion, S., & Pemminat, S. (2023). Sodium-glucose cotransporter 2 (SGLT2) inhibitors: Benefits versus risk. *Cureus*, 15(1), e33939.

Katherine, A., & Clark, A. (2023). The use of sodium-glucose cotransporter 2 inhibitors in heart failure with reduced or preserved ejection fraction: New guidelines hot off the press and directly into guidelines. *Postgraduate Medical Journal*, 99, 1052-1057.

Khawaja, M., Stefan, D., & Butter, J. (2023). SGLT-2 inhibitors in heart failure: A review of current evidence. *International Journal of Heart Failure*, 5(2), 82-90.

Lee, S. A., & Riella, L. V. (2024). Narrative Review of Immunomodulatory and Anti-inflammatory Effects of Sodium-Glucose Cotransporter 2 Inhibitors: Unveiling Novel Therapeutic Frontiers. *Kidney International Reports*, 9, 1601-1613.

Li, J., Zhou, L., & Gong, H. (2022). New insights and advances of sodium-glucose cotransporter 2 inhibitors in heart failure. *Frontier Cardiovascular Medicine*, 9, 903902.

Mahaffey, K. W., Neal, B., Perkovic, V., de Zeeuw, D., Fulcher, G., Erondu, N., Shaw, W., Fabbrini, E., Sun, T., Li, Q., Patel, S., Desai, M., Matthews, D. R., (2018). Canagliflozin for primary and secondary prevention of cardiovascular events: Results from the CANVAS Program (Canagliflozin Cardiovascular Assessment Study). *Circulation*, 137(4), 323-334.

Mosenzon, O., Wiviott, S. D., Cahn, A., Rozenberg, A., Yanuv, I., Goodrich, E. L., Murphy, S. A., Bhatt, D. L., Leiter, L. A., McGuire, D. K., Wilding, J. P. H., Gause-Nilsson, I. A. M., Fredriksson, M., Johansson, P. A., Langkilde, A. M., Sabatine, M. S., & Raz, I. (2019). Effects of dapagliflozin on development and progression of kidney disease in patients with type 2 diabetes: an analysis from the DECLARE-TIMI 58 randomized trial. *Lancet Diabetes Endocrinol*, 7(8), 606-617.

Pabel, S., Hamdani, N., Luedde, M., & Sossalla, S. (2021). SGLT2 Inhibitors and Their Mode of Action in Heart Failure Has the Mystery Been Unravelled? *Current Heart Failure Reports*, 18, 315-328.

Rosenstock, J., Aggarwal, N., Polidori, D., Zhao, Y., Arbit, D., Usiskin, K., & Canovatchel, W. (2013). Efficacy and safety of canagliflozin versus placebo in subjects with type 2 diabetes on background metformin monotherapy: a randomized clinical trial. *Diabetologia*, 56(2), 2582-2592.

Salvatore, T., Galiero, R., Caturano, A., Rinaldi, L., Martino, A., Albanese, G., Salvo, J., Epifani, R., Marfella, R., & Docimo, G. (2022) An Overview of the Cardiorenal Protective Mechanisms of SGLT2 Inhibitors. *International Journal of Molecular Sciences*, 23, 3651.

Sayour, A., Olah, A., Ruppert, M., Barta, B., Merkely, B., & Radovits, T. (2024). Efect of pharmacological selectivity of SGLT2 inhibitors on cardiovascular outcomes in patients with type 2 diabetes: a meta-analysis. *Scientific Reports*, 14, 2188.

Tang, J., Lifang, Y., Yan, Q., Zhang, X., Wang, L. (2022). Effects of Sodium-Glucose Cotransporter 2 inhibitors on water and sodium metabolism. *Frontiers in pharmacology*, 13, 800490.

Wanner, C., Inzucchi, S. E., Lachin, J. M., Fitchett, D., von Eynatten, M., Mattheus, M., Johansen, O. E., Woerle, H. J., Broedl, U. C., & Zinman, B. (2016). Empagliflozin and progression of kidney disease in type 2 diabetes. *New England Journal of Medicine*, 375(4), 323-334.

Young, F. C., Farnoudi, N., Chen, J., & Shubrook, J. H. (2023). Exploring SGLT-2 Inhibitors: Benefits beyond the Glucose-Lowering Effect What is new in 2023? *Endocrines*, 4, 630-655.

Zelniker, T. A., & Braunwald, E. (2018). Cardiovascular and renal effects of sodium-glucose co-transporter 2 inhibitors in type 2 diabetes: a comprehensive review of cardiovascular outcome trials. *Lancet*, 392(10164), 31-39.

Zinman, B., Wanner, C., Lachin, J. M., Fitchett, D., Bluhmki, E., Hantel, S., Mattheus, M., Devins, T., Johansen, O. E., Woerle, H. J., & Broedl, U. C. (2023). Empagliflozin, cardiovascular outcomes, and mortality in type 2 diabetes. *New England Journal of Medicine*, 389(22), 2105-2117.

Chapter 10

SGLT2 Inhibitors from Natural Sources

Kashmira K. Malusare[1,*]
Sachin P. Borikar[1]
Dipali N. Tapre[2]
and Shirish P. Jain[1]
[1]Department of Pharmacology, Rajarshi Shahu College of Pharmacy, Buldhana, Maharashtra, India
[2]Department of Pharmaceutical Chemistry, Rajarshi Shahu College of Pharmacy, Buldhana, Maharashtra, India

Abstract

Managing type 2 diabetes mellitus with insulin and oral hypoglycemics can be challenging, as many patients struggle to consistently achieve and maintain target blood glucose levels. As a result, there is an ongoing demand for new therapeutic drugs that offer a better balance between benefits and risks. Under normal physiological conditions, nearly all filtered glucose is reabsorbed in the proximal tubule of the nephron, mainly by the sodium-glucose cotransporter 2 (SGLT2). SGLT2 inhibitors are a modern class of oral antidiabetic agents that lower blood glucose by promoting its excretion through urine, independent of insulin secretion or activity. SGLT2 inhibitors effectively reduce blood glucose and show promise for managing diabetes-related comorbidities. Numerous studies have shown that plant extracts and their active phytonutrients possess various antidiabetic effects. Phlorizin, the first naturally occurring SGLT2 inhibitor, is a bitter compound found in the root bark, leaves, shoots, and fruit of the apple tree, making it an important natural source for the development of SGLT2 inhibitors. Other natural sources, such as *Sophora flavescens*, *Acer nikoense*, *Alstonia macrophylla*, *Gnetum gnemon*, *Schisandra chinensis*, and *Phyllanthus emblica*, also exhibit SGLT2 inhibitory effects. In addition to phlorizin, natural compounds such as chlorogenic acid, quercetin, kaempferol, kurarinone, and sophoraflavanone have been studied for their ability to improve blood glucose regulation. Further research is needed to clarify the mechanisms by which these natural compounds help manage type 2 diabetes mellitus and its related comorbidities. Given their established safety profiles, these natural compounds have strong potential as foundational elements in the development of SGLT2 inhibitors.

---

* Corresponding Author's Email: kashmiramalusare55@gmail.com

In: Receptor-Targeted Therapies in Diabetes Mellitus
Editors: Ajmer Singh Grewal, Neelam Singh, Swati Verma et al.
ISBN: 979-8-89530-587-4

Keywords: SGLT-2 inhibitors, diabetes mellitus, natural sources, phlorizin, phytochemicals, T2DM

Abbreviations

AMPK	Adenosine monophosphate activated protein kinase
GLP-1	Glucagon like peptide-1
GLUT	Glucose transporter
IL	Interleukin
PHF	Polyherbal formulations
PPAR-γ	Peroxisome proliferated activated receptor γ
RAS	renin-angiotensin system
SGLT1	Sodium glucose co-transporter-1
SGLT2	Sodium glucose co-transporter-2
SGOT	Serum glutamic oxaloacetic transaminase
SGPT	Serum glutamic pyruvic transaminase
T2DM	Type-2 diabetes mellitus
TNF-α	Tumour necrosis factor-α
WHO	World Health Organization

Introduction

Diabetes remains a major global health challenge, requiring coordinated efforts among biopharmaceutical companies, device manufacturers, patients, and society to address its growing morbidity and mortality (De Pascalis et al. 2021). Sodium-glucose cotransporter 2 (SGLT2) inhibitors represent a promising class of medications for managing hyperglycemia by inhibiting glucose reabsorption in the kidneys. This inhibition increases glucose excretion in the urine, effectively lowering blood glucose and glycosylated hemoglobin levels (Nauck et al. 2014). Common SGLT2 inhibitors, such as dapagliflozin, canagliflozin, and empagliflozin, also offer cardioprotective and renoprotective benefits, as demonstrated in extensive trials, even in non-diabetic patients. Additionally, SGLT2 inhibitors act as indirect antioxidants, reducing oxidative stress associated with high blood glucose. They may also help manage inflammation by affecting the renin-angiotensin system (RAS), enhancing tissue perfusion, and restoring redox balance (Tsai et al. 2021). The kidneys play a crucial role in maintaining glucose homeostasis by filtering approximately 180 liters of plasma daily, with a glucose concentration around 90 mg/dL. In individuals with normal glucose tolerance, all filtered glucose is reabsorbed in the proximal tubule, leaving no glucose in the urine (Abdul-Ghani & DeFronzo, 2008). Glucose reabsorption is regulated by SGLTs, particularly SGLT1 and SGLT2. SGLT1, a high-affinity transporter located partially in the kidney, aids in glucose reabsorption, while SGLT2, a low-affinity transporter primarily found in the kidneys, plays a significant role in the proximal tubule. Genetic mutations in the SGLT1 gene can lead to glucose/galactose malabsorption, whereas inhibition of SGLT2 reduces glucose reabsorption, resulting in glycosuria (Vaidya & Goyal, 2010). Interest in natural SGLT2 inhibitors is growing, with phlorizin, a compound initially extracted from apple tree bark, recognized as an early natural SGLT2 inhibitor. It promotes urinary glucose excretion by blocking renal glucose reabsorption. However, due to limitations with phlorizin's stability and bioavailability, synthetic analogs have been developed by pharmaceutical companies to improve efficacy (Choi et al. 2016). Facilitated glucose transporters (GLUTs) also contribute to glucose movement across membranes in various organs, including the proximal renal tubule, small intestine, and blood-brain barrier, complementing the glucose-regulating functions of SGLTs (Marsenic, 2009).

Phlorizin as the First Naturally Occurring SGLT-2 Inhibitor

Phlorizin is a glycoside, a naturally occurring compound belonging to the polyphenol family, and is classified as a chalcone, a type of organic molecule. This compound, found in various plants, particularly apples, has been shown to increase the excretion of glucose in urine (Salehi et al. 2023). Phlorizin is the predominant phenolic-glucoside in apple trees (root bark, shoots, and foliage). It has been used for medicinal purposes and physiological research for over 150 years. In 1835, French chemists isolated phlorizin from apple tree bark. Based on its bitter taste and the antipyretic properties of similar plant extracts, such as those from willow and cinchona trees, phlorizin was initially thought to have potential in treating fevers and infectious diseases, particularly malaria. When ingested, phlorizin caused glycosuria, a condition where glucose is excreted in the urine. This led to the hypothesis that phlorizin could mimic the symptoms of diabetes mellitus, which is characterized by polyuria (excessive urination) and persistent glucose in the urine. As researchers observed, administering phlorizin to dogs resulted in glycosuria, polyuria, and weight loss symptoms that resembled those seen in diabetic humans. This led to the idea that phlorizin could be used to model diabetes in animals. In the 1930s, Homer Smith developed a method to intravenously administer phlorizin to induce glycosuria in patients without pre-existing conditions. This technique significantly contributed to the understanding of renal hemodynamics and metabolic transport processes in the kidney's tubules. Smith's research also demonstrated that intravenous phlorizin administration posed no significant safety risks in humans. In the 1970s, LaVeen conducted studies to further evaluate the safety of intravenous phlorizin in humans. The research aimed to explore the potential of phlorizin in treating malignancies by inhibiting glucose uptake by cancer cells (Ehrenkranz et al. 2005). Phlorizin inhibits glucose absorption in the small intestine and blocks glucose reabsorption in the kidneys, specifically at the luminal membrane of brush border cells in the proximal tubules. The compound's ability to obstruct sugar transport across membranes led to the identification of the SGLT mechanism. Phlorizin has been shown to effectively inhibit both SGLT-1 and SGLT-2, key transporters involved in glucose reabsorption (Blaschek, 2017).

Natural SGLT-2 Inhibitors

Acer nikoense

The Aceraceae family includes Acer nikoense, a species native to Asia. Traditional Japanese medicine used preparations from its stem and branches to treat hepatic and ophthalmic disorders. Researchers have investigated the effects of four molecules derived from the bark of

Acer nikoense and sixteen analogous compounds on the efficacy of SGLT inhibitors. Among them, two cyclic diarylheptanoids, acerogenin A (9) and acerogenin B (10), showed significant inhibition of SGLT1 [IC50 (μM): 9: 20.0; 10: 26.0] and SGLT2 [IC50 (μM): 9: 94.0; 10: 43.0]. In contrast, several isolated compounds, particularly an acyclic diarylheptanoid, exhibited minimal inhibition of both SGLT transporters. Inhibition of SGLT leads to reduced blood glucose levels. The analysis of bark extracts revealed various polyphenolic compounds, including diarylheptanoids like acerogenin and acerosides. The cyclic diarylheptanoids, acerogenin A and acerogenin B, are present in the methanol extract of Acer nikoense bark. These compounds function by selectively inhibiting the sodium-glucose transporter. The researchers found that the extent of this inhibitory effect may be influenced by the configuration of the sugar groups and the stereochemistry of the molecules (Eszter et al. 2017).

Alstonia macrophylla

Alstonia macrophylla, a perennial plant from the Apocynaceae family, is native to Southeast Asia. Various regions have utilized different parts of the plant in traditional medicine. Preparations from the leaves and stems of A. macrophylla have been employed to treat gastrointestinal and dermatological conditions, with the leaves also demonstrating anticholinergic effects. Phytochemical analysis revealed the presence of tannins, flavonoids, and triterpenoids in the plant. The alkaloids of A. macrophylla, including alstiphyllanines, picraline, and ajmaline, exhibit SGLT2 inhibitory properties. Methanolic extracts of A. macrophylla also demonstrate antibacterial activity. The crude leaf extracts show analgesic, antipyretic, and anti-inflammatory properties. Additionally, extracts from the root bark of A. macrophylla display cytotoxic and anti-cancer effects, with certain extracts showing cytotoxic activity against various cell lines. Furthermore, A. macrophylla has been found to exhibit acetylcholinesterase activity. Its extracts act as free radical scavengers, possess antioxidant capabilities, and demonstrate anti-inflammatory activities (Mokat & Kharat, 2023).

Pyllanthus emblica

Phyllanthus emblica, a species from the Phyllanthaceae family, is widely distributed in Bangladesh and central India. Commonly known as Amla, it is renowned for its diverse pharmacological activities, including antioxidant, antifungal, antibacterial, anti-allergic, antiviral, anticancer, and antidiabetic effects. The plant exerts its antidiabetic properties by suppressing glycogenolysis, hepatic gluconeogenesis, and intestinal glucose absorption. Additionally, it enhances insulin production and promotes glucose utilization throughout the body. In Southeast Asia, traditional medicine extensively uses P. emblica fruits to treat conditions such as diabetes, cough, asthma, and pneumonia. Common diabetes treatments include SGLT2 inhibitors, GLP-1 receptor agonists, and peroxisome proliferator-activated receptor-gamma (PPAR-γ) activators. GLP-1 receptor agonists, in particular, increase insulin secretion and inhibit glucagon release from the pancreas. Regular consumption of a mixture of *P. emblica* fruit juice and bitter gourd juice over two months has demonstrated significant antidiabetic benefits, including alleviation of diabetes-related ocular complications. The phytochemicals in *P. emblica* are considered less toxic, benign, and non-harmful. Researchers have identified compounds such as estradiol, quercetin, and ellagic acid in P. emblica, which may help individuals with diabetes by targeting GLP-1(Sharma et al. 2020).

Aspalathus linearis

Aspalathus linearis, commonly known as Rooibos, is indigenous to South Africa and is recognized for its potential therapeutic properties, particularly in treating type 2 diabetes mellitus (T2DM) and related conditions. The presence of flavonoids and C-glucosyl dihydrochalcones in Rooibos contributes significantly to its beneficial effects. Aspalathin, a key bioactive compound in Rooibos, plays a critical role in regulating blood glucose levels by activating AMP-activated protein kinase (AMPK) and facilitating the translocation of GLUT4 to target tissues. Additionally, aspalathin suppresses the gene expression of hepatic enzymes involved in glucose and lipid production, highlighting its potential anti-diabetic properties. Research has demonstrated that aspalathin significantly reduces mitochondrial dysfunction and insulin resistance by decreasing the production of pro-inflammatory mediators such as protein kinase C-theta, IL-6, and TNF-α. Previous studies have shown that aspalathin can modulate the insulin receptor substrate 1 (IRS-1) and insulin receptor signaling pathways by inhibiting protein tyrosine phosphatases. This inhibition helps reduce hyperuricemia and enhance glucosuria through the inhibition of SGLT2. Aspalathin, a C-linked glucosyl dihydrochalcone, is a naturally occurring compound in Rooibos, commonly consumed as herbal tea worldwide. Besides its anti-diabetic properties, aspalathin exhibits various pharmacological effects, including antimutagenic, anti-inflammatory, antithrombotic, and xanthine oxidase inhibitory activities. Studies suggest that aspalathin may help prevent the progression of metabolic disorders and lower the risk of cardiovascular complications in individuals with diabetes (Salehi et al. 2023; Chaudhary et al. 2021).

Quercetin

Quercetin has been extensively studied for its broad spectrum of medicinal properties, including its ability to lower elevated blood glucose levels. It helps manage hyperglycemia, high cholesterol, hypertension, and oxidative damage, thereby reducing the risk of cardiovascular diseases. Quercetin regulates blood glucose levels by enhancing glucose tolerance and improving pancreatic β-cell function through several mechanisms, including the activation of AMPK. AMPK plays a crucial role in regulating GLUT4 expression in adipose tissue and skeletal muscles, thereby improving glucose uptake and metabolism. Additionally, quercetin reduces GLUT2 expression and intestinal glucose absorption, limiting glucose uptake from the gut. It also suppresses the release of pro-inflammatory mediators such as TNF-α, IL-1, IL-4, IL-6, and IL-8, thereby protecting pancreatic β-cells from damage. These actions enhance insulin sensitivity and stimulate insulin production by promoting the regeneration of pancreatic β-cells. These effects make quercetin a promising compound in the management of T2DM. Ongoing research is exploring the potential of quercetin as a treatment for diabetes. Further studies, including animal experiments and clinical trials, are essential to fully understand its efficacy in reducing blood glucose levels and improving insulin production in individuals with T2DM. These investigations will also help elucidate the molecular mechanisms underlying its therapeutic effects (Ansari et al. 2022). A study investigated the effects of quercetin-4-glucoside (spiraeoside) and quercetin-3-glucoside (isoquercitrin) on the absorption of Methyl-D-glucopyranoside (MDG), an indigestible sugar analog. Both glucosides were found to significantly reduce MDG absorption by inhibiting SGLT1. In contrast, quercetin-3-rhamnoglucoside and aglycone quercetin showed no effect. These findings suggest that the transport of quercetin glucosides across the intestinal brush-border membrane is unlikely.

Further research is needed to identify novel quercetin glucosides with potential SGLT2 inhibitory properties (Salehi et al. 2023).

Sophora flavescens

Sophora flavescens, a cornerstone of traditional Chinese medicine, is widely used to treat various conditions, including leucorrhoea, diarrhea, jaundice, scabies, fever, pyogenic skin infections, edema, and general discomfort. The plant's root, commonly known as „Kushen," has long been recognized for its therapeutic properties. In a study by Sato et al. researchers evaluated the potential of nine compounds derived from the dried root of S. flavescens to inhibit SGLT activity. Among these, two isoflavonoid compounds, maackiain and formononetin, were found to selectively antagonize SGLT2 without affecting SGLT1. Further investigation into the structure-activity relationship (SAR) of these compounds revealed that a hydroxyl functional group is critical for the effective inhibition of SGLT2 activity by isoflavonoids. Additionally, two sophoraflavanone compounds, G and (-)-kurarinone, demonstrated remarkable specificity, with IC50 values of 4.1 μM and 1.7 μM for SGLT2 and 18.7 μM and 10.4 μM for SGLT1, respectively. Sato and colleagues also identified seven flavonoids and a 5-lavandulyl chalcone from S. flavescens as potent inhibitors of both SGLT1 and SGLT2, showing greater effectiveness in inhibiting SGLT2. The study highlighted the importance of the lavandulyl group, positioned at either C-8 or C-5 in chalcone, in enhancing SGLT1 inhibition. This group was present in chalcone 5 and flavanones 5, 6, and 8. The findings suggest that the lavandulyl group significantly improves the ability of flavanones to inhibit SGLT1. For isoflavonoids to inhibit SGLT2, and for lavandulyl flavanones to be effective, the presence of a hydroxyl group is essential. Furthermore, adding methoxy groups at the C-5 position of the flavanone molecule could enhance their inhibitory effects on SGLTs. These findings underscore the potential of these compounds as novel SGLT inhibitors, offering promising therapeutic avenues for diabetes treatment (Salehi et al. 2023).

Vitexin

Vitexin and isovitexin are bioactive compounds commonly found in various medicinal herbs, particularly in traditional Chinese medicine. Vitexin, also known as apigenin-8-C-glucoside, has gained attention for its wide range of therapeutic properties, including analgesic, neuroprotective, anticancer, antioxidant, and anti-inflammatory effects. Its isomer, isovitexin (apigenin-6-C-glucoside), is also recognized for its diverse physiological benefits. Due to their similar structures and complementary properties, vitexin and isovitexin are often studied together (Mustapha & Taib, 2023). One of the most promising properties of vitexin is its hypoglycemic effect, making it a potential candidate for diabetes treatment. Studies have demonstrated that administering vitexin and isovitexin to non-diabetic animals significantly reduces postprandial blood sugar levels, suggesting their therapeutic potential in managing diabetes. Vitexin has been shown to inhibit the activity of SGLT2, a key protein involved in glucose reabsorption in the kidneys, thereby lowering blood glucose levels. Supporting these findings, a platform developed using pharmacophore modeling to scan Indonesian plant databases identified cucumber A, cucumber B, and vitexin as compounds with SGLT2 inhibitory effects. These results further highlight vitexin's potential as an effective agent in diabetes therapy, particularly through its role in regulating glucose levels by targeting SGLT2 (Salehi et al. 2023).

Gnetum gnemonoides

Gnetum gnemonoides, a tropical liana native to Southeast Asia and the Pacific islands, including New Guinea, the Bismarck Archipelago, Indonesia, Malaysia, and the Philippines, has not been extensively studied for its medicinal properties. However, stilbenes derived from Gnetum gnemonoides have demonstrated various biological activities, including antioxidant, hepatoprotective, enzyme inhibitory, and antibacterial effects. Notably, the stilbenes gneyulins A and B, extracted from the outer bark of Gnetum gnemonoides, exhibit modest inhibitory effects on both SGLT1 and SGLT2. In contrast, dihydroflavone-C-glycosides, specifically noidesols A and B, showed no impact on SGLT activity. These findings indicate that certain compounds from Gnetum gnemonoides, particularly stilbenes like gneyulins A and B, may hold potential as SGLT inhibitors, supporting their possible use in diabetes treatment or related therapies (Salehi et al. 2023).

Polyherbal mixture

A holistic approach to managing diabetes and its complications emphasizes combining conventional and alternative treatments, often utilizing multiple plant-based therapies to enhance efficacy and minimize side effects. This polyherbal strategy is considered more effective than relying on a single herb. Aimil Pharmaceuticals, with approval from the AYUSH Ministry of the Indian government, has introduced BGR-34, a polyherbal formulation designed to regulate blood glucose levels. A comprehensive review and meta-analysis by Suvarna and colleagues demonstrated that polyherbal formulations effectively reduce blood glucose levels in individuals with T2DM. In a recent study, a polyherbal formulation (PHF) comprising seven *Rungia cinerea*, *Andrographis roxburghiana*, *Cinnamomum Pereira*, *Curcuma longa*, *Datura indica*, *Trigonella sinensis*, and *Sphaeranthus glabrawas* shown to significantly lower glucose levels by inhibiting SGLT2. Additionally, treatment with PHF in rats substantially reduced cholesterol, triglycerides, bilirubin, SGOT, and SGPT levels. Toxicological and histological evaluations confirmed the safety of the formulation. These findings suggest that PHF may serve as an effective antihyperglycemic agent in animal models, offering promising potential as a therapeutic option for diabetes management (Salehi et al. 2023).

Efficacy of Phytochemicals for Diabetes Treatment

With the rising prevalence of diabetes, patients are increasingly turning to traditional herbs as a treatment option, either as standalone remedies or in conjunction with conventional therapies. The widespread use of herbal medicines for diabetes management has prompted regulatory bodies to consider implementing stricter guidelines to ensure their safe and standardized use. This is particularly important due to the potential interactions between herbs and pharmaceuticals, highlighting the need for increased public awareness about the safety of herbal treatments (Ahmadi et al. 2021). The World Health Organization (WHO) has endorsed traditional botanical therapies for diabetes due to their non-toxic nature, effectiveness, low incidence of side effects, and compatibility with oral medications. In recent years, various plant sources have yielded numerous phytochemicals with antidiabetic properties, including flavonoids, alkaloids, peptidoglycans, amino acids, glycosides, glycolipids, polysaccharides, saponins, and dietary fibers. These compounds have demonstrated potential as hypoglycemic agents, offering alternative or complementary treatment options to conventional medications (Salehi et al. 2023). Researchers have documented the efficacy of natural compounds in managing diabetes and its complications. Medicinal plants contain beneficial secondary metabolites, such as essential oils, sterols, triterpenoids, saponins, carotenoids, alkaloids, flavonoids, phenolic acids, tannins, and coumarins, which mimic insulin effects and show promise as potential antidiabetic drugs (Teoh & Das, 2018).

Therapeutic Potential of Naturally Occurring SGLT2 Inhibitors

The use of natural resources, including various botanicals, has long been a cornerstone of traditional medicine worldwide and has significantly contributed to modern pharmaceutical development. Approximately 25% of globally prescribed pharmaceuticals are derived from medicinal plants. Many individuals use herbs as their primary treatment or as a supplement to conventional medicines. In some countries, herbal medicines remain the only affordable or accessible healthcare option. With the growing reliance on herbal remedies, it is crucial to ensure these products are safe and contain the designated active ingredients. Consumers must have access to scientifically validated information regarding appropriate dosages, usage limitations, and effectiveness. Global harmonization of regulations governing herbal remedies is essential to support ethical extraction, distribution, and safe public use. Although herbs are often perceived as naturally safe, they can cause adverse effects, particularly when used in unregulated dosages or combined with other medications.

Rationale for SGLT2 Inhibitors to Address Toxicity of Existing Drugs

Diabetes often arises from either insufficient insulin production or decreased insulin sensitivity. Although various antihyperglycemic drugs are available, their side effects underscore the urgent need for safer treatment options. SGLT2 inhibitors represent a promising class of antidiabetic drugs that lower blood glucose levels by inhibiting glucose reabsorption in the kidneys, thereby promoting urinary glucose excretion. These inhibitors are generally well-tolerated, with minimal adverse effects, and have demonstrated therapeutic benefits for cardiovascular and renal conditions, particularly in diabetic patients. Preclinical studies have also highlighted the antioxidant potential of SGLT2 inhibitors in managing diabetes, cardiovascular diseases, and nephropathy. Their ability to maintain redox balance further underscores their therapeutic value. Continued research is essential to deepen our understanding of the pathogenesis of these diseases and to identify new targets that may work synergistically with SGLT2 inhibitors (Tsai et al. 2021).

Recent Advances in the Discovery of SGLT2 Inhibitors from Natural Sources

In recent years, significant progress has been made in developing SGLT2 inhibitors, with numerous studies examining their effectiveness in managing type 2 diabetes and evaluating their real-world impact and safety profile. SGLT2 inhibitors offer several advantages over traditional treatments, including a lower risk of hypoglycemia and modest weight reduction, which is particularly beneficial for overweight or obese individuals. This novel class of drugs has also been shown to prevent heart failure in both diabetic and non-diabetic patients and to slow the progression of renal function decline in individuals with diabetic nephropathy. One of the distinguishing features of SGLT2 inhibitors is their insulin-independent glucose-lowering mechanism, enabling effective glycemic control without a significant risk of hypoglycemia. Recent research, particularly post-2018, has confirmed the safety of SGLT2 inhibitors, reinforcing their value as reliable treatment options for both type 1 and type 2 diabetes. These drugs are well-tolerated and effective, whether used as monotherapies or in combination with other treatments, making them a versatile and valuable addition to diabetes management strategies (Tsai et al. 2021).

Conclusion

The management of T2DM remains a significant challenge, as many patients struggle to achieve and maintain optimal blood glucose levels. This has driven ongoing efforts to develop novel therapeutic medications that provide an ideal balance between efficacy and safety. While a wide range of antidiabetic drugs is available, many are associated with toxicity, and single-agent therapies often prove inadequate in controlling the progression of diabetes and its related comorbidities. Our investigation focuses on plants with potential SGLT2 inhibitory activity, highlighting the crucial role of these inhibitors in managing diabetes and its complications. SGLT2 inhibitors have emerged as a pivotal therapeutic target, particularly in addressing hypertension in diabetic patients. Further, comprehensive research and detailed botanical studies are essential to identify the active constituents responsible for these effects in plants. Such discoveries could pave the way for innovative and effective treatment options for diabetes and its associated health challenges.

References

Abdul-Ghani, M. A., & DeFronzo, R. A. (2008). Inhibition of renal glucose reabsorption: a novel strategy for achieving glucose control in type 2 diabetes mellitus. *Endocrine Practice*, 14(6), 782-790.

Ahmadi, S., Rafiey, H., Sajjadi, H., Nosrati Nejad, F., Ahmadi, N., Yoosefi, M., Irandoost, S. F., & Farzadfar, F. (2021). Trend and pattern of using herbal medicines among people who are aware of their diabetes mellitus: Results from National STEPs Surveys in 2005 to 2011 in Iran. *Journal of Diabetes & Metabolic Disorders*, 20(2), 1319–1325.

Ansari, P., Choudhury, S. T., Seidel, V., Rahman, A. B., Aziz, M. A., Richi, A. E., Rahman, A., Jafrin, U. H., Hannan, J. M. A., & Abdel-Wahab, Y. H. A. (2022). Therapeutic potential of quercetin in the management of type-2 diabetes mellitus. *Life*, 12(8), 1146.

Gaikwad, S. B., Mohan, G. K., & Rani, M. S. (2014). Phytochemicals for diabetes management. *Pharmaceutical Crops*, 5, 11-28.

Blaschek, W. (2017). Natural products as lead compounds for sodium glucose cotransporter (SGLT) inhibitors. *Planta Medica*, 83(12/13), 985-993.

Chaudhary, S. K., Sandasi, M., Makolo, F., van Heerden, F. R., & Viljoen, A. M. (2021). Aspalathin: A rare dietary dihydrochalcone from Aspalathus linearis (rooibos tea). *Phytochemistry Reviews*, 20, 1161-1192.

Choi, C. I. (2016). Sodium-glucose cotransporter 2 (SGLT2) inhibitors from natural products: discovery of next-generation antihyperglycemic agents. *Molecules*, 21(9), 1136.

De Pascalis, A., Cianciolo, G., Capelli, I., Brunori, G., & La Manna, G. (2021). SGLT2 inhibitors, sodium and off-target effects: an overview. *Journal of Nephrology*, 34, 673-680.

Ehrenkranz, J. R., Lewis, N. G., Kahn, R. C., & Roth, J. (2005). Phlorizin: A review. *Diabetes/Metabolism Research and Reviews*, 21(1), 31-38.

Riethmüller, E. (2017). Recovery of new diarylheptanoid sources in Betulaceae: Characterisation of the phenolic profile of Corylus species by HPLC-ESI-MS methods (PhD Dissertation). Semmelweis Egyetem - Központi Könyvtár.

Manoj, A., Das, S., Kunnath Ramachandran, A., Alex, A. T., & Joseph, A. (2020). SGLT2 inhibitors, an accomplished development in field of medicinal chemistry: an extensive review. *Future Medicinal Chemistry*, 12(21), 1961-1990.

Marsenic, O. (2009). Glucose control by the kidney: an emerging target in diabetes. *American Journal of Kidney Diseases*, 53(5), 875-883.

Mokat, D. N., & Kharat, T. (2023). Phytochemical and pharmacological potential of Hard Milkwood, Alstonia macrophylla Wall. ex G. Don. *In Phytochemical Composition and Pharmacy of Medicinal Plants*: 2-volume set (p. 123).

Moradi-Marjaneh, R., Paseban, M., & Sahebkar, A. (2019). Natural products with SGLT2 inhibitory activity: Possibilities of application for the treatment of diabetes. *Phytotherapy Research*, 33(10), 2518-2530.

Mustapha, M., & Taib, C. N. M. (2022). Beneficial role of Vitexin in Parkinson's disease. *Malaysian Journal of Medical Sciences*, 30(2), 8-25.

Nauck, M. A. (2014). Update on developments with SGLT2 inhibitors in the management of type 2 diabetes. *Drug Design, Development and Therapy*, 8, 1380-1380.

Rosenwasser, R. F., Sultan, S., Sutton, D., Choksi, R., & Epstein, B. J. (2013). SGLT-2 inhibitors and their potential in the treatment of diabetes. *Diabetes, metabolic syndrome and obesity: targets and therapy*, 6, 453-467.

Salehi, M., Rayatpisheh, N., Salehi, M., & Mardanparvar, H. (2023). Phytochemicals with sodium-glucose co-transporter inhibitory effects for the management of diabetes; a narrative review on recent findings. *Journal of Renal Endocrinology*, 9(1), e25095-e25095.

Sharma, P., Joshi, T., Joshi, T., Chandra, S., & Tamta, S. (2020). In silico screening of potential antidiabetic phytochemicals from Phyllanthus emblica against therapeutic targets of type 2 diabetes. *Journal of Ethnopharmacology*, 248, 112268.

Teoh, S. L., & Das, S. (2018). Phytochemicals and their effective role in the treatment of diabetes mellitus: a short review. *Phytochemistry Reviews*, 17, 1111-1128.

Tsai, K. F., Chen, Y. L., Chiou, T. T. Y., Chu, T. H., Li, L. C., Ng, H. Y., Lee, W. C., & Lee, C. T. (2021). Emergence of SGLT2 inhibitors as powerful antioxidants in human diseases. *Antioxidants*, 10(8), 1166.

Vaidya, H. B., & Goyal, R. K. (2010). Exploring newer target sodium glucose transporter 2 for the treatment of diabetes mellitus. *Mini Reviews in Medicinal Chemistry*, 10(10), 905-913.

Chapter 11

Harnessing SIRT1: Innovative Approaches to Glucose Metabolism and Diabetes Management

Sanket Seksaria[1,2]
Bramhajit Chatterjee[1]
Pranshul Sethi[2,3]
Somnath Dey[2,4]
and Satyam Mal[1,*]
[1]Department of Pharmaceutical Technology, Brainware University, Barasat, Kolkata, West Bengal, India
[2]Chitkara College of Pharmacy, Chitkara University, Punjab, India
[3]Department of Pharmacology, College of Pharmacy, Shri Venkateshwara University, Gajraula, Uttar Pradesh, India
[4]School of Pharmacy, Techno India University, Bidhannagar, Kolkata, West Bengal, India

Abstract

The global epidemiological trajectory of diabetes mellitus is on a concerning rise and is projected to become the seventh leading cause of mortality shortly. Central to this trend is SIRT1, a critical nuclear protein that orchestrates a range of cellular and molecular processes while regulating energy and glucose metabolism through NAD+-dependent deacetylation mechanisms. Calorie restriction has emerged as a promising strategy for delaying aging and mitigating various diseases, including diabetes mellitus. SIRT1 plays a vital role in regulating insulin secretion from pancreatic β cells, protecting them from inflammation, apoptosis, mitochondrial dysfunction, and oxidative stress. In the context of type 2 diabetes mellitus (T2DM), where insulin resistance is a major contributing factor, SIRT1 enhances insulin sensitivity and promotes glucose uptake by precisely modulating the insulin signaling cascade. Furthermore, SIRT1 interacts with downstream effectors such as FOXO and PGC-1α, as well as crosstalk pathways like AMPK, PI3K/AKT, p38 MAPK, and NF-κB, offering protection against the microvascular and macrovascular complications induced by hyperglycemia. Various pharmacological and non-pharmacological approaches have been developed within the therapeutic landscape to activate SIRT1, underscoring its potential as a promising target for effective diabetes management.

---

* Corresponding Author's Email: satyam.mal26@gmail.com

In: Receptor-Targeted Therapies in Diabetes Mellitus
Editors: Ajmer Singh Grewal, Neelam Singh, Swati Verma et al.
ISBN: 979-8-89530-587-4

Keywords: Diabetes mellitus, SIRT1, insulin resistance, secondary complications, PGC-1α, AMPK

Abbreviations

AGE	Advanced Glycation End Products
AKT	Protein Kinase B
AMPK	AMP-Activated Protein Kinase
DN	Diabetic Nephropathy
ECM	Extracellular Matrix
ER	Endoplasmic Reticulum
FOXO	Forkhead Box Protein O
GFR	Glomerular Filtration Rate
ICAM-1	Intercellular Adhesion Molecule 1
IL	Interleukin
JNK	c-Jun N-terminal Kinase
MAPK	Mitogen-Activated Protein Kinase
mTOR	Mechanistic Target of Rapamycin
NAD+	Nicotinamide Adenine Dinucleotide
NF-κB	Nuclear Factor Kappa B
PI3K	Phosphoinositide 3-Kinase
PPAR	Peroxisome Proliferator-Activated Receptor
ROS	Reactive Oxygen Species
SIRT1	Silent Information Regulator 1
SMAD	Sma and Mad Proteins (regulatory proteins in TGF-β signaling)
STAC	Sirtuin-Activating Compound
T1DM	Type 1 Diabetes Mellitus
T2DM	Type 2 Diabetes Mellitus
TNF-α	Tumor Necrosis Factor Alpha
VCAM-1	Vascular Cell Adhesion Molecule 1

Introduction

Sirtuins, also known as silent information regulator 2 (Sir2) proteins, are NAD+-dependent protein deacetylases found in organisms ranging from bacteria to humans. These enzymes regulate a variety of biological processes in eukaryotes, including transcriptional repression, recombination, the cell division cycle, microtubule organization, and cellular responses to DNA damage (Juan et al. 2023). They are also implicated in the molecular mechanisms underlying aging. Mammalian homologs of yeast Sir2, commonly referred to as class III protein deacetylases or sirtuins, consist of seven conserved isotypes (SIRT1–SIRT7). Among these, SIRT1, SIRT6, and SIRT7 are predominantly localized in the nucleus; SIRT2 is primarily found in the cytoplasm; and SIRT3, SIRT4, and SIRT5 are mainly located in the mitochondria (Michishita et al. 2005). Sirtuin 1 (SIRT1), one of the most extensively studied members of the sirtuin family, is a NAD+-dependent deacetylase that facilitates chromatin silencing and transcriptional repression in response to the cell's energy state. This protein family includes several promising therapeutic targets (Bazyluk et al. 2019). The first sirtuin, Sir2, was identified approximately 40 years ago in the budding yeast Saccharomyces cerevisiae. Before its discovery, it was referred to as the mating-type regulator 1 protein (Rine et al. 1979). In the late 1990s, research demonstrated that Sir2 played a critical role in preventing genomic instability, thereby extending the lifespan of yeast. The absence of Sir2 significantly reduced yeast lifespan, while introducing an additional copy of the Sir2 gene increased it by approximately 40%. Subsequent studies revealed that Sir2 exhibited NAD+-dependent histone deacetylase (HDAC) enzymatic activity. This discovery established a molecular framework linking NAD+-dependent histone deacetylation to aging and genomic silencing in yeast, with potential implications for metabolic processes in higher eukaryotes (Imai et al. 2000). Since their discovery, sirtuins have garnered considerable attention. While it would take volumes to cover all aspects of the sirtuin family, the most extensively studied member is SIRT1, the original deacetylase in this class and a homolog of yeast's silent information regulator Sir2. Early research in yeast identified Sir2/SIRT1 as a longevity enhancer and promoter of genomic stability. As a result, SIRT1 has been linked to a wide range of conditions, including neurodegeneration, cancer, metabolic syndrome, brain plasticity, aging, and numerous other human diseases (Stünkel & Campbell, 2011). The detailed structure of SIRT1, determined through crystallographic analysis, reveals that the protein consists of 747 amino acids, forming a catalytic domain with extended N- and C-terminal regions. This domain includes a Rossmann-fold that binds the NAD+ molecule, which is essential for SIRT1's activity, and is divided into small and large lobes. Key residues, such as Gly415, Glu416, Lys444, and Arg446, are critical for substrate binding, forming hydrogen bonds with the substrate peptide. The acetyl-lysine side chain fits into a hydrophobic pocket formed by Phe414, Leu418, and Val445, with His363 and Phe297 flanking the acetyl group (Dai et al. 2015).

SIRT1 and Metabolic Disorders

SIRT1 plays a significant role in regulating glucose metabolism in both type 1 and type 2 diabetes. In T1DM, SIRT1 enhances beta-cell survival and function, potentially leading to increased insulin production. In type 2 diabetes, SIRT1 contributes to better blood glucose management and metabolic health by reducing inflammation and improving insulin sensitivity (Lu et al. 2023).

Role of SIRT1 in the Management of T1DM

Recent studies highlight the therapeutic potential of SIRT1 in managing T1DM. As a NAD+-dependent deacetylase, SIRT1 plays a crucial role in regulating insulin sensitivity, inflammation, and glucose metabolism, impacting several pathways vital for glucose homeostasis. In T1DM, which is characterized by the autoimmune destruction of pancreatic β-cells, leading to insufficient insulin production and chronic hyperglycemia, SIRT1 helps maintain β-cell activity and increases insulin production, addressing key challenges in diabetes management (Al-Khaldi & Sultan, 2019). The primary mechanism through which SIRT1 affects insulin secretion is via its deacetylase activity, which modifies transcription factors and co-regulators involved in insulin gene expression. SIRT1 activates PGC-1α, a key regulator of mitochondrial biogenesis and function, thereby promoting β-cell health. Additionally, SIRT1 enhances the activity of FOXO1, a transcription factor crucial for insulin signaling and glucose metabolism, by deacetylating it, which boosts insulin sensitivity and glucose uptake (Wang et al. 2021a). SIRT1's anti-inflammatory effects are also crucial for T1DM management. Chronic inflammation, a hallmark of T1DM, exacerbates insulin resistance and β-cell degeneration. SIRT1 reduces inflammation by deacetylating NF-κB, a transcription factor that regulates the release of pro-inflammatory cytokines. This reduction in inflammation protects β-cells from autoimmune damage and improves overall metabolic health (Wang et al. 2021b). Preclinical studies have shown that SIRT1 activators, like resveratrol and its derivatives, can enhance SIRT1 activity and improve metabolic outcomes in diabetes models. These compounds also possess antioxidant properties, which protect β-cells from oxidative stress. Clinical trials are underway to evaluate the effectiveness of these activators in humans, to translate these promising findings into practical treatments (Wang et al. 2021c). Given its potential to improve β-cell function, reduce inflammation, and increase insulin production, SIRT1 is a promising target for T1DM treatment.

Role of SIRT1 in the Management of T2DM

Studies investigating SIRT1's function in T2DM suggest that the protein may serve as an important therapeutic target. As a NAD+-dependent deacetylase, SIRT1 plays a critical role in regulating inflammation, insulin sensitivity, and glucose metabolism. Activation of SIRT1 has been shown to improve insulin resistance, enhance mitochondrial function, and reduce oxidative stress—key factors in managing T2DM. SIRT1 suppresses inflammation, enhances hepatic glucose and lipid metabolism, and regulates insulin secretion and β-cell protection (Kitada & Koya, 2013a). SIRT1 also influences circadian rhythms, which in turn affects metabolic activities. Additionally, it regulates the release of adiponectin, a hormone that controls blood sugar levels and fatty acid breakdown. By improving mitochondrial biogenesis and function, SIRT1 reduces reactive oxygen species (ROS) generation and alleviates oxidative stress. This reduction in oxidative stress is crucial for enhancing insulin signaling pathways and overall cellular function. SIRT1's ability to improve mitochondrial activity and reduce oxidative stress makes it vital for managing T2DM. Therapeutic strategies targeting SIRT1 aim to mimic the benefits of calorie restriction, which is known to delay the onset of age-related diseases such as T2DM and insulin resistance (Ding et al. 2024). By enhancing mitochondrial biogenesis and function, SIRT1 inhibits ROS generation, thereby mitigating oxidative stress and its harmful effects on insulin signaling. This comprehensive approach highlights SIRT1's significance in T2DM management and its potential for the development of novel therapies to treat the diseases (Kitada & Koya, 2013b).

Impact of SIRT1 in the Management of Diabetes-Associated Microvascular Complications

Role of SIRT1 in Diabetic Retinopathy (DR)

One of the debilitating secondary complications of chronic hyperglycemia is DR, which is a leading cause of permanent blindness and impaired vision in individuals with diabetes. Prolonged poor blood sugar control and metabolic dysregulation result in changes to retinal blood flow, damage to the retinal vasculature, ischemia, and, ultimately, blindness. Several pathological factors, including high glucose-induced inflammatory processes, apoptosis, oxidative stress, mitochondrial dysfunction, and the accumulation of AGEs, significantly contribute to the development of DR (Wang & Lo, 2018). Chronic hyperglycemia reduces SIRT1 expression, accelerating the pathogenesis of DR. This leads to increased inflammation, with elevated pro-inflammatory cytokines such as tumor necrosis factor (TNF-α), interleukin-6 (IL-6), interleukin-1 (IL-1), and leukocyte adhesion molecules, causing damage to retinal epithelial cells. These processes are primarily mediated by the overactivation of the NF-κB pathway (Karbasforooshan & Karimi, 2018). Additionally, hyperglycemia reduces intracellular NAD+ levels, leading to decreased SIRT1 and PPAR-α expression. This reduction exacerbates inflammation and activates the NF-κB pathway, contributing to retinal endothelial cell dysfunction (Strycharz et al. 2018). Moreover, high glucose levels induce mitochondrial dysfunction and oxidative stress, primarily mediated by SIRT1 downregulation through certain microRNAs. This cascade of events promotes the accumulation of vascular endothelial growth factor (VEGF) and fibronectin in retinal cells, leading to endothelial hyperpermeability (Nebbioso et al. 2022). Additionally, fibrosis, a major contributor to the progression of DR, is driven by poor glycemic control. This condition impairs SIRT1-mediated deacetylation of the SMAD protein, leading to the upregulation of TGF-β and increased deposition of extracellular matrix components, endothelin, and matrix metalloproteinases in retinal cells. These changes affect blood flow, cause vessel dysfunction, and promote fibrosis (Wang et al. 2022).

Role of SIRT1 in Diabetic Nephropathy (DN)

DN is a chronic and progressive complication of both T1DM and T2DM. It is characterized by a series of stages, beginning with normoalbuminuria, progressing to hyperfiltration, microalbuminuria, and macroalbuminuria, and eventually leading to a reduced glomerular filtration rate (GFR). In the most severe cases, DN can progress to end-stage renal failure, requiring dialysis, particularly in T1DM (Schena & Gesualdo, 2005). The development of DN in T2DM is more complex due to the long-term presence of insulin resistance and additional comorbidities, such as hypertension. Histological studies of DN reveal distinct morphological changes, including a reduction in podocyte numbers, mesangial expansion, glomerulosclerosis, glomerular basement membrane thickening, and damage to tubular epithelial cells. Mesangial expansion and glomerulosclerosis are primarily driven by mesangial cell proliferation, hypertrophy, and phenotypic changes. These processes lead to the excessive accumulation of mesangial matrix, which contributes to a decline in GFR and reduced renal function (Choi et al. 2011). Furthermore, in diabetic kidneys, tubular epithelial cells may undergo hypertrophy, apoptosis, inflammation, or transformation into mesenchymal cells. Chronic hyperglycemia also stimulates tubular interstitial cells to accumulate fibroblasts and fibronectin, leading to severe fibrosis and further renal deformation (Xu et al. 2023).

Impact of SIRT1 in the Management of Diabetes-Associated Macrovascular Complications

Cardiovascular complications, including cardiomyopathy, coronary artery disease, and heart failure, are among the most common and serious secondary complications associated with chronic hyperglycemia. These complications significantly increase the mortality risk in diabetic patients. The structural and functional integrity of the heart is severely affected by a range of pathological processes triggered by chronic high glucose levels, including mitochondrial dysfunction, oxidative stress, inflammation, apoptosis, endoplasmic reticulum (ER) stress, fibrosis, and altered post-translational protein modifications (Shah et al. 2022). Hyperglycemia leads to increased production of ROS, which results in heightened oxidative stress. This, in turn, triggers the expression of pro-apoptotic proteins in cardiac cells, contributing to the activation of the MAPK pathway, particularly the c-Jun N-terminal kinase (JNK) and P38 pathways. These interactions damage cardiac myocytes and promote ischemic reperfusion injury (Watanabe et al. 2010). Increased SIRT1 expression offers protection to cardiac myocytes by alleviating ROS-induced oxidative stress and apoptosis. SIRT1 interacts with the extracellular signal-regulated kinase (ERK) pathway and downregulates MAPK expression, thereby mitigating cardiac cell damage (Luo et al. 2019). The heart, which requires a significant amount of energy, is particularly vulnerable to dysfunction under chronic hyperglycemia due to the accumulation of AGEs. These AGEs impair the Na+/K+/ATPase pump, which is crucial for energy metabolism, and exacerbate ER stress. Additionally, a reduction in AMPK expression plays a key role in the progression of diabetic cardiomyopathy. AMPK downregulation leads to decreased SIRT1 and peroxisome proliferator-activated receptor gamma coactivator-1 α (PGC-1α) expression, impairing mitochondrial biogenesis and promoting left ventricular hypertrophy (Yao et al. 2021). Furthermore, reduced SIRT1 expression in the context of hyperglycemia enhances oxidative stress and inflammation in cardiomyocytes through the activation of the NF-κB pathway. Myocyte fibrosis, a prominent feature of diabetic cardiomyopathy, is largely driven by high glucose-induced activation of the TGF-β/SMAD pathway via acetylation of the P300 protein. Research indicates that SIRT1, through the deacetylation of P300, inhibits TGF-β activation, thereby preventing fibrosis and attenuating the progression of cardiomyopathy (Liu et al. 2023).

Clinical and Preclinical Prospective of SIRT1 Activators

DM is a chronic metabolic disorder characterized by hyperglycemia due to impaired insulin secretion or action, leading to long-term complications such as cardiovascular disease, neuropathy, nephropathy, and retinopathy. Targeting SIRT1 has emerged as a promising strategy for the management of DM. SIRT1 regulates glucose and lipid metabolism, inflammation, and insulin sensitivity, making it a key target for potential therapeutic interventions (Fiorino et al. 2018).

Mechanisms of SIRT1 in Metabolism

SIRT1 plays a vital role in metabolic regulation by deacetylating key transcription factors and coactivators that govern glucose and lipid metabolism. One of its primary targets is peroxisome proliferator-activated receptor-gamma coactivator 1-alpha (PGC-1α), a central regulator of mitochondrial biogenesis and oxidative metabolism. Through deacetylation, SIRT1 enhances PGC-1α activity, promoting mitochondrial function and energy expenditure, which is essential for maintaining cellular energy homeostasis. Additionally, SIRT1 modulates the activity of forkhead box protein O1 (FOXO1) and p53, both of which are involved in gluconeogenesis and insulin sensitivity. By deacetylating these transcription factors, SIRT1 helps regulate glucose production in the liver and promotes insulin sensitivity, thereby improving metabolic control. SIRT1 activation also exerts anti-inflammatory effects by inhibiting the activity of NF-κB, a key mediator of inflammation and a contributor to insulin resistance. This ability to suppress NF-κB activity is particularly significant in the context of metabolic diseases like T2DM, where chronic inflammation exacerbates insulin resistance (Milne & Denu, 2008).

Preclinical Studies of SIRT1 Activators

Preclinical studies provide compelling evidence supporting the role of SIRT1 activators in improving metabolic parameters associated with diabetes. Resveratrol, a naturally occurring polyphenol found in grapes and red wine, is one of the most extensively studied SIRT1 activators. In animal models of T2DM, resveratrol has been shown to enhance insulin sensitivity, lower blood glucose levels, and reduce oxidative stress and inflammation (Table 1).

Table 1. SIRT1 activators and their role in the management of diabetes mellitus and related complications

SIRT1 Activators	Role in Diabetes and Associated Complications	References
Nicotinamide Riboside	Improves mitochondrial dysfunction via activation of the SIRT1/PGC-1α/PPAR α pathway in db/db mouse models of T2DM	(Trammell et al. 2016)
Resveratrol and its derivatives	Decreases blood glucose levels, improves lipid profile, increases insulin sensitivity, enhances mitochondrial biogenesis, and regulates the downstream transcription factors of SIRT1 to prevent secondary complications.	(Huang et al. 2020)
Quercetin	Exhibits anti-hyperglycemic, anti-inflammatory, and anti-apoptotic activities.	(Ansari et al. 2022)
Berberine	Decreases hepatic gluconeogenesis, improves energy metabolism, and exhibits antioxidant and anti-inflammatory actions.	(Dong et al. 2012)
Curcumin	Improves diabetes-associated cardiovascular complications through antifibrotic, antioxidant, and anti-apoptotic actions.	(Pivari et al. 2019)
Metformin	Decreases blood glucose levels, hepatic gluconeogenesis, and protects organs by activating the SIRT1/FoxO1 autophagic signaling pathway. Also decreases oxidative stress, inflammation, and apoptosis induced by hyperglycemia.	(Cuyàs et al. 2018)

Research indicates that resveratrol improves glucose homeostasis by activating SIRT1, which enhances mitochondrial function and increases fatty acid oxidation (Lagouge et al. 2006). In addition to resveratrol, synthetic SIRT1 activators such as SRT1720 and SRT2104 have demonstrated promising effects in preclinical models. These small molecules directly activate SIRT1, mimicking the beneficial effects of resveratrol. In diabetic mice, SRT1720 has been shown to lower fasting glucose levels, improve glucose tolerance, and reduce markers of inflammation. These findings suggest that SRT1720 and similar compounds hold significant potential as therapeutic agents for diabetes management, offering an innovative approach to enhancing insulin sensitivity, reducing hepatic steatosis, and improving lipid metabolism (Mitchell et al. 2014).

Clinical Prospective of SIRT1 Activators

Despite the promising results in preclinical studies, the translation of SIRT1 activators into clinical practice has been challenging. Clinical trials with resveratrol in diabetic patients have yielded mixed results. Some studies have reported improvements in glycemic control, insulin sensitivity, and cardiovascular function, while others have shown minimal or no benefit. The variability in outcomes may be due to differences in study design, patient populations, and dosages used (Poulsen et al. 2013).

Non-Pharmacological Approaches to Manage Diabetes Mellitus via SIRT1 Activation

DM is a major global health challenge, marked by chronic hyperglycemia and insulin resistance, leading to significant morbidity and mortality. While pharmacological interventions remain central to its management, non-pharmacological approaches are gaining recognition for their potential in modulating metabolic pathways, particularly through the activation of SIRT1. SIRT1 plays a critical role in regulating cellular processes such as metabolism, aging, and stress resistance. Activation of SIRT1 has been linked to improved insulin sensitivity, better glucose homeostasis, and reduced inflammation, positioning it as a promising target for managing diabetes through lifestyle interventions, including dietary changes and physical activity (Houtkooper et al. 2012).

Caloric Restriction and Intermittent Fasting

Caloric restriction (CR) and intermittent fasting (IF) are non-pharmacological interventions that have demonstrated the ability to activate SIRT1 and improve metabolic health. CR involves reducing calorie intake without causing malnutrition, and it has been consistently shown to enhance SIRT1 activity. This activation is thought to be facilitated by increased NAD+ levels, a cofactor required for SIRT1's enzymatic function, leading to improved insulin sensitivity and glucose metabolism. Similarly, intermittent fasting, which alternates between periods of eating and fasting, has also been found to activate SIRT1. Studies suggest that IF enhances mitochondrial function, reduces oxidative stress, and improves insulin sensitivity, with SIRT1 playing a key role in these benefits. For instance, research has shown that fasting-induced SIRT1 activation improves insulin sensitivity and boosts glucose uptake in peripheral tissues (Canto & Auwerx, 2009).

Exercise

Physical activity is another effective non-pharmacological approach to activating SIRT1. Regular exercise has been shown to increase SIRT1 expression in critical tissues such as skeletal muscle, liver, and adipose tissue, which play key roles in glucose and lipid metabolism. Exercise-induced activation of SIRT1 contributes to enhanced mitochondrial biogenesis, improved insulin sensitivity, and reduced inflammation. For instance, a study demonstrated that endurance exercise increases SIRT1 expression in skeletal muscles, leading to improved insulin sensitivity and glucose uptake. Moreover, the combination of exercise with dietary interventions like CR can have a synergistic effect, further enhancing SIRT1 activity and improving metabolic health in individuals with diabetes (Ferrara et al. 2008).

Diet and Nutritional Interventions

Diet plays a crucial role in modulating SIRT1 activity. Nutritional components such as polyphenols, found in foods like grapes, berries, and green tea, have been shown to activate SIRT1. Resveratrol, a polyphenol present in red wine, is a well-known SIRT1 activator that mimics the effects of caloric restriction. Dietary interventions that include these SIRT1-activating compounds can enhance metabolic health and potentially reduce the risk of developing diabetes or help manage its progression. Furthermore, a diet rich in omega-3 fatty acids, found in fish oil, has been shown to increase SIRT1 expression and improve insulin sensitivity. These dietary strategies are not only beneficial for diabetes management but also for overall metabolic health (Dyck et al. 2006).

Stress Management and Sleep

Chronic stress and poor sleep are associated with metabolic dysregulation and insulin resistance. Managing stress through techniques such as meditation, yoga, and adequate sleep can positively influence SIRT1 activity. A study found that improved sleep quality is associated with increased SIRT1 expression, leading to better glucose regulation and insulin sensitivity (Yehuda et al. 2009).

Future Directions

Future research into SIRT1-based therapies for diabetes focuses on developing potent, selective, and safe activators to address the metabolic dysfunction associated with the disease. While natural compounds like resveratrol show promise, issues with bioavailability and dosage limitations highlight the need for next-generation SIRT1 activators with enhanced pharmacokinetics and safety profiles. An expanded understanding of the molecular pathways influenced by SIRT1 will support drug development. Beyond glucose metabolism, SIRT1 also regulates lipid metabolism and mitochondrial function and interacts with other metabolic regulators such as AMPK, PPARs, and FOXO1. Unraveling these mechanisms may identify additional therapeutic targets, allowing the creation of more precise SIRT1 modulators that specifically impact desired pathways. Combination therapies also hold promise. By targeting multiple metabolic pathways simultaneously, therapies that include SIRT1 activators alongside insulin sensitizers, anti-inflammatory agents, or GLP-1 receptor agonists could provide superior outcomes. Such multi-targeted approaches may improve glucose control, insulin sensitivity, and inflammation management compared to single-agent treatments, offering a more comprehensive strategy for managing diabetes. Personalized medicine is pivotal in SIRT1-based therapy development, as genetic variations can influence a patient's response to treatments. Genetic profiling and pharmacogenomics could help tailor SIRT1-targeted therapies, enhancing effectiveness and minimizing side effects. As genetic sequencing becomes more accessible, treatment protocols could increasingly incorporate genetic data, allowing clinicians to customize interventions based on individual genetic profiles. Bringing SIRT1 activators to the market will require navigating scientific, technological, and regulatory challenges. Addressing toxicity, safety, and pharmacokinetics through rigorous preclinical studies is essential before large-scale clinical trials can establish efficacy in diverse populations. Regulatory processes demand solid evidence of safety and efficacy, highlighting the need for substantial investment from public and private sectors. Clear regulatory guidelines for SIRT1-based therapies will be critical, particularly as SIRT1 activation remains a relatively novel approach in diabetes management. Ensuring patient-centricity in drug development is also vital. Patients' needs, adherence factors, and lifestyle compatibility should shape the development of SIRT1-targeted therapies. Medications with complex administration or high side effects may hinder adherence, while treatments designed with patient feedback can enhance long-term usability. By aligning therapy design with real-world patient preferences, companies can develop treatments that are both effective and practical. Funding and collaboration will drive progress in SIRT1-based research. Partnerships among public institutions, pharmaceutical companies, and healthcare providers will accelerate preclinical findings' translation to clinical applications. Policy support and philanthropic funding focused on diabetes and metabolic diseases can further stimulate innovation. Finally, research into SIRT1's broader therapeutic potential across diseases such as obesity, cardiovascular disorders, and neurodegenerative conditions could yield new insights. Tissue-specific SIRT1 activation, particularly in the liver, muscle, and adipose tissue, may present another frontier for therapeutic advancement.

Conclusion

In conclusion, SIRT1 stands out as a promising target for addressing glucose metabolism and the broader metabolic challenges of diabetes mellitus. Advances in understanding its structure, regulatory pathways, and effects on metabolic health provide a solid framework for developing innovative therapies. Integrating SIRT1-targeted treatments into current diabetes management approaches offers potential for improved patient outcomes, especially in preventing long-term complications and enhancing overall metabolic health. As research evolves, the transformative potential of SIRT1-based therapies in diabetes care becomes more apparent, bringing hope for more effective, tailored interventions for the management of this complex disease.

References

Al-Khaldi, G., & Sultan, S. (2019). Role of SIRT1 in the regulation of β-cell function in diabetes mellitus. *Diabetes Research and Clinical Practice*, 149, 144–150.

Ansari, M. A., Khan, A., Khan, M. S., Ahmad, S., Ahmad, F., & Baig, M. H. (2022). Quercetin alleviates hyperglycemia, oxidative stress, inflammation, and apoptosis in diabetic rats by regulating insulin signaling, NF-κB, and MAPK pathways. *Biomedicine & Pharmacotherapy*, 146, 112529.

Bazyluk, A., Wiczkowski, W., & Bukowska, M. (2019). SIRT1—A promising target in metabolic diseases. *Biochimica et Biophysica Acta*, 1865(6), 1319-1330.

Canto, C., & Auwerx, J. (2009). Calorie restriction: Is AMPK a key sensor and effector? *Physiology*, 24(6), 362-371.

Choi, Y. J., Kim, S. T., & Kim, D. W. (2011). Histological changes in diabetic nephropathy and the effect of SIRT1 activation on renal function. *Journal of Diabetes Research*, 2011, 876538.

Cuyàs, E., Verdura, S., Llorach-Parés, L., Fernández-Arroyo, S., Joven, J., Martin-Castillo, B., & Menendez, J. A. (2018). Metformin is a direct SIRT1-activating compound: Computational modeling and experimental validation. *Frontiers in Endocrinology*, 9, 657.

Dai, H., Case, A., Riera, T. V., Considine, T., & Hubbard, B. P. (2015). Crystallographic structure of SIRT1 and its interactions with the human mitochondrial network. *Nature Structural & Molecular Biology*, 22(5), 416–423.

Ding, S., Yang, G., & Wang, Y. (2024). Role of SIRT1 in glucose metabolism and insulin resistance: New insights into therapeutic strategies. *Journal of Diabetes Research*, 2024, 238564.

Dong, H., Wang, N., Zhao, L., & Lu, F. (2012). Berberine in the treatment of type 2 diabetes mellitus: A systemic review and meta-analysis. *Evidence-Based Complementary and Alternative Medicine*, 2012, 591654.

Dyck, D. J., Peters, S. J., Wendling, P. S., Chesley, A., Harger, R. N., & Bonen, A. (2006). Regulation of muscle palmitate oxidation by muscle activity and fatty acid availability. *American Journal of Physiology-Endocrinology and Metabolism*, 290(4), E619-E627.

Ferrara, C. M., Goldberg, A. P., Ortmeyer, H. K., Ryan, A. S., & Davy, K. P. (2008). Regular exercise and the effects of lipid metabolism. *Journal of Applied Physiology*, 104(5), 1503-1512.

Fiorino, E., Giudici, M., Ferrari, A., Mitro, N., & Caruso, D. (2018). Control of SIRT1 activity by lipid metabolism: Implications in non-alcoholic fatty liver disease. *Frontiers in Pharmacology*, 9, 872.

Houtkooper, R. H., Pirinen, E., & Auwerx, J. (2012). Sirtuins as regulators of metabolism and healthspan. *Nature Reviews Molecular Cell Biology*, 13(4), 225-238.

Huang, D., Liu, M., Jiang, Y., & Yang, X. (2020). Resveratrol mitigates insulin resistance and mitochondrial dysfunction in type 2 diabetes by activating SIRT1 and modulating mitochondrial function. *Journal of Nutritional Biochemistry*, 82, 108241.

Imai, S., Armstrong, C. M., Kaeberlein, M., & Guarente, L. (2000). Transcriptional silencing and longevity protein Sir2 is an NAD-dependent histone deacetylase. *Nature*, 403(6771), 795–800.

Juan, C. A., Pérez, T., & Lozano, R. (2023). Sirtuin modulation and regulation of cellular processes. *Molecular Cell*, 72(8), 1091–1099.

Karbasforooshan, H., & Karimi, G. (2018). The role of SIRT1 in diabetic retinopathy. *BioFactors*, 44(3), 261-267.

Kitada, M., & Koya, D. (2013a). SIRT1: A potential therapeutic target for type 2 diabetes and its complications. *Endocrine, Metabolic & Immune Disorders - Drug Targets*, 13(4), 416–425.

Kitada, M., & Koya, D. (2013b). The use of SIRT1 activators as therapeutic agents for diabetes and its complications. *Diabetes Research and Clinical Practice*, 101(1), 54–61.

Lagouge, M., Argmann, C., Gerhart-Hines, Z., Meziane, H., Lerin, C., Daussin, F., Messadeq, N., Milne, J., Lambert, P., Elliott, P., Geny, B., Laakso, M., Puigserver, P., & Auwerx, J. (2006). Resveratrol improves mitochondrial function and protects against metabolic disease by activating SIRT1 and PGC-1α. *Cell*, 127(6), 1109 1122.

Liu, W., Luo, H., & Xu, M. (2023). Role of SIRT1 in diabetic cardiomyopathy: Molecular mechanisms and therapeutic strategies. *Diabetes & Vascular Disease Research*, 20(1), 12-19.

Liu, X., Wang, Y., Zhang, Z., & Ma, X. (2020). SIRT1 regulates AMPK/mTOR/Akt pathway to prevent glomerular basement thickening in diabetic nephropathy. *Nephrology Dialysis Transplantation*, 35(7), 1124-1135.

Lu, Q., Tan, Y., & Wu, L. (2023). SIRT1 in metabolic health and insulin secretion. *Diabetes Care*, 46(2), 153–165.

Luo, T., Liu, Z., & Ma, Z. (2019). SIRT1 activation protects cardiac cells by mitigating ROS-mediated apoptosis in diabetic cardiomyopathy. *Journal of Molecular and Cellular Cardiology*, 131, 113-124.

Ma, Z., Liu, Z., & Yao, T. (2019). The role of SIRT1 activation in ameliorating renal cell injury in diabetic nephropathy. *Kidney International*, 96(3), 521-532.

Michishita, E., Park, J. Y., Burneskis, J. M., Barrett, J. C., & Horikawa, I. (2005). Evolutionarily conserved and nonconserved cellular localizations and functions of human SIRT proteins. *Molecular Biology of the Cell*, 16(10), 4623-4635.

Milne, J. C., & Denu, J. M. (2008). The Sirtuin family: Therapeutic targets to treat diseases of aging. *Current Opinion in Chemical Biology*, 12(1), 11-17.

Mitchell, S. J., Martin-Montalvo, A., Mercken, E. M., Palacios, H. H., Ward, T. M., Abulwerdi, G., Minor, R. K., Vlasuk, G. P., Ellis, J. L., Sinclair, D. A., Dawson, J., Allison, D. B., Zhang, Y., Becker, K. G., Bernier, M., & de Cabo, R. (2014). The SIRT1 activator SRT1720 extends lifespan and improves health of mice fed a standard diet. *Cell Reports*, 6(5), 836-843.

Nebbioso, A., Sirignano, E., & Molinari, A. M. (2022). SIRT1 in diabetic retinopathy: A focus on VEGF regulation and retinal permeability. *International Journal of Molecular Sciences*, 23(15), 8716.

Pivari, F., Mingione, A., Brasacchio, C., & Soldati, L. (2019). Curcumin and type 2 diabetes mellitus: Prevention and treatment. *Nutrients*, 11(8), 1837.

Poulsen, M. M., Vestergaard, P. F., Clasen, B. F., Radko, Y., Christensen, L. P., Stødkilde-Jørgensen, H., Møller, N., Jessen, N., Pedersen, S. B., & Jørgensen, J. O. L. (2013). High-dose resveratrol supplementation in obese men: an investigator-initiated, randomized, placebo-controlled clinical trial of substrate metabolism, insulin sensitivity, and body composition. *Diabetes*, 62(4), 1186-1195.

Rine, J., & Herskowitz, I. (1979). Mating type interconversion in yeast: The role of the silent mating type loci HML and HMR. *Cell*, 27(1), 25-35.

Schena, F. P., & Gesualdo, L. (2005). Pathogenetic mechanisms of diabetic nephropathy. *Journal of the American Society of Nephrology*, 16(Suppl 1), S30-S33.

Shah, A., Mehta, N., & Jain, M. (2022). Oxidative stress and diabetic cardiomyopathy: Role of SIRT1 and MAPK pathways. *Diabetes Research and Clinical Practice*, 187, 109896.

Strycharz, J., Drzewoski, J., & Szemraj, J. (2018). SIRT1 and its role in regulating the function of retinal cells under high glucose conditions. *Experimental Eye Research*, 176, 135-145.

Stünkel, W., & Campbell, R. M. (2011). Sirtuin 1 (SIRT1): Mechanisms and diverse roles in the regulation of metabolism and inflammation. *Biochimica et Biophysica Acta (BBA) - Molecular Basis of Disease*, 1812(8), 1456-1464.

Trammell, S. A. J., Schmidt, M. S., Weidemann, B. J., Redpath, P., Jaksch, F., Dellinger, R. W., Li, Z., Abel, E. D., Migaud, M. E., & Brenner, C. (2016). Nicotinamide riboside is uniquely and orally bioavailable in mice and humans. *Nature Communications*, 7, 12948.

Wang, M., Wu, Y., & Zhang, X. (2022). The role of SIRT1 and fibrosis in diabetic retinopathy. *Biomedicine & Pharmacotherapy*, 146, 112524.

Wang, W., & Lo, A. C. Y. (2018). Diabetic retinopathy: Pathophysiology and treatments. *International Journal of Molecular Sciences*, 19(6), 1816.

Wang, X., Zhang, Y., & Zhao, T. (2021a). Role of SIRT1 in β-cell function and insulin secretion in diabetes mellitus. *Journal of Molecular Endocrinology*, 66(3), 179–190.

Wang, X., Zhao, T., & Liu, Y. (2021b). SIRT1 and its role in inflammation in diabetes. *Current Diabetes Reports*, 21(10), 112–124.

Wang, X., Zhao, T., Liu, Y., & Zhang, Y. (2021c). Potential therapeutic role of SIRT1 activators in diabetes. *Frontiers in Endocrinology*, 12, 678954.

Watanabe, K., Liu, H., & Matsui, M. (2010). Role of MAPK and oxidative stress in cardiac apoptosis and fibrosis during diabetes. *Journal of Molecular and Cellular Cardiology*, 48(3), 751-760.

Yao, T., Wang, X., & Liu, Z. (2021). AMPK pathway regulation by SIRT1 in diabetic cardiomyopathy and mitochondrial function. *Cardiovascular Diabetology*, 20(1), 152.

Yehuda, R., Golier, J. A., & Kaufman, S. (2009). Circadian regulation of glucocorticoid feedback inhibition by the SIRT1-FOXO pathway. *Journal of Clinical Endocrinology & Metabolism*, 94(10), 4068-4074.

Chapter 12

Adenosine Monophosphate Activated Protein Kinase (AMPK): A Master Regulator of Energy Balance

Narinderpal Kaur*
Shiwali Sharma
Shivali Bisht
and Suhani Thakur
Chitkara University School of Pharmacy, Chitkara University, Himachal Pradesh, India

Abstract

Adenosine triphosphate is known to be the energy currency of the body. Adenosine heterotrimeric enzyme is responsible for both energy-constructive and energy-destructive pathways to maintain intracellular energy balance in the body. Apart from its role in maintaining homeostasis, it also plays an immensely important role in some diseases such as cardiovascular disease, renal injury, cancer, etc. Adenosine monophosphate-activated protein kinase forms an interconnection between a series of chemical reactions and the regulation of muscle mass. Adenosine monophosphate protein kinase (AMPK) checks the level of basal energy. It gets stimulated via the addition of a phosphate groups in specific substrate or compound while levels of energy are not high. It permits balancing the level of equilibrium in the body as well as enhancing the metabolic reactions in order to produce energy currency for cells. AMPK is known as the master regulator of energy balance. This chapter provides an overview of the synchronization, structure of AMPK, its regulation, role in metabolism, and influence on various organs, including the kidney, heart, and brain.

Keywords: adenosine monophosphate protein kinase, homeostasis, renal injury, bone regulation, tumours, memory, health, research

* Corresponding Author's Email: narinderpal.kaur@chitkarauniversity.edu.in

In: Receptor-Targeted Therapies in Diabetes Mellitus
Editors: Ajmer Singh Grewal, Neelam Singh, Swati Verma et al.
ISBN: 979-8-89530-587-4

Abbreviations

Acetyl CO A	Acetyl coenzyme A
AML	Acute myeloid leukemia
AMPK	Adenosine Monophosphate Protein Kinase
AVP	Arginine Vasopressor
CAMP	Cyclic Adenosine Monophosphate
GAA	Guanidino acetic acid
IGF	Insulin like growth factor
IP3R	Inositol 1,4,5-triphospahte receptor
MSC	Mesenchymal stem cells
mtDNA	Mitochondrial Di Ribo Nucleic Acid
mTOR	Mammalian target of rapamycin
PGC	Peroxisome proliferator-activated gamma coactivator
RIPK1	Receptor-Interacting Serine/Threonine Kinase 1
SIRT	Sirtuin; ULK: Unc-51-like Kinase

Introduction

Adenosine monophosphate-activated protein kinase plays a crucial role in maintaining the homeostasis of both the somatic and autonomic nervous systems. It is primarily involved in sensitizing the adenine nucleotide, which is activated in response to low cellular energy. The activation of AMPK ensures synchronized energy regulation. AMPK promotes the attachment of phosphate groups to molecules or ions and enhances photo-sensing receptors. Additionally, it plays a key role in signaling metabolic modulation and neuronal cell death, contributing to both pathophysiology and therapeutic approaches (Kalra et al. 2023). Adenosine monophosphate-activated protein kinase (AMPK) is a member of the highly conserved eukaryotic protein family. It is expressed in various tissues, including the brain, heart, and skeletal muscles. As a macromolecule, it consists of three subunits: a catalytic α subunit and two regulatory subunits, β and γ. Each subunit has two or more isoforms (α1, α2, β1, β2, γ1, γ2, and γ3), which are functionally similar but have distinct amino acid sequences. These isoforms are widely expressed across different tissues and subcellular compartments. AMPK is activated when cellular energy levels are low, acting to inhibit anabolic (energy-storing) metabolic pathways while promoting catabolic (energy-releasing) processes. For example, it facilitates glucose uptake and beta-oxidation of fatty acids to generate adenosine triphosphate (ATP), thereby restoring cellular energy balance (Chen et al. 2020). Recent studies have revealed that, in addition to its primary function of inhibiting anabolic pathways and promoting catabolic pathways, adenosine monophosphate-activated protein kinase (AMPK) acts as a potential sensitizer and stimulator for both oxidative and reductive processes. AMPK also plays a critical role in regulating cardiac function, thereby mitigating related illnesses. Its role in health and disease is highly significant. Moreover, AMPK influences cytoplasmic metabolism over extended periods by targeting genetic regulators. Activated AMPK stabilizes energy levels by either increasing ATP production or reducing ATP consumption. The overall effect of AMPK includes inhibition of cholesterol and triglyceride synthesis, regulation of insulin secretion by pancreatic beta cells, and suppression of adipocyte lipogenesis. Dysregulation of AMPK is frequently associated with metabolic disorders such as obesity, diabetes mellitus, cancer, and cardiovascular diseases (Wu et al. 2020). AMPK activity is heightened to maintain metabolic homeostasis during stress conditions. However, prolonged exposure to stress factors may lead to cell necrosis. The mechanisms by which AMPK governs cell necrosis remain unclear. Research indicates that AMPK-induced phosphorylation regulates cellular responses to stress and reveals a previously unrecognized role for the AMPK-RIPK1 axis in metabolism, cell necrosis, and inflammation (Zhang et al. 2023). AMPK is considered an amalgamate compound being composed of one catalytic subunit, α, and two regulative subunits, β and γ. Energization of AMPK is persuaded by an elevated ratio of energy currencies, i.e., AMP, ATP, or ADP (Zhu and Han, 2022). The objective of this chapter is to provide a comprehensive overview of AMPK, exploring its structure, regulatory mechanisms, and critical role in maintaining cellular energy balance. The chapter also examines AMPK's influence on metabolic pathways and its impact on various organs, including the heart, kidney, and brain.

Adenosine Monophosphate Activated Protein Kinase

Structure of AMPK

AMPK is a macromolecule composed of three subunits: an enzymatic α-subunit, a scaffolding β-subunit, and a regulatory γ-subunit. In humans, the α- and β-subunits each have two isoforms (α1, α2 and β1, β2), while the γ-subunit has three isoforms (γ1, γ2, and γ3). These isoforms combine to produce 12 distinct forms of AMPK, which vary in expression and regulation across different tissues. The α-subunit contains the kinase domain and a crucial residue that is phosphorylated by upstream kinases. This α-subunit is essential, as the knockout of AMPKα1 and AMPKα2 in mice is lethal. The β-subunit includes a glycogen-binding domain, enabling AMPK to interact with glycogen stores. The γ-subunit allows AMPK to respond to fluctuations in AMP, ADP, and ATP levels, with four key molecular regions facilitating AMPK binding to adenine nucleotides (Wu et al. 2020).

Regulation of AMPK

AMPK is activated through mechanisms sensitive to changes in ATP and AMP concentrations. When cellular energy is depleted, the increase in AMP triggers AMPK activation, primarily through phosphorylation at specific substrate residues. This energy-sensitive regulation occurs across various tissues, including adipose tissue, skeletal muscle, and smooth muscle. AMPK activation involves three main processes: phosphorylation, inhibition of dephosphorylation (the removal of phosphate groups), and alterations in its allosteric site to enhance enzyme activity. Additionally, AMPK regulation is influenced by protein degradation processes mediated by interactions between AMPK and DNA fragments (Rodríguez et al. 2021).

Role of AMPK in Metabolism

AMPK maintains cellular homeostasis by reducing ATP consumption in certain processes, such as fat synthesis gene transcription, ribosomal RNA production, and the synthesis of ribosomal proteins and fatty acids. Simultaneously, it enhances energy-generating pathways like fatty acid oxidation, glucose uptake, and autophagy, ensuring ATP availability during periods of high energy demand. The synthesis of AMP is crucial for balancing the body's internal environment with external energy requirements. AMPK plays a key role in regulating glucose levels and modulating metabolism through various pathways influenced by external factors, such as pH, workload, and physiological signals, which increase AMPK activity and improve metabolic efficiency. Research has shown that AMPK promotes glycolysis, particularly in white blood cells, by transferring phosphate groups to specific molecules, thereby enhancing metabolic activity (Haran et al. 2022). Additionally, AMPK activation through oxidative stress initiates phosphorylation of various compounds, converting them to active biochemical forms and influencing both translation and transcription processes (Malik et al. 2023).

Role of AMPK in Kidney

AMP acts as a key intermediary in intracellular signal transduction, directing physiological functions throughout the body. Disruptions in AMP function can lead to diseases such as renal disease, diabetes mellitus, and hypertension, all of which increase the risk of chronic kidney disease. AMP levels are regulated by specific proteins, including those influenced by arginine vasopressin (AVP); however, excessive AVP activation is associated with the progression of chronic kidney disease (Sholokh et al. 2021). Maintaining cellular self-degradation, or autophagy, is essential for optimal renal function. AMPK promotes the expression of ULK1 (unc-51-like autophagy-activating kinase 1) and inhibits mTOR activity, thereby supporting autophagy. Activation of AMPK also reduces macrophage infiltration, mitigates oxidative stress, and modulates macrophage degradation. These roles underscore the potential of AMPK agonists in the treatment of renal disease (Zhu & Han, 2022).

AMPK and Cancer

Malignancy, resulting from abnormal and excessive cellular proliferation that invades and destroys surrounding tissues and organs, is caused by the uncontrolled growth of cancer cells. Recent studies highlight the active role of AMPK in both malignant tumors and normal cellular metabolism. Further research and human trials are essential to better understand the role of AMPK in cancer cell metabolism, uncover its related signaling pathways, and develop novel activators that may hold promise for cancer treatment (Choi et al. 2023). As a key regulator of cellular metabolic reactions, AMPK plays an important role in suppressing tumor growth and managing cellular responses to metabolic stress. The role of AMPK in response to chemotherapeutic treatments has been examined in solid tumors, including its effects on acute myelogenous leukemia (AML) cells, which exhibit varied responses to hormone therapy; however, the underlying mechanisms are not fully understood. AMPK also plays a significant role in maintaining gut health. Beyond enhancing intestinal barrier function and nutrient absorption, it suppresses colorectal carcinogenesis and reduces intestinal inflammation. In cases of gut cancer, AMPK pathway activity is often diminished (Al-Ishaq et al. 2020). Research indicates that AMPK function can be impaired by hormone therapy in certain AML cells. Experimental studies on solid tumors have shown that AMPK is activated by hormone therapy, which also influences the DNA damage response. AML cells lacking active AMPK display higher resistance to treatment and show less DNA damage response compared to normal cells, which are more responsive to treatment (Ghiraldeli et al. 2022).

Role of AMPK in Bone Regeneration and Metabolic Bone Disorders

Bone defects and related diseases often stem from inadequate bone regeneration, necessitating new therapeutic approaches for trauma patients. Recent studies have identified that AMPK and ULK1 form a novel autophagy-related pathway that applies mechanical tension to promote osteoblastogenesis. Findings suggest that combining mesenchymal stem cells (MSCs) embedded in hydrogels with negative pressure wound therapy significantly enhances bone healing in rat models with critical-size calvarial defects (Zhang et al. 2022). High sugar intake, such as fructose, is linked to metabolic disorders and negatively impacts bone health. As a dynamic organ, bone tissue continuously remodels, but studies show that fructose not only reduces bone mineral density but also increases fat accumulation in bone marrow. AMPK is crucial in managing bone fat levels, and research has demonstrated that fructose accelerates bone loss and marrow adipose tissue buildup by inhibiting AMPK activation in bone marrow MSCs (BMMSCs) (Yan et al. 2024).

AMPK and Lipolysis

The hydrolysis of fats is a critical pathway for maintaining energy balance, and regulating lipolysis in adipose tissue is a promising therapeutic target for metabolism-related diseases. AMPK plays a vital role in lipid metabolism and is a potential target for the treatment of diabetes mellitus and obesity (Boone-Villa et al. 2022). Interestingly, arriheuk-mediated PGC-1α expression stimulates mitochondrial production of compounds by promoting the addition of a phosphate group to AMPK and enhancing SIRT1 expression in specialized connective tissue containing fat. Additionally, it suppresses the accumulation of fat-laden cells in adipose tissue at various sites in the body, promoting browning through the AMPK- and SIRT1-associated pathways. These findings strongly suggest that arriheuk extract modulates lipid metabolism in 3T3-L1 white adipose cells by activating the AMPK/SIRT1 pathway, indicating its potential as a functional food to combat obesity. (Yoon et al. 2023).

AMPK's Involvement in Brain

The etiology of inflammation plays a crucial role in the development of various brain disorders. Numerous studies have shown that indole derivatives exhibit anti-inflammatory effects, aiding in the recovery from several diseases. These derivatives help alleviate brain swelling, behavioral changes, internal nerve damage, and basal cell inflammation. Overall, significant changes are observed in various research models, such as inhibiting inflammation through the stimulation of AMPK (Jin et al. 2022). It is well-established that AMPK plays a key role in sensitization, particularly in nerve cells, where it is crucial for restoring long-term memory. Memory retention is a stepwise process involving the transmission of nerve signals across synapses. Discovered in the mid-1990s, AMPK plays a significant role in memory formation, interacting with other factors as well. Research suggests that AMPK not only activates protein kinases but also regulates protein-mediated transmission, which is essential for memory retention and signal transmission. AMPK plays a specific, stepwise role in each of these processes (Naz et al. 2022). The use of neohesperidin dihydrochalcone has been linked to an increase in programmed cell death and AMPK activation. However, prolonged administration, whether in small or large doses, may have adverse effects on both the brain and the body (Jiang et al. 2022). Glycogen degradation, a natural process facilitated by the lysosomal enzyme GAA, is also influenced by cyclic adenosine monophosphate (cAMP). Short-term glycogen depletion promotes the breakdown of molecules, reconnecting cellular metabolic reactions by reducing glucose breakdown and enhancing AMPK activity. This also improves the metabolism of fatty acids and glutamine amino acids (Heden et al. 2022).

AMPK and Muscles

The mitochondrion, often referred to as the powerhouse of the cell, is a crucial organelle in the body, especially in skeletal muscles. It plays a significant role in various processes related to growth, development, and regeneration. AMPK acts as a key regulator, modulating these processes. AMPK is considered a growth regulator, particularly in metabolic functions, by influencing the concentration gradients of potential energy sources. The basic structural and functional unit of the body, the cell, is involved in essential processes where ATP is converted into AMP, generating free energy. When ATP concentrations within cells fluctuate, AMPK helps regulate the body's energy balance, ensuring proper cellular function (Jiang et al. 2023).

AMP-Protein Kinase and Mutation

Morbid variations in the human mitochondrial genome (mtDNA) are associated with numerous injury-related conditions affecting the brain, spinal cord, and peripheral nerves. These mutations also result in defects in personal and developmental growth, although the underlying mechanisms remain poorly understood. Monitoring AMPK plays a crucial role in addressing the issues arising from mitochondrial DNA mutations, as demonstrated in Caenorhabditis elegans models. Such mutations can lead to a complete loss or reduction of various cellular functions, including osmotic regulation, compound synthesis, sensory perception, movement, cognitive abilities, and increased inactivity during embryonic development. Mitochondrial DNA variations reduce cellular energy levels, with AMPK, forkhead box class O (FOXO) transcription factors, and the inositol 1,4,5-trisphosphate receptor (IP3R) pathway serving as key modulators of these defects (Zhang et al. 2023).

AMPK and Antidepressants

Autophagy, a critical process for the stepwise degradation of cellular components, is frequently altered in various diseases, including those involving plaque accumulation and nerve transmission disorders. Studies suggest that selective serotonin reuptake inhibitors (SSRIs), a class of drugs commonly used to treat depression, also function as inducers of autophagy. Notably, basal cells often lack specific expressions necessary to activate AMP-activated protein kinase (AMPK). The therapeutic potential of these antidepressant drugs is highly promising, providing significant benefits in managing neurodegenerative diseases (Hwang et al. 2021).

AMPK and Cold Stress

It has been suggested that the phosphate ester of the nucleoside adenosine plays a crucial role in mitigating the effects of cold stress on intestinal health. Studies have explored the impact of conditions that impair the body's ability to maintain normal temperature, influencing developmental processes, agglutinin biochemistry, and AMPK activity in broilers. Developmental activity was monitored, and agglutinogen accumulation was analyzed. Furthermore, intestinal mucosa samples were examined to identify amino acid chains in occluding junctions, thermal exhaustion, and the activation of proteins and enzymes involved in cellular energy regulation (Zhou et al. 2021).

Inhibition of AMPK Leading to High Cholesterol Level Promoting Insulin Resistance

The ester of phosphoric acid with the nucleoside adenosine plays a critical role in maintaining numerous neural transmission pathways associated with the catabolism and anabolism of fatty acids and glycogen. Many research studies suggest that the addition of a phosphate group to a substrate and the inhibition of specific enzymes in this process suppress the formation of cholesterol. AMPK-mediated nerve transmission is, by itself, sufficient to regulate all metabolic cycles in the body under favorable conditions, such as a balanced and proportional diet. AMPK also plays a vital role in supporting immunity and serves as a key regulator of the immune system (Samimi et al. 2019). The adenosine nucleoside has been extensively recognized for its role in immunity-mediated injuries, marked by significant white blood cell infiltration in the hepatic duct, elevated alanine aminotransferase levels, and considerable proliferation of self-antigens. It supports the normal immune function of tract cells and provides protection against autoimmune renal damage (Zhu et al. 2021).

AMPK's Role in Hunger, Satiety, and Energy Metabolism

The neural centers in the thalamus (or diencephalon), which monitor metabolic reactions, play a significant role in regulating food intake and maintaining energy balance. These centers respond to variations in nutrients and peptides, such as ghrelin and fat-derived proteins, which strongly influence hunger and satiety. Modulation of these peptides affects hunger, cravings, and satisfaction responses, thereby controlling food consumption. This critical regulator of energy balance is further influenced by orexigenic signals, such as ghrelin, which is chemically activated and plays a crucial role in modulating glycolysis and fatty acid oxidation. Additionally, chemicals derived from the cannabis plant or other organisms can activate adenine nucleosides. Estrogen, a female sex hormone, along with fat-derived hormones and peptide hormones released by pancreatic beta cells, which help maintain blood glucose levels, inhibits AMPK activity (Hurtado-Carneiro et al. 2020). Emerging evidence reveals that AMPK, the enzyme responsible for maintaining energy balance, plays a key role in regulating hunger, as well as the anabolic and catabolic effects of various protein-based substances. Several studies have demonstrated that the activation or inhibition of AMPK significantly influences food consumption. Diets high in fat content led to obesity and disrupt the activity of this vital energy regulator in the hypothalamus and skeletal muscles. It is hypothesized that higher energy intake reduces AMPK expression, resulting in significant weight gain, while lower energy intake elicits the opposite response (Hu et al. 2019).

Conclusion

The heterotrimeric structure of AMPK consists of an alpha catalytic subunit and two regulatory subunits, β and γ. This enzyme is present in all eukaryotic organisms with nucleated cells, with the α subunit playing a catalytic role. AMPKα2 is activated through a process that involves both alterations at the enzyme's binding site and enhanced phosphorylation. Nearly all eukaryotic cells carry the genetic code for the 5' AMP-activated protein kinase enzyme, except for intracellular parasites. These parasites, which spend the majority of their lifecycle inside a host organism, rely on the host's regulatory mechanisms for energy balance. Under normal conditions, energy intake and expenditure are tightly linked, maintaining energy balance and regulating body weight. However, variations in energy consumption and expenditure, such as those associated with weight loss, can disrupt this coordination, often leading to the restoration of the original body weight.

References

Al-Ishaq, R. K., Overy, A. J., & Büsselberg, D. (2020). Phytochemicals and gastrointestinal cancer: cellular mechanisms and effects to change cancer progression. *Biomolecules*, 10(1), 105.

Boone-Villa, D., Ventura-Sobrevilla, J., Aguilera-Mendez, A., & Jiménez-Villarreal, J. (2022). The effect of adenosine monophosphate-activated protein kinase on lipolysis in adipose tissue: an historical and comprehensive review. *Archives of Physiology and Biochemistry*, 128(1), 7-23.

Chen, H., Vanhoutte, P. M., & Leung, S. W. S. (2020). Vascular adenosine monophosphate-activated protein kinase: enhancer, brake or both? *Basic & Clinical Pharmacology & Toxicology*, 127(2), 81-91.

Choi, H. K., Park, S. H., Lee, J., & Hwang, J. T. (2023). Review of Patents for Anticancer Agents Targeting Adenosine Monophosphate-Activated Protein Kinase. *Journal of Medicinal Food*, 26(9), 605-615.

Ghiraldeli, L., Anderson, R., Pladna, K., & Pardee, T. S. (2022). Adenosine monophosphate activated protein kinase (AMPK) enhances chemotherapy response in acute myeloid leukemia (AML). *Cancer Letters*, 535, 215659.

Heden, T. D., Chow, L. S., Hughey, C. C., & Mashek, D. G. (2022). Regulation and role of glycophagy in skeletal muscle energy metabolism. *Autophagy*, 18(5), 1078-1089.

Hu, X., Wang, Y., Sheikhahmadi, A., Li, X., Buyse, J., Lin, H., & Song, Z. (2019). Effects of dietary energy level on appetite and central adenosine monophosphate-activated protein kinase (AMPK) in broilers. *Journal of Animal Science*, 97(11), 4488-4495.

Hurtado-Carneiro, V., Pérez-García, A., Alvarez, E., & Sanz, C. (2020). PAS kinase: A nutrient and energy sensor „master key" in the response to fasting/feeding conditions. *Frontiers in Endocrinology*, 11, 594053.

Hwang, H. Y., Shim, J. S., Kim, D., & Kwon, H. J. (2021). Antidepressant drug sertraline modulates AMPK-MTOR signaling-mediated autophagy via targeting mitochondrial VDAC1 protein. *Autophagy*, 17(10), 2783-2799.

Jiang, W., Hu, C., Chen, Y., Li, Y., Sun, X., Wu, H., Yang, R., Tang, Y., Niu, F., Wei, W., Sun, C., & Han, T. (2023). Dysregulation of the microbiota-brain axis during long-term exposure to polystyrene nanoplastics in rats and the protective role of dihydrocaffeic acid. *Science of the Total Environment*, 874, 162101.

Jin, L., Jin, F., Guo, S., Liu, W., Wei, B., Fan, H., Li, G., Zhang, X., Su, S., Li, R., Fang, D., Duan, C., & Li, X. (2022). Metformin inhibits NLR family pyrin domain containing 3 (NLRP)-relevant neuroinflammation via an adenosine-5′-monophosphate-activated protein kinase (AMPK)-dependent pathway to alleviate early brain injury after subarachnoid hemorrhage in mice. *Frontiers in Pharmacology*, 13, 796616.

Kalra, P., Khan, H., Singh, T. G., & Grewal, A. K. (2023). Mechanistic insights on impact of Adenosine monophosphate-activated protein kinase (AMPK) mediated signalling pathways on cerebral ischemic injury. *Neuroscience Research*, 190, 17-28.

Malik, N., Ferreira, B. I., Hollstein, P. E., Curtis, S. D., Trefts, E., Weiser Novak, S., Yu, J., Gilson, R., Hellberg, K., Fang, L., Sheridan, A., Hah, N., Shadel, G. S., Manor, U., & Shaw, R. J. (2023). Induction of lysosomal and mitochondrial biogenesis by AMPK phosphorylation of FNIP1. *Science*, 380(6642), eabj5559.

Muraleedharan, R., & Dasgupta, B. (2022). AMPK in the brain: its roles in glucose and neural metabolism. *The FEBS Journal*, 289(8), 2247-2262.

Naz, S., Mahmood, T., Ahsan, F., Rizvi, A. A., & Shamim, A. (2022). Repercussion of cAMP and EPAC in Memory and Signaling. *Drug Research*, 72(2), 65-71.

Rodríguez, C., Muñoz, M., Contreras, C., & Prieto, D. (2021). AMPK, metabolism, and vascular function. *The FEBS Journal*, 288(12), 3746-3771.

Samimi, Z., Kardideh, B., Zafari, P., Bahrehmand, F., Roghani, S. A., & Taghadosi, M. (2019). The impaired gene expression of adenosine monophosphate-activated kinase (AMPK), a key metabolic enzyme in leukocytes of newly diagnosed rheumatoid arthritis patients. *Molecular biology reports*, 46, 6353-6360.

Sholokh, A., & Klussmann, E. (2021). Local cyclic adenosine monophosphate signalling cascades—Roles and targets in chronic kidney disease. *Acta Physiologica*, 232(1), e13641.

Wu, S., & Zou, M. H. (2020). AMPK, mitochondrial function, and cardiovascular disease. *International Journal of Molecular Sciences*, 21(14), 4987.

Yan, Y., Li, M., Lin, J., Ji, Y., Wang, K., Yan, D., Shen, Y., Wang, W., Huang, Z., Jiang, H., Sun, H., & Qi, L. (2022). Adenosine monophosphate activated protein kinase contributes to skeletal muscle health through the control of mitochondrial function. *Frontiers in Pharmacology*, 13, 947387.

Yan, Z., Du, J., Zhao, R., Liu, X., Xu, J., Guo, L., & Liu, Y. (2024). Fructose Potentiates Bone Loss and Marrow Adipose Tissue Accumulation by Inhibiting Adenosine 5′-Monophosphate-Activated Protein Kinase in Mesenchymal Stem Cells. *Stem Cells*, 42(4), 374-384.

Yoon, Y., Park, M. K., Kim, K. H., & Lee, G. H. (2023). Black wheat extracts (arriheuk) regulate adipogenesis and lipolysis via adenosine monophosphate (AMP) activated protein kinase (AMPK)/sirtuin 1 (SIRT1) signaling pathways. *Foods*, 12(14), 2727.

Zhang, H., Zhu, Y., Suehiro, Y., Mitani, S., & Xue, D. (2023). AMPK–FOXO–IP3R signaling pathway mediates neurological and developmental defects caused by mitochondrial DNA mutations. *Proceedings of the National Academy of Sciences*, 120(36), e2302490120.

Zhang, S., Xie, Y., Yan, F., Zhang, Y., Yang, Z., Chen, Z., Zhao, Y., Huang, Z., Cai, L., & Deng, Z. (2022). Negative pressure wound therapy improves bone regeneration by promoting osteogenic differentiation via the AMPK-ULK1-autophagy axis. *Autophagy*, 18(9), 2229-2245.

Zhang, T., Xu, D., Trefts, E., Lv, M., Inuzuka, H., Song, G., Liu, M., Lu, J., Liu, J., Chu, C., Wang, M., Wang, H., Meng, H., Liu, H., Zhuang, Y., Xie, X., Dang, F., Guan, D., Men, Y., Jiang, S., Jiang, C., Dai, X., Liu, J., Wang, Z., Yan, P., Wang, J., Tu, Z., Babuta, M., Erickson, E., Hillis, A. L., Dibble, C. C., Asara, J. M., Szabo, G., Sicinski, P., Miao, J., Lee, Y., Pan, L., Shaw, R. J., Yuan, J., & Wei, W. (2023). Metabolic orchestration of cell death by AMPK-mediated phosphorylation of RIPK1. Science, 380(6652), 1372–1380.

Zhou, H. J., Kong, L. L., Zhu, L. X., Hu, X. Y., Busye, J., & Song, Z. G. (2021). Effects of cold stress on growth performance, serum biochemistry, intestinal barrier molecules, and adenosine monophosphate-activated protein kinase in broilers. *Animal*, 15(3), 100138.

Zhu, H., Liu, Z., An, J., Zhang, M., Qiu, Y., & Zou, M. H. (2021). Activation of AMPKα1 is essential for regulatory T cell function and autoimmune liver disease prevention. *Cellular & Molecular Immunology*, 18(12), 2609-2617.

Zhu, N., & Han, M. (2022). Roles of adenosine monophosphate-activated protein kinase (AMPK) in the kidney. *Chinese Medical Journal*, 135(4), 488-490.

Chapter 13

Muscarinic Acetylcholine Receptors (mAchRs): Modulating Insulin Secretion

Asavari V. Mahajan[1,*]
Sachin P. Borikar[2]
Deepali N. Tapre[3]
Kashmira K. Malusare[2]
and Shirish P. Jain[2]
[1]Department of Pharmaceutics, Dr. L. H. Hiranandani College of Pharmacy, Ulhasnagar, Maharashtra, India
[2]Department of Pharmacology, Rajarshi Shahu College of Pharmacy, Buldhana, Maharashtra, India
[3]Department of Pharmaceutical Chemistry, Rajarshi Shahu College of Pharmacy, Buldhana, Maharashtra, India

Abstract

Muscarinic acetylcholine (mACh) receptor activity regulates several essential physiological processes. The presence of M3 mACh receptors (mAChRs; M1-M5), which are linked to G proteins in the Gq family, in pancreatic β-cells has been previously reported. The ability of pancreatic β-cells to secrete insulin is significantly influenced by mAChRs, especially the M3 subtype. Through various processes, activation of these receptors by ACh or other muscarinic agonists increases the amount of insulin released in response to glucose. The complex regulation of insulin release in response to food intake is made possible by these G protein-coupled receptors, which bind to acetylcholine generated from parasympathetic nerve terminals. Insulin-containing vesicles are exocytosed when M3 receptor activation raises intracellular calcium levels through the phospholipase C (PLC), inositol trisphosphate (IP3), and diacylglycerol (DAG) signaling cascade. On the other hand, M2 receptors typically lower cyclic AMP (cAMP) levels, inhibiting insulin release. There are important clinical considerations regarding mAChRs' involvement in insulin secretion, especially in the management of diabetes. Recognizing the distinct functions and mechanisms of various mAChR subtypes serves as a foundation for developing tailored pharmaceutical treatments intended to augment or regulate insulin release. In addition to highlighting their potential as therapeutic targets for diabetes treatment, this chapter

* Corresponding Author's Email: asavari.mahajan@dlhhcop.org

In: Receptor-Targeted Therapies in Diabetes Mellitus
Editors: Ajmer Singh Grewal, Neelam Singh, Swati Verma et al.
ISBN: 979-8-89530-587-4

examines the current understanding of mAChRs in pancreatic β-cells and their role in regulating insulin secretion for diabetes management.

Keywords: muscarinic acetylcholine receptors; mAChRs, GPCRs, M3 receptor, acetylcholine, insulin secretion, diabetes management

Abbreviations

Ach	Acetylcholine
cAMP	cyclic AMP
CNS	Central nervous system
DAG	diacylglycerol
ER	Endoplasmic reticulum
GPCRs	G protein couple receptors
IP3	Inositol trisphosphate
mAChRs	Muscarinic acetylcholine receptors
Ach	Acetylcholine
PKC	Protein kinase C
PLC	Phospholipase C
T2D	Type 2 diabetes

Introduction

The inability of glucose to sufficiently trigger insulin secretion from pancreatic cells is a fundamental characteristic of type 2 diabetes (T2D) (Moller, 2001; Borikar et al. 2017). Typically, hyperglycemia arises as pancreatic β-cells gradually lose their ability to compensate for increasing insulin resistance. Even in the absence of elevated glucose levels, drugs like sulfonylureas can stimulate insulin release. Ideally, anti-diabetic medications would enhance insulin release in a glucose-dependent manner (Moller, 2001). Certain neurotransmitters and hormones, such as acetylcholine, are known to influence glucose-dependent insulin secretion. During the pre-absorptive phase, intrapancreatic parasympathetic (vagal) nerve terminals release acetylcholine. Although smaller in amount than the insulin released after food intake, this acetylcholine-mediated phase of insulin secretion plays a significant role in maintaining normal glucose tolerance (Ahren, 2000). In pancreatic β-cells, muscarinic acetylcholine receptors (mAChRs), specifically the M3 receptor subtype, regulate insulin secretion and glucose balance. Activation of M3 receptors triggers the phospholipase C (PLC) pathway, which mobilizes intracellular calcium and facilitates insulin release through the exocytosis of insulin molecules (Boschero et al. 1995; Igarashi-Hisayoshi et al. 2023). This process integrates glucose-stimulated insulin production with input from the parasympathetic nervous system, highlighting the physiological importance of mAChRs in maintaining metabolic homeostasis. mAChRs play a key role in understanding diabetes mellitus by influencing insulin resistance and impaired glucose tolerance. Current research focuses on modulating insulin secretion via mAChRs. Proper regulation of insulin release by pancreatic β-cells is essential for maintaining blood glucose homeostasis. While glucose and other nutrients are primary regulators, other factors, including neurotransmitters and hormones, also influence insulin release. Insulin secretion by β-cells in the pancreatic islets of Langerhans is tightly regulated by glucose and other nutrients in the bloodstream, and acetylcholine (ACh) from parasympathetic cholinergic input is a well-known regulatory factor (Honey et al. 1980; Brown, 2019). Although cholinergic regulation of insulin release has long been recognized, only recently has the regulatory mechanism, specifically the identity of the primary cholinergic receptor subtype involved, been identified (Haam and Yakel, 2017).

Muscarinic Acetylcholine Receptors

ACh is a neurotransmitter that activates mAChRs, a type of G-protein-coupled receptor (GPCR). These receptors play a vital role in regulating various physiological processes, including glandular secretion, heart rate, and smooth muscle contraction, and are distributed throughout both the peripheral and central nervous systems (Verma et al. 2018). mAChRs are essential for regulating glucose metabolism and insulin secretion, particularly in the context of diabetes treatment. There are five cholinergic muscarinic receptor subtypes, labeled M1 to M5. When activated by acetylcholine, the M3 subtype on pancreatic beta cells predominantly enhances insulin production. By increasing insulin release and modulating beta cell function, mAChRs in T2D help counteract insulin resistance (Moller, 2001; Igarashi-Hisayoshi et al. 2023). In terms of therapeutic potential, agonists that target these receptors may boost insulin secretion, while cholinergic drugs could improve insulin sensitivity and glucose metabolism. Current research aims to enhance glucose regulation in diabetic patients by developing combination therapies and precision medicine approaches. These strategies focus on minimizing side effects and optimizing treatment outcomes through the creation of specific mAChR modulators.

Structure and Function of mAChRs

mAChRs are a class of GPCRs activated by the neurotransmitter acetylcholine. This receptor family mediates various physiological functions, such as glandular secretion, heart rate regulation, smooth muscle contraction, and memory formation (Kumar, 2013). Structurally, mAChRs consist of a single polypeptide chain that spans the cell membrane seven times, forming seven transmembrane alpha-helices linked by extracellular and intracellular loops. When ACh binds to a receptor in a pocket created by the transmembrane helices, the extracellular loops and N-terminal domain facilitate ligand binding. The intracellular loops and C-terminal domain interact with G proteins and other intracellular signaling molecules. Each of the five known mAChR subtypes (M1 to M5) is encoded by a distinct gene, and these subtypes vary in their functional roles and tissue distribution (Thal et al. 2016). The five highly conserved subtypes (M1R to M5R) share 82-92% sequence similarity and 64-82% sequence identity in their transmembrane regions. Despite their structural similarities, each mAChR subtype associates with different heterotrimeric GTP-binding proteins (G proteins) and is distributed in distinct tissues, enabling unique signaling functions.

Importance of mAchRs in Various Physiological Processes

mAChRs play an essential role in numerous physiological functions and are particularly influential in the pathogenesis and management of diabetes through their impact on insulin production, glucose metabolism, and overall metabolic balance (Postic et al. 1999; Fernández-Cabezudo et al. 2019). In pancreatic β-cells, the M3 subtype of mAChRs stimulates insulin secretion in response to glucose. Acetylcholine released by the parasympathetic nervous system binds to these receptors to enhance insulin release and regulate blood glucose levels (Gilon and Henquin, 2001). mAChRs also support glucose homeostasis by influencing glycogenolysis and gluconeogenesis in the liver and by facilitating glucose uptake in peripheral tissues like muscle and fat, thereby improving insulin sensitivity and lowering blood glucose levels (Postic et al. 1999). Additionally, mAChRs affect gastrointestinal function by regulating the rate of gastric emptying, which can modulate postprandial blood glucose levels. Slower gastric emptying may benefit diabetic patients by reducing glucose absorption and helping to control post-meal blood sugar spikes (Zhu et al. 2019; Igarashi-Hisayoshi et al. 2023). Cardiovascular health and inflammation, both crucial in diabetes management, are also influenced by mAChRs, particularly the M2 and M3 subtypes, which regulate heart rate and vascular tone, potentially reducing cardiovascular risks associated with diabetes. Meanwhile, the M1 and M3 subtypes play a role in modulating inflammatory responses, a hallmark of diabetes, and may impact insulin resistance and β-cell function by contributing to the chronic low-grade inflammation observed in diabetic patients (Zhu et al. 2019; Satin and Kinard, 1998).

Muscarinic Acetylcholine Receptors in Pancreatic Beta Cells

Pancreatic β-cells

Pancreatic β-cells, located in the islets of Langerhans scattered throughout the pancreas, are vital for regulating blood glucose levels through their production and secretion of insulin. These small, polygonal cells make up approximately 65 to 80 percent of the islet cell population. When blood glucose levels rise, glucose transporter 2 (GLUT2) facilitates glucose entry into β-cells, where it is metabolized to generate ATP (Kumar, 2013). This process leads to cell depolarization, closing ATP-sensitive potassium channels and opening voltage-dependent calcium channels. The resulting influx of calcium ions triggers the release of insulin-containing vesicles into the bloodstream through exocytosis. Insulin then promotes glucose uptake by tissues and inhibits hepatic glucose production, maintaining glucose homeostasis. Dysfunction of β-cells is a key factor in diabetes: type 1 diabetes arises from immune-mediated destruction of these cells, while type 2 diabetes involves impaired β-cell function coupled with increased insulin resistance (Stringer et al. 2015).

Expression of mAChRs in β-cells

mAChRs are divided into five subtypes, M1 through M5, with M1, M3, and M5 being particularly relevant to pancreatic β-cells. Although M1 receptors are less common, they influence insulin secretion, especially when blood glucose levels are high. M3 receptors are the most prevalent subtype in β-cells and play a crucial role in insulin secretion. When activated by acetylcholine, they stimulate phospholipase C (PLC), leading to intracellular calcium release and triggering insulin exocytosis. Dysfunction or reduced expression of M3 receptors is associated with impaired insulin production, a key factor in T2D. Although M5 receptors are expressed at lower levels in β-cells compared to M3 receptors, they also have potential as therapeutic targets for managing conditions like diabetes mellitus, where insulin regulation is disrupted (Kulkarni et al. 1999; Wess, 1996).

Types of mAChRs Receptor (M1, M2, M3, M4 and M5)

mAChRs have a variety of functions in controlling physiological processes throughout the body. The neurological, cardiovascular, and gastrointestinal systems are affected by a range of disorders and ailments, making mAChRs important candidates for therapeutic interventions due to their tissue-specific distributions and unique signaling pathways (Hurst et al. 2013; Kruse et al. 2014; Borikar et al. 2024). Table 1 provides a comprehensive summary of the different types of mAChRs based on their location, function, mechanism, and effect on blood sugar levels.

Table 1 Summary of the different types of mAChRs

Receptor name	Location	Function	Mechanism	Effect on blood sugar level
M1	CNS, gastric parietal cells	Cognitive function, gastric acid secretion	Gq protein, activates PLC, increases IP3 and DAG, and increases intracellular Ca^{2+}	Decrease blood glucose level
M2	Heart, CNS	Decreases heart rate, decreases contractility, CNS effects	Gi protein, inhibits adenylate cyclase, decreases cAMP, opens K^+ channels, inhibits Ca^{2+} channels	Maintain baseline of insulin into body
M3	Smooth muscles (e.g., bladder, GI tract), exocrine glands	Smooth muscle contraction, glandular secretion	Gq protein, activates PLC, increases IP3 and DAG, and increases intracellular Ca^{2+}	Decrease blood glucose level
M4	CNS	Modulation of neurotransmitter release	Gi protein, inhibits adenylate cyclase, decreases cAMP	Maintain baseline of insulin into body
M5	CNS	Modulation of dopamine release	Gq protein, activates PLC, increases IP3 and DAG, and increases intracellular Ca^{2+}	Decrease blood glucose level

Metabolic Roles of β-cell Muscarinic Acetylcholine Receptors

Pancreatic β-cells, particularly those with M3 subtype mAChRs, play a central role in glucose homeostasis and insulin regulation. When acetylcholine binds to these receptors, it activates PLC, triggering a signaling cascade that increases diacylglycerol and inositol trisphosphate levels, which raises intracellular calcium levels (Kruse et al. 2014; Ito et al. 2019). Elevated calcium is crucial for promoting the exocytosis of insulin granules, thereby enhancing insulin release (Kahn, 2001). Dysregulation in mAChR signaling can lead to insufficient insulin secretion and impaired glucose regulation, contributing to diabetes and other metabolic disorders. Understanding the detailed mechanisms of β-cell mAChR function provides valuable insights into potential therapeutic strategies for boosting insulin production and managing diabetes, highlighting their essential role in maintaining metabolic balance (Moller, 2001; Gilon and Henquin, 2001; Öz-Arslan et al. 2024).

Roles of Different Muscarinic Receptors in β Cell Functions, Signalling in Insulin Secretion and Glucose Homeostasis

Insulin and glucagon work in tandem to maintain blood glucose levels, with mAChRs on pancreatic β-cells playing a key role in the tightly regulated pathways involved in insulin secretion and glucose homeostasis. Among these mAChRs, the M1 and M3 subtypes are most crucial for insulin secretion, binding ACh released by parasympathetic nerve terminals onto β-cells. When these receptors engage with Gq proteins, they activate PLC, which subsequently hydrolyzes phosphatidylinositol 4,5-bisphosphate to produce inositol trisphosphate (IP3) and diacylglycerol (DAG) (Kruse et al. 2014). IP3 binds to receptors on the endoplasmic reticulum (ER), releasing calcium ions (Ca^{2+}) into the cytoplasm. This calcium release from the ER opens voltage-dependent calcium channels (VDCCs) in the plasma membrane, allowing additional calcium influx from the extracellular space, which sustains the elevated intracellular calcium required for insulin exocytosis (Dalle et al. 2024). Meanwhile, M2 and M4 muscarinic receptors, through their interaction with Gi proteins, reduce adenylate cyclase activity, lower cAMP levels, and decrease protein kinase A (PKA) activity, all of which modulate insulin release.

Mechanisms of Insulin Secretion Modulation Muscarinic Acetylcholine Receptors

Physiological Role of mAchRs in Regulating Insulin Release

Promising therapeutic strategies for diabetes focus on enhancing insulin production and promoting the proliferation of pancreatic β-cells, processes that are regulated by signals from the vagal nerve. Pancreatic β-cells express GPCRs, including GPR40, which plays a significant role in augmenting glucose-stimulated insulin secretion (GSIS) in response to medium- or long-chain fatty acids. GPR40 agonists have emerged as potential therapeutic targets for treating T2D (Yamada et al. 2016). The pancreas, vital for regulating nutritional homeostasis, operates through distinct autonomic mechanisms controlling its endocrine and exocrine functions. Experimental evidence indicates that the parasympathetic and sympathetic nervous systems exert opposing effects on insulin secretion. During feeding, parasympathetic neural activity stimulates insulin production, whereas sympathetic activity during stress inhibits insulin release (Chandra & Liddle, 2020).

Signaling Pathways Activated by M3 Receptors

GPCRs facilitate the exchange of guanine nucleotides on Gαβγ heterotrimers, which include Gq family G proteins, thereby activating the PLCβ enzyme. The interaction between PLCβ and intermediate scaffolds often leads to the formation of physical complexes with GPCRs, enhancing the signaling process (Belmonte et al. 1998). Additionally, PLC plays a crucial role in regulating the efficacy of muscarinic receptor signaling through its GTPase-accelerating action, which kinetically scaffolds Gq to a GPCR, modulating the signaling process (Kan et al. 2014). The PLC family consists of six subfamily members that hydrolyze phosphatidylinositol 4,5-bisphosphate to generate two critical secondary messengers, IP3 and DAG, which are responsible for various cellular mechanisms. Table 2 presents the isoforms of PLC, their functions, and expressions (Sternweis & Smrcka, 1992). Glucose is the primary physiological trigger for insulin release, but acetylcholine plays a crucial role as an enhancer in insulin production. IP3 and DAG are key secondary messengers that mediate various biological activities. The potency and efficacy of potent agonists are similar in their ability to mobilize calcium ions (Ca2+) and induce IP3 synthesis. DAG, formed when phosphatidylinositol 4,5-bisphosphate (PIP2) is broken down by agonist stimulation, further enhances the enzyme's sensitivity (Owusu et al. 2020). The presence of extracellular calcium is necessary for the enhanced release of insulin induced by carbamoylcholine (CbCh) in pancreatic islets. Insulin is secreted by pancreatic β-cells through exocytosis, a process that depends on calcium ions and involves the release of secretory granules (Abdel-Latif, 1997). Glucose triggers a rapid rise in intracellular calcium concentration ($[Ca^{2+}]i$), primarily by facilitating the entry of calcium ions. Under normal physiological conditions, glucose can also stimulate the release of calcium ions from intracellular stores by promoting the breakdown of membrane phospholipids and the production of IP3, a potent trigger for calcium release (Sánchez-Andrés et al. 1988; Carvalho et al. 2018).

Table 2. PLC isoforms with functions and their expressions

PLC isoform	Functions/ Expressions
PLC- β1	It occurs in the cardiovascular system as well as the neural system, mostly in the cerebral cortex and hippocampus.
PLC-β2	Reflected in platelets and hematopoietic cells, which has the ability to control chemotaxis.
PLC-β3	Found in the liver, brain, cardiovascular system and parotid gland.
PLC- β4	It is mainly found in cerebellum and retina for photo transduction.
PLC-γ1	Produced by fibroblast growth factor, hepatocyte growth factor, epidermal growth factor, and platelet-derived growth factor.
PLC δ1	This PLC isoform is important for homeostasis and tissue metabolism.
PLC δ2	Plays essential roles in different tissue types and cells.

Inhibitory Role of M2 Receptors

Insulin is believed to play a crucial role in the development of airway inflammation. Furthermore, reduced function of M2 muscarinic receptors in neurons leads to heightened sensitivity to stimuli, a process regulated by insulin in the lungs. In individuals with diabetes, M2 muscarinic receptor function is impaired, with both high- and low-affinity regions of these receptors exhibiting increased binding affinity for antagonists in diabetic tissues (Abdel-Latif, 1997; Coulson et al. 2004).

Physiological and Pathophysiological Implications

Insulin Resistance and Impaired Glucose Tolerance

Insulin resistance is a key factor in the development of various metabolic diseases, including T2D. It occurs when insulin-targeted tissues become less responsive to normal insulin levels. As a primary and widespread contributor to metabolic disorders, insulin resistance represents a critical therapeutic target for managing conditions like diabetes. However, the precise mechanisms underlying insulin resistance remain unclear and are yet to be universally agreed upon (Lee et al. 2022).

Altered Parasympathetic Tone and Its Impact on Insulin Secretion

The central nervous system (CNS) plays a crucial role in regulating islet hormone release, cell development, and energy balance. Reduced parasympathetic function in individuals with diabetes and pre-diabetes has been linked to elevated HbA1c levels and aging. Interestingly, mild inflammatory markers do not appear to weaken the association between impaired glucose metabolism and parasympathetic nervous system activity (Hadad et al. 2022).

Therapeutic Potential and Current Research Findings

Pharmacological Modulation of mAchRs

Research on mAChR antagonists and subtype-specific mAChR activators highlights the critical role of the muscarinic cholinergic system in regulating normal cognitive function. These studies suggest that modulating mAChRs could provide a potential approach to reversing cognitive deficits commonly observed in neurological and psychiatric conditions, including schizophrenia and Alzheimer's disease (AD). This promising avenue of research offers hope for developing novel therapeutic strategies aimed at improving cognitive function in these disorders (Danao et al. 2021; Borikar et al. 2024).

Potential Therapies Targeting M3 Receptors

Medications targeting M3 receptors hold significant promise for diabetes treatment by enhancing insulin release from pancreatic β-cells. Selective M3 receptor agonists are being developed to specifically activate these receptors, thereby increasing insulin secretion without impacting other tissues or causing excessive side effects. Both animal studies and clinical trials have demonstrated that these agonists can improve insulin sensitivity and glucose tolerance

(Weston-Green et al. 2013; Bubser et al. 2012). Furthermore, the synergistic effects of combination therapies—such as M3 receptor agonists paired with other diabetes treatments like GLP-1 agonists and DPP-4 inhibitors—are being investigated to achieve even better glycemic control (Azua et al. 2011).

M2 Receptor Antagonists in Insulin Regulation

M2 receptor antagonists offer a promising approach for regulating insulin secretion and may serve as a valuable therapeutic option for managing diabetes. Unlike M3 receptors, which facilitate insulin release, M2 receptors inhibit insulin secretion from pancreatic β-cells. By blocking these inhibitory signals, M2 receptor antagonists can enhance insulin production, thereby improving glucose tolerance and overall glycemic control (Weston-Green et al. 2013; Grasiolli et al. 2007). Recent studies have demonstrated that M2 receptor antagonists can enhance insulin release in preclinical models, underscoring their potential as a treatment for diabetes. However, to minimize side effects, it is crucial to develop selective M2 receptor antagonists that specifically target β-cells without disrupting other cholinergic functions (Vasincu et al. 2023). As research advances, these antagonists may emerge as an essential component of diabetes therapy, particularly for patients with inadequate insulin production (Grasiolli et al. 2007).

Conclusion

mAChRs play a vital role in modulating insulin secretion and maintaining glucose homeostasis, with each subtype contributing distinctively. The M3 receptor is particularly critical for enhancing glucose-stimulated insulin secretion via key signaling pathways that increase intracellular calcium levels and promote insulin exocytosis. These pathways involve PLC, IP3, and DAG. Conversely, M2 receptors generally inhibit insulin release, underscoring the intricate balance of mAChR activity within the endocrine pancreas. A comprehensive understanding of these pathways is essential for elucidating their roles in both normal physiology and pathological conditions such as diabetes mellitus, where receptor dysregulation contributes to reduced insulin production and impaired glucose tolerance. Pharmacological modulation of mAChRs either by enhancing M3 receptor activity or inhibiting M2 receptor activity offers a promising approach to managing diabetes.

References

Abdel-Latif, A. A. (1997). The polyphosphoinositide signaling system. In *Principles of Medical Biology* (Vol. 7, pp. 469-486). Elsevier.

Ahrén, B. (2000). Autonomic regulation of islet hormone secretion–implications for health and disease. *Diabetologia*, 43(4), 393-410.

Azua, I. R., Gautam, D., Guettier, J. M., & Wess, J. (2011). Novel insights into the function of β-cell M3 muscarinic acetylcholine receptors: Therapeutic implications. *Trends in Endocrinology & Metabolism*, 22(2), 74-80.

Babic, T., & Travagli, R. A. (2016). Neural control of the pancreas. *Pancreapedia: The Exocrine Pancreas Knowledge Base.*

Balakrishnan, S., Mathew, J., Antony, S., & Paulose, C. S. (2009). Muscarinic M1, M3 receptors function in the brainstem of streptozotocin induced diabetic rats: Their role in insulin secretion from the pancreatic islets as a function of age. *European Journal of Pharmacology*, 608(1-3), 14-22.

Belmonte, K. E., Fryer, A. D., & Costello, R. W. (1998). Role of insulin in antigen-induced airway eosinophilia and neuronal M2 muscarinic receptor dysfunction. *Journal of Applied Physiology*, 85(5), 1708-1718.

Borikar, S. P., Kallewar, N. G., Mahapatra, D. K., & Dumore, N. G. (2018). Dried flower powder combination of Clitoria ternatea and Punica granatum demonstrated analogous anti-hyperglycemic potential as compared with standard drug metformin: *In vivo* study in Sprague Dawley rats. *Journal of Applied Pharmaceutical Science*, 8(11), 075-079.

Borikar, S. P., Kallewar, N. G., Mahapatra, D. K., Dumore, N. G., & Danao, K. R. (2017). Combined flower decoction of Clitoria ternatea and Punica granatum expressed comparable hypoglycemic activity with that of metformin: *In vivo* study. *International Journal of Pharmaceutical Sciences and Research*, 2(5), 4-7.

Borikar, S. P., Sonawane, D. S., Tapre, D. N., & Jain, S. P. (2024). Exploring the neuropharmacological potential of empagliflozin on nootropic and scopolamine-induced amnesic model of Alzheimer's like conditions in rats. *International Journal of Neuroscience*, 2024, 1-13.

Boschero, A. C., Szpak-Glasman, M., Carneiro, E. M., Bordin, S., Paul, I., Rojas, E., & Atwater, I. (1995). Oxotremorine-m potentiation of glucose-induced insulin release from rat islets involves M3 muscarinic receptors. *American Journal of Physiology-Endocrinology and Metabolism*, 268(2), E336-E342.

Brown, D. A. (2019). Acetylcholine and cholinergic receptors. *Brain and Neuroscience Advances*, 3, 2398212818820506.

Bubser, M., Byun, N., Wood, M. R., & Jones, C. K. (2012). Muscarinic receptor pharmacology and circuitry for the modulation of cognition. *Muscarinic Receptors*, 208, 121-166.

Carvalho, D. S., de Almeida, A. A., Borges, A. F., & Campos, D. V. (2018). Treatments for diabetes mellitus type II: new perspectives regarding the possible role of calcium and cAMP interaction. *European Journal of Pharmacology*, 830, 9-16.

Chandra, R., & Liddle, R. A. (2020). *Regulation of pancreatic secretion.* Pancreapedia: The Exocrine Pancreas Knowledge Base.

Coulson, F. R., Jacoby, D. B., & Fryer, A. D. (2004). Insulin regulates neuronal M2 muscarinic receptor function in the ileum of diabetic rats. *Journal of Pharmacology and Experimental Therapeutics*, 308(2), 760-766.

Dalle, S., & Abderrahmani, A. (2024). Receptors and Signaling Pathways Controlling Beta-Cell Function and Survival as Targets for Anti-Diabetic Therapeutic Strategies. *Cells*, 13(15), 1244.

Danao, K., Kodape, Y., Mahapatra, D., Borikar, S., & Karande, N. (2021). Highlights on synthetic, natural, and hybrid cholinesterase inhibitors for effective treatment of Alzheimer's disease: A review. *International Journal of Current Research and Review*, 13(11), 27.

Fernández-Cabezudo, M. J., George, J. A., Bashir, G., Mohamed, Y. A., Al-Mansori, A., Qureshi, M. M., & Al-Ramadi, B. K. (2019). Involvement of acetylcholine receptors in cholinergic pathway-mediated protection against autoimmune diabetes. *Frontiers in Immunology*, 10, 1038.

Gautam, D., Han, S. J., Heard, T. S., Cui, Y., Miller, G., Bloodworth, L., & Wess, J. (2005). Cholinergic stimulation of amylase secretion from pancreatic acinar cells studied with muscarinic acetylcholine receptor mutant mice. *Journal of Pharmacology and Experimental Therapeutics*, 313(3), 995-1002.

Gautam, D., Jeon, J., Li, J. H., Han, S. J., Hamdan, F. F., Cui, Y., & Wess, J. (2008). Metabolic roles of the M3 muscarinic acetylcholine receptor studied with M3 receptor mutant mice: A review. *Journal of Receptors and Signal Transduction*, 28(1-2), 93-108.

Gilon, P., & Henquin, J. C. (2001). Mechanisms and physiological significance of the cholinergic control of pancreatic β-cell function. *Endocrine Reviews*, 22(5), 565-604.

Grassiolli, S., Gravena, C., & de Freitas Mathias, P. C. (2007). Muscarinic M2 receptor is active on pancreatic islets from hypothalamic obese rat. *European Journal of Pharmacology*, 556(1-3), 223-228.

Haam, J., & Yakel, J. L. (2017). Cholinergic modulation of the hippocampal region and memory function. *Journal of Neurochemistry*, 142, 111-121.

Hadad, R., Akobe, S. F., Weber, P., Madsen, C. V., Larsen, B. S., Madsbad, S., Nielsen, O. W., Dominguez, M. H., Haugaard, S. B., & Sajadieh, A. (2022). Parasympathetic tonus in type 2 diabetes and pre-diabetes and its clinical implications. *Scientific Reports*, 12(1), 18020.

Honey, R. N., & Weir, G. C. (1980). Acetylcholine stimulates insulin, glucagon, and somatostatin release in the perfused chicken pancreas. *Endocrinology*, 107(4), 1065-1068.

Hurst, R., Rollema, H., & Bertrand, D. (2013). Nicotinic acetylcholine receptors: From basic science to therapeutics. *Pharmacology & Therapeutics*, 137(1), 22-54.

Igarashi-Hisayoshi, Y., Ihara, E., Bai, X., Higashi, C., Ikeda, H., Tanaka, Y., & Ogawa, Y. (2023). Determination of Region-Specific Roles of the M3 Muscarinic Acetylcholine Receptor in Gastrointestinal Motility. *Digestive Diseases and Sciences*, 68(2), 439-450.

Ito, Y., Kaji, M., Sakamoto, E., & Terauchi, Y. (2019). The beneficial effects of a muscarinic agonist on pancreatic β-cells. *Scientific Reports*, 9(1), 16180.

Kahn, S. E. (2001). The importance of β-cell failure in the development and progression of type 2 diabetes. *The Journal of Clinical Endocrinology & Metabolism*, 86(9), 4047-4058.

Kan, W., Adjobo-Hermans, M., Burroughs, M., Faibis, G., Malik, S., Tall, G. G., & Smrcka, A. V. (2014). M3 muscarinic receptor interaction with phospholipase C β3 determines its signaling efficiency. *Journal of Biological Chemistry*, 289(16), 11206-11218.

Kruse, A. C., Kobilka, B. K., Gautam, D., Sexton, P. M., Christopoulos, A., & Wess, J. (2014). Muscarinic acetylcholine receptors: novel opportunities for drug development. *Nature Reviews Drug Discovery*, 13(7), 549-560.

Kulkarni, R. N., Brüning, J. C., Winnay, J. N., Postic, C., Magnuson, M. A., & Kahn, C. R. (1999). Tissue-specific knockout of the insulin receptor in pancreatic β cells creates an insulin secretory defect similar to that in type 2 diabetes. *Cell*, 96(3), 329-339.

Kumar, A., Goel, M. K., Jain, R. B., Khanna, P., & Chaudhary, V. (2013). India towards diabetes control: Key issues. *The Australasian Medical Journal*, 6(10), 524.

Lee, S. H., Park, S. Y., & Choi, C. S. (2022). Insulin resistance: from mechanisms to therapeutic strategies. *Diabetes & Metabolism Journal*, 46(1), 15-37.

Moller, D. E. (2001). New drug targets for type 2 diabetes and the metabolic syndrome. *Nature*, 414(6865), 821-827.

Owusu Obeng, E., Rusciano, I., Marvi, M. V., Fazio, A., Ratti, S., Follo, M. Y., Xian, J., Manzoli, L., Billi, A. M., Mongiorgi, S., Ramazzotti, G., & Cocco, L. (2020). Phosphoinositide-dependent signaling in cancer: a focus on phospholipase C isozymes. International Journal of Molecular Sciences, 21(7), 2581.

Öz-Arslan, D., Durer, Z. A., & Kan, B. (2024). G protein-coupled receptor-mediated autophagy in health and disease. *British Journal of Pharmacology*, online ahead of print.

Postic, C., Shiota, M., Niswender, K. D., Jetton, T. L., Chen, Y., Moates, J. M., & Magnuson, M. A. (1999). Dual roles for glucokinase in glucose homeostasis as determined by liver and pancreatic β cell-specific gene knock-outs using Cre recombinase. *Journal of Biological Chemistry*, 274(1), 305-315.

Renuka, T. R., Robinson, R., & Paulose, C. S. (2006). Increased insulin secretion by muscarinic M1 and M3 receptor function from rat pancreatic islets *in vitro*. *Neurochemical Research*, 31, 313-320.

Sánchez-Andrés, J. V., Ripoll, C., & Soria, B. (1988). Evidence that muscarinic potentiation of insulin release is initiated by an early transient calcium entry. *FEBS Letters*, 231(1), 143-147.

Satin, L. S., & Kinard, T. A. (1998). Neurotransmitters and their receptors in the islets of Langerhans of the pancreas: what messages do acetylcholine, glutamate, and GABA transmit? *Endocrine*, 8, 213-223.

Sternweis, P. C., & Smrcka, A. V. (1992). Regulation of phospholipase C by G proteins. *Trends in Biochemical Sciences*, 17(12), 502-506.

Stringer, D. M., Zahradka, P., & Taylor, C. G. (2015). Glucose transporters: cellular links to hyperglycemia in insulin resistance and diabetes. *Nutrition Reviews*, 73(3), 140-154.

Vasincu, A., Rusu, R. N., Ababei, D. C., Neamţu, M., Arcan, O. D., Macadan, I., & Bild, V. (2023). Exploring the therapeutic potential of cannabinoid receptor antagonists in inflammation, diabetes mellitus, and obesity. *Biomedicines*, 11(6), 1667.

Verma, S., Kumar, A., Tripathi, T., & Kumar, A. (2018). Muscarinic and nicotinic acetylcholine receptor agonists: current scenario in Alzheimer's disease therapy. *Journal of Pharmacy and Pharmacology*, 70(8), 985-993.

Wess, J. (1996). Molecular biology of muscarinic acetylcholine receptors. *Critical Reviews in Neurobiology*, 10(1), 69-99.

Weston-Green, K., Huang, X. F., & Deng, C. (2013). Second generation antipsychotic-induced type 2 diabetes: a role for the muscarinic M3 receptor. *CNS Drugs*, 27, 1069-1080.

Yamada, H., Yoshida, M., Ito, K., Dezaki, K., Yada, T., Ishikawa, S. E., & Kakei, M. (2016). Potentiation of glucose-stimulated insulin secretion by the GPR40–PLC–TRPC pathway in pancreatic β-cells. *Scientific Reports*, 6(1), 25912.

Zhu, L., Rossi, M., Cohen, A., Pham, J., Zheng, H., Dattaroy, D., & Wess, J. (2019). Allosteric modulation of β-cell M3 muscarinic acetylcholine receptors greatly improves glucose homeostasis in lean and obese mice. *Proceedings of the National Academy of Sciences*, 116(37), 18684-18690.

Chapter 14

Fructose 1,6-Bisphosphatase: Role, Mechanism and Therapeutic Potential

Yash Janve[1,*]
Jagdish Kakadiya[1]
and Kamalpreet Kaur[2]
[1]Department of Pharmacology, Parul Institute of Pharmaceutical Education and Research, Parul University, Limda, Vadodara, Gujarat, India
[2]Guru Gobind Singh College of Pharmacy, Yamuna Nagar, Haryana, India

Abstract

Fructose 1,6-bisphosphatase (FBPase) plays a key role in the metabolic process of gluconeogenesis, which involves the synthesis of glucose from substrates other than carbohydrates. FBPase catalyzes the hydrolysis of fructose 1,6-bisphosphate (FBP) to fructose 6-phosphate and inorganic phosphate, a critical step that bypasses the irreversible reaction of phosphofructokinase in glycolysis. This regulation helps maintain metabolic control, with fructose 2,6-bisphosphate and AMP acting as key regulators of FBPase activity in response to the cell's energy status, balancing glycolysis and gluconeogenesis. FBPase is a homotetrameric enzyme, with each of its four subunits contributing to the formation of a new catalytic site on the active site. The enzyme's structure and phosphorylation status tightly regulate glucose biosynthesis, ensuring precise metabolic control. In metabolic diseases like diabetes mellitus, characterized by hyperglycemia due to increased gluconeogenesis, elevated FBPase activity has been implicated. Given its critical role, FBPase is an attractive target for modulating blood glucose levels in therapeutic interventions. Small molecule inhibitors (SMIs) of FBPase have shown potential as a new approach for diabetes management in preclinical models. These inhibitors can enhance glycemic control in conjunction with other treatments by suppressing hepatic glucose production. Moreover, further understanding of FBPase's role and regulation, along with research into its inhibitors, could lead to improved strategies for managing metabolic disorders.

Keywords: gluconeogenesis, fructose 1,6-bisphoshatase, FBPase, diabetes, enzyme inhibition, metabolic regulation, hyperglycemia

---

* Corresponding Author's Email: yash.subhashjanve@gmail.com

In: Receptor-Targeted Therapies in Diabetes Mellitus
Editors: Ajmer Singh Grewal, Neelam Singh, Swati Verma et al.
ISBN: 979-8-89530-587-4

Abbreviations

AMP	Adenosine Monophosphate
ATP	Adenosine Triphosphate
cAMP	Cyclic AMP
DDS	Drug Delivery System
DHAP	Dihydroxyacetone Phosphate
F2,6BP	Fructose 2,6-bisphosphate
FBP	Fructose 1,6-bisphosphate
FBPase	Fructose 1,6-bisphosphatase
G6Pase	Glucose-6-Phosphatase
PEPCK	Phosphoenolpyruvate Carboxykinase
PFK-2	Phosphofructokinase-2
PKA	Protein Kinase A
PTH	Parathyroid Hormone
SMIs	Small Molecule Inhibitors

Introduction

Fructose 1,6-bisphosphatase (FBPase) is a key enzyme in the gluconeogenic pathway (Timson, 2019). It is responsible for converting fructose-1,6-bisphosphate (FBP) to fructose-6-phosphate, a reaction that enables the production of glucose from non-carbohydrate substrates. This process ensures a continuous supply of glucose to vital organs, such as the brain and red blood cells, particularly during fasting or intense physical activity when glycogen stores are depleted. FBPase bypasses the irreversible step of glycolysis catalyzed by phosphofructokinase (PFK), hydrolyzing FBP into fructose-6-phosphate and inorganic phosphate, thereby supporting gluconeogenesis, the body's natural mechanism for glucose production (Kuznetsova et al. 2010). The regulation of FBPase is critical due to its central role in gluconeogenesis (Icard et al. 2021). The enzyme is tightly controlled by cellular energy status indicators. Key regulators include fructose 2,6-bisphosphate (F2,6BP) and adenosine monophosphate (AMP). F2,6BP, which is controlled by the bifunctional enzyme phosphofructokinase-2/fructose-2,6-bisphosphatase (PFK-2/FBPase-2), is a potent allosteric inhibitor of FBPase. High levels of F2,6BP inhibit FBPase, promoting glycolysis and limiting gluconeogenesis, while low levels of F2,6BP enhance FBPase activity, favoring gluconeogenesis. Additionally, AMP inhibits FBPase activity when cellular energy is low, thereby preventing glucose production during energy-deficient states. Understanding the regulation of FBPase is especially important in the context of metabolic disorders such as diabetes mellitus. Hyperglycemia, a hallmark of diabetes, is linked to alterations in FBPase activity. In type 1 diabetes, insulin deficiency leads to uncontrolled gluconeogenesis and elevated FBPase activity. In type 2 diabetes, impaired regulation of gluconeogenesis results in sustained hyperglycemia, with elevated FBPase activity contributing to the persistence of high blood glucose levels (Xu et al. 2021). Targeting FBPase with small molecule inhibitors (SMIs) offers a promising therapeutic approach for managing diabetes and controlling blood glucose levels. These inhibitors selectively target FBPase to reduce hepatic glucose production, thereby lowering blood glucose levels.

Preclinical studies have demonstrated the efficacy of FBPase inhibitors in animal models, suggesting their potential as adjunctive therapies alongside current treatments. This presents an alternative strategy for managing hyperglycemia (Gizak et al. 2013). This chapter will explore the structure, regulation, and activity of FBPase, focusing on its role in glucose metabolism. It will also discuss the therapeutic potential of FBPase inhibitors and the impact of FBPase dysregulation in the development of diabetes mellitus. The aim is to provide a comprehensive overview of FBPase's involvement in metabolic processes and its potential for therapeutic intervention in metabolic diseases.

Structure and Functions of Fructose 1,6-Bisphosphatase

Molecular Structure

FBPase is a homotetramer, composed of four similar subunits, each contributing to the formation of the enzyme's active site (Pirovich et al. 2021). The quaternary structure is crucial for regulating the enzyme's activity. The active sites are located at the interfaces between subunits, and control over the catalytic process is exerted through these sites. Structural stability is maintained by various non-covalent interactions, including hydrophobic interactions, non-specific ionic interactions, and hydrogen bonding. Advanced techniques such as NMR spectroscopy and X-ray crystallography have been pivotal in determining the precise positioning of subunits and identifying regulatory and catalytic residues. The hydrolysis reaction that drives gluconeogenesis occurs within the catalytic domain of FBPase. Each subunit of the enzyme consists of 331 amino acids in humans. The active site of FBPase includes a metal ion, typically Mg^{2+}, which is crucial for transition state stabilization and enhancing the catalytic process. Additionally, a binding pocket for FBP is present, facilitating substrate interaction. Structural analysis has revealed several conserved residues essential for catalysis, particularly those involved in substrate binding and transition state formation. Any alteration in these key residues can significantly impact the enzyme's activity (Bu et al. 2018). FBPase's regulation is further influenced by its homotetrameric structure. The presence of covalent subunits plays a role in its regulatory mechanisms. The enzyme's functionality is intricately linked to interactions at the allosteric regulation site. Allosteric effectors can induce conformational shifts, causing the enzyme to move between different states based on cellular conditions. Due to its structural flexibility, FBPase can rapidly adjust to changes in the cellular environment, ensuring that gluconeogenesis remains tightly controlled (Bu et al. 2018).

Mechanism of Action

FBPase plays a critical role in gluconeogenesis by catalyzing the conversion of FBP into fructose-6-phosphate and inorganic phosphate. This reaction is particularly important during fasting or carbohydrate scarcity, such as during intense physical activity, when glucose stores are low. FBPase's structure and catalytic function are highly regulated to efficiently maintain metabolic balance (Park et al. 2020). FBPase relies on a metal ion, typically Mg^{2+}, within its active site to facilitate a two-step hydrolysis process, stabilizing the transition state and enhancing the reaction rate. The Mg^{2+} ion is crucial for enzyme function, as it stabilizes the developing negative charges and interacts with the phosphate groups on FBP. This coordination supports substrate binding and precise positioning within the active site.

The reaction begins with the formation of a transient enzyme-substrate complex between FBP and FBPase. Upon binding FBP, the enzyme undergoes a conformational shift, repositioning essential catalytic residues to interact more effectively with the substrate. This shift ensures that the metal ion and substrate are optimally positioned for catalysis. In the subsequent step, the complex breaks down to release fructose-6-phosphate and inorganic phosphate. Catalysis is facilitated by primary and secondary amines in the active site, along with the metal ion. The phosphate ester bond is cleaved by an enzyme-activated water molecule, which initiates a nucleophilic attack on the phosphate group. Throughout this process, the metal ion stabilizes the negative charges created, ensuring an efficient and timely reaction. The precise synchronization of these stages is essential for effective gluconeogenesis (Gupta et al. 2021).

Regulatory Mechanisms

FBPase activity, essential for maintaining metabolic homeostasis, is regulated by multiple feedback mechanisms. Two key allosteric effectors in this regulation are F2,6BP and AMP. F2,6BP acts as a competitive inhibitor of FBPase by binding to an allosteric site, which reduces the enzyme's affinity for FBP and induces a conformational change. This regulation is crucial as it prevents a futile cycle of simultaneous glucose synthesis and breakdown, effectively stalling gluconeogenesis when glycolysis is prioritized. AMP, another important regulator of FBPase, signals low cellular energy levels and acts as a competitive inhibitor by binding to an allosteric site on the enzyme. This inhibition ensures that glucose synthesis is limited to conditions where energy is needed, such as during fasting or intense physical exertion. By restricting gluconeogenesis to times of necessity, AMP helps maintain energy balance within the cell (Hanson and Owen, 2013).

Therapeutic Implications

Developing effective therapeutic inhibitors for FBPase requires a thorough understanding of the enzyme's structure and regulatory mechanisms. In diabetes mellitus, FBPase is overexpressed, contributing to hyperglycemia, which makes it a promising target for anti-diabetic drugs. *In vitro* studies suggest that SMIs of FBPase could slow glucose production in the liver, helping to regulate blood sugar levels in diabetic patients. Depending on the level of inhibition needed, FBPase inhibitors can be designed to target either the enzyme's active site or its allosteric site. Insights from structural studies have facilitated the development of more selective and potent inhibitors. These inhibitors may enhance patient outcomes by offering an additional means of blood glucose control alongside traditional diabetes treatments. FBPase plays a fundamental role in gluconeogenesis, and its structure and function are intricately designed to ensure efficient glucose production, which is essential for metabolic stability. Its regulation through allosteric effectors, along with the metabolic imbalances seen in disorders like diabetes, underscores the enzyme's therapeutic potential. Although some aspects of

FBPase's structure and function remain unclear, ongoing research into these areas is advancing the development of pharmacological inhibitors that could significantly aid in managing metabolic disorders (Kaur et al. 2017).

Regulation of FBPase

Allosteric Regulation

FBPase activity is finely tuned by various metabolites that reflect the cell's energy charge, modulating the enzyme through allosteric regulation. A major endogenous inhibitor of FBPase is F2,6BP, which decreases FBPase activity and ensures that glycolysis and gluconeogenesis do not occur simultaneously. Elevated levels of F2,6BP encourage glycolysis and inhibit gluconeogenesis by both suppressing FBPase and enhancing PFK activity. Conversely, when F2,6BP levels are low, FBPase activity rises, facilitating gluconeogenesis. Another critical regulator is AMP, which binds to an allosteric site on FBPase, inhibiting it. During low-energy states, AMP levels increase, signaling the need to conserve glucose by halting its synthesis. AMP prevents unnecessary glucose production when rapid energy is required through glycolysis, thereby inhibiting FBPase. Together, F2,6BP and AMP align FBPase activity with the cell's energy needs. Additionally, citrate plays a regulatory role by activating FBPase when energy levels are high. This action prompts gluconeogenesis, allowing the conversion of surplus metabolites into glucose for storage or other biosynthetic pathways (Yang et al. 2016).

Hormonal Regulation

FBPase regulation is also influenced by hormonal signals that align the body's metabolic processes with physiological needs. Insulin, released in response to elevated blood glucose levels, suppresses FBPase production and activity (Berg, 2019). By promoting glucose uptake and glycolysis in tissues, insulin reduces the need for gluconeogenesis, thus helping to manage blood glucose levels and counteract hyperglycemia through FBPase inhibition. In contrast, glucagon, released during fasting or low blood glucose levels, promotes gluconeogenesis by upregulating both FBPase expression and activity. This hormone aids in sustaining blood glucose homeostasis by stimulating the formation of glucose from non-carbohydrate sources when energy reserves are low. Cortisol, a glucocorticoid hormone, also affects FBPase regulation, particularly under stress or fasting conditions, when its levels rise. Cortisol enhances FBPase and other gluconeogenic enzymes, ensuring sufficient glucose availability to meet the body's increased energy demands during stress. Thus, the interplay between insulin, glucagon, and cortisol finely regulates FBPase, reflecting the enzyme's crucial role in maintaining glucose homeostasis across varying physiological states (Berg, 2019).

FBPase in Gluconeogenesis and Glycolysis

Role in Gluconeogenesis

FBPase is a crucial enzyme in gluconeogenesis, the process that forms glucose from non-carbohydrate molecules. This enzyme plays a key role during fasting, prolonged physical activity, or low carbohydrate intake, when the body needs to produce glucose for energy. A primary regulatory step in gluconeogenesis is the hydrolysis of FBP by FBPase, which releases fructose 6-phosphate and inorganic phosphate. This step bypasses the irreversible glycolytic reaction catalyzed by PFK and allows glucose synthesis from precursors like lactate, glycerol, and certain amino acids. FBPase is regulated by various hormonal signals that adjust its activity based on the body's energy needs. During periods of low blood sugar, the pancreas releases glucagon, which promotes gluconeogenesis. In liver cells, glucagon increases cAMP levels, activating PKA. PKA reduces F2,6BP levels, an allosteric inhibitor of FBPase, by phosphorylating and inhibiting PFK-2. This reduction in F2,6BP enhances FBPase activity, facilitating glucose production. Similarly, the stress hormone cortisol increases the expression of FBPase and other gluconeogenic enzymes, boosting glucose availability in stressful or fasting conditions. Conversely, insulin suppresses FBPase activity in response to high blood glucose, reducing gluconeogenesis while enhancing glucose uptake and storage. Insulin stimulates phosphoprotein phosphatases, which dephosphorylate PFK-2, increasing F2,6BP levels. High F2,6BP concentrations inhibit FBPase, ensuring that glucose is stored rather than produced unnecessarily. Insulin thus promotes glycogen formation and helps maintain blood glucose levels within a healthy range. FBPase is also regulated by cellular energy status and substrate availability. High concentrations of substrates such as lactate, glycerol, and amino acids can stimulate gluconeogenesis. Lactate, a byproduct of anaerobic glycolysis, is transported to the liver, where it is converted to pyruvate and incorporated into the gluconeogenic pathway. Glycerol, released during triglyceride breakdown, is phosphorylated to form DHAP, another gluconeogenic intermediate. Additionally, alanine is converted to pyruvate through transamination, further fueling gluconeogenesis. The cell's energy status, as indicated by AMP and ATP levels, also regulates FBPase. High AMP levels, signaling low energy, bind to an allosteric site on FBPase, inhibiting it and preventing excess glucose production when energy is scarce. This mechanism directs glucose toward glycolysis and oxidative phosphorylation to produce ATP. Conversely, a high ATP/low AMP ratio signals a high-energy state, promoting glucose synthesis and storage through gluconeogenesis (Gupta et al. 2024).

Interaction with Glycolysis

Glycolysis and gluconeogenesis must be reciprocally regulated to maintain metabolic balance. This means that glycolysis, the breakdown of glucose to produce energy, must counterbalance gluconeogenesis, the synthesis of glucose from non-carbohydrate sources. This reciprocal control prevents these processes from occurring simultaneously in the same cell, thus avoiding energy waste. Key enzymes, including FBPase (in gluconeogenesis) and PFK (in glycolysis), are central to this regulation. F2,6BP, a potent allosteric effector, promotes glycolysis by activating PFK while inhibiting FBPase, ensuring that only one pathway is active at a time. The regulation of these enzymes is also influenced by sex hormones and other hormonal and metabolic signals. For instance, elevated AMP levels, indicative of low cellular energy, enhance glycolysis to prioritize energy production and further suppress gluconeogenesis. Hormones such as glucagon and insulin play key roles in regulating these pathways. Glucagon, released during fasting, promotes gluconeogenesis by stimulating FBPase and inhibiting PFK. In contrast, insulin, secreted in response to high blood glucose, enhances glycolysis by activating PFK and inhibiting FBPase, supporting glucose utilization over synthesis. This intricate hormonal regulation maintains metabolic homeostasis by promoting glucose production during fasting and its utilization during feeding. Additional hormones, such as parathyroid hormone (PTH), alongside insulin, contribute to the fine-tuning of FBPase and PFK activities, aligning with the body's energy requirements. This coordination allows cells to alternate effectively between glucose synthesis and utilization, depending on energy demands and substrate availability (Li et al. 2022).

FBPase and Metabolic Diseases

Diabetes mellitus is a chronic metabolic disorder characterized by hyperglycemia due to insufficient insulin, impaired insulin action, or both. This condition often affects gluconeogenesis, leading to elevated blood glucose levels. FBPase plays a crucial role in gluconeogenesis, and its activity is typically regulated by insulin. In type 1 diabetes, where insulin production is insufficient, unregulated gluconeogenesis occurs due to the lack of insulin's inhibitory effect on FBPase, significantly increasing the risk of hyperglycemia. Since the body cannot adequately regulate glucose production, patients with type 1 diabetes rely on insulin therapy for glycemic control. In type 2 diabetes, insulin's effectiveness is reduced, leading to insufficient suppression of gluconeogenesis and increased FBPase activity. This condition exacerbates hyperglycemia, as the liver continues to produce glucose despite high blood sugar levels. Studies indicate that excessive FBPase activity in the liver is a key factor in the dysregulation of glucose in diabetes, making FBPase an attractive target for antidiabetic therapies. Inhibiting FBPase has been proposed as a strategy to reduce hepatic glucose production and improve blood glucose control. SMIs targeting FBPase have shown promise in preclinical studies, lowering blood glucose levels by reducing gluconeogenesis. This approach could complement existing diabetes treatments, enhancing glycemic management for patients. Given FBPase's role in gluconeogenesis, effective and selective FBPase inhibitors hold significant potential for improving diabetes management (Xu et al. 2020).

Therapeutic Potential of FBPase Inhibitors

The development SMIs targeting FBPase is a promising approach for diabetes treatment, aiming to reduce blood glucose levels. These inhibitors have shown encouraging results in prediabetic models, improving glycemic control. To design effective FBPase inhibitors, understanding the enzyme's structure and function is essential. Potent inhibitors have been discovered through computational modeling, structure-based drug design, and high-throughput screening of chemical databases, leading to the identification of several compounds with strong FBPase inhibition. However, selectivity remains a significant challenge in developing these inhibitors. To maximize therapeutic efficacy and minimize side effects, inhibitors must selectively target FBPase without affecting other phosphatases or enzymes involved in gluconeogenesis. Achieving greater selectivity and potency in FBPase inhibitors will enhance their potential for diabetes treatment (Zhang et al. 2019).

Future Directions

The future of FBPase research is likely to focus on identifying novel inhibitors with improved safety profiles and efficacy (Rines et al. 2016). Computational modeling and structural biology will remain essential for the development and optimization of these inhibitors. A deeper understanding of the enzyme's structure and function will be crucial for designing more selective and potent inhibitors. The incorporation of FBPase inhibitors into existing diabetic treatments could enhance clinical outcomes, offering an additional approach to glucose regulation. In combination with insulin or other oral antidiabetic agents, FBPase inhibitors may improve glucose control and mitigate complications. Future research exploring combination therapies targeting different aspects of gluconeogenesis, such as PEPCK or G6Pase, could provide new perspectives in diabetes treatment. Evaluating the combined effects of FBPase inhibitors and current antidiabetic drugs could offer a comprehensive strategy for managing blood sugar levels. Long-term studies are necessary to assess the impact of FBPase inhibitors on overall health, insulin resistance, and glycemic control in diabetes patients. Additionally, understanding the role of FBPase in various tissues, including the liver, kidneys, and adipose tissue, is crucial (Kaur et al. 2017).

Conclusion

FBPase plays a crucial role in gluconeogenesis, helping regulate blood glucose levels. Metabolic flexibility is influenced by several factors, including the modulation of FBPase by hormones and allosteric effectors. In diabetes mellitus, elevated FBPase activity contributes to hyperglycemia, making it a rational target for treatment. SMIs of FBPase have shown promise in preclinical models, offering a novel approach to diabetes management. Further research on FBPase will deepen our understanding and pave the way for developing new therapies for metabolic diseases.

References

Berg, J. M., Tymoczko, J. L., Gatto, G. J., & Stryer, L. (2019). *Biochemistry* (9th ed.). Macmillan.

Bu, P., Chen, K. Y., Xiang, K., Johnson, C., Crown, S. B., Rakhilin, N., Ai, Y., Wang, L., Xi, R., Astapova, I., Han, Y., Li, J., Barth, B. B., Lu, M., Gao, Z., Mines, R., Zhang, L., Herman, M., Hsu, D., Zhang, G. F., & Shen, X. (2018). Aldolase B-mediated fructose metabolism drives metabolic reprogramming of colon cancer liver metastasis. *Cell Metabolism*, 27(6), 1249–1262.

Gizak, A., Mazurek, J., Wozniak, M., Maciaszczyk-Dziubinska, E., & Rakus, D. (2013). Destabilization of fructose 1,6-bisphosphatase–Z-line interactions is a mechanism of gluconeogenesis down-regulation *in vivo*. *Biochimica et Biophysica Acta (BBA) - Molecular Cell Research*, 1833(3), 622–628.

Gupta, A., Varma, A., & Storey, K. B. (2021). New insights to regulation of fructose-1,6-bisphosphatase during anoxia in red-eared slider, Trachemys scripta elegans. *Biomolecules*, 11(10), 1548.

Gupta, A., Varma, A., & Storey, K. (2024). FBPase controls gluconeogenesis: New insights to regulation of fructose 1,6 bisphosphatase during anoxia in red-eared slider, Trachemys scripta elegans. *Authorea*, 1(1), 1–3.

Icard, P., Alifano, M., Donnadieu, E., & Simula, L. (2021). Fructose-1,6-bisphosphate promotes PI3K and glycolysis in T cells? *Trends in Endocrinology & Metabolism*, 32(8), 540–543.

Kaur, R., Dahiya, L., & Kumar, M. (2017). Fructose-1,6-bisphosphatase inhibitors: A new valid approach for management of type 2 diabetes mellitus. *European Journal of Medicinal Chemistry*, 141, 473–505.

Kuznetsova, E., Xu, L., Singer, A., Brown, G., Dong, A., Flick, R., Cui, H., Cuff, M., Joachimiak, A., Savchenko, A., & Yakunin, A. F. (2010). Structure and activity of the metal-independent fructose-1,6-bisphosphatase YK23 from Saccharomyces cerevisiae. *Journal of Biological Chemistry*, 285, 21049–21059.

Li, C. H., Chan, M. H., & Chang, Y. C. (2022). The role of fructose 1,6-bisphosphate-mediated glycolysis/gluconeogenesis genes in cancer prognosis. *Aging*, 14(7), 3233–3258.

Park, H. J., Jang, H. R., Park, S. Y., Kim, Y. B., Lee, H. Y., & Choi, C. S. (2020). The essential role of fructose-1,6-bisphosphatase 2 enzyme in thermal homeostasis upon cold stress. *Experimental & Molecular Medicine*, 52, 485–496.

Pirovich, D. B., Da'dara, A. A., & Skelly, P. J. (2021). Multifunctional fructose 1,6-bisphosphate aldolase as a therapeutic target. *Frontiers in Molecular Biosciences*, 8, 719678.

Rines, A. K., Sharabi, K., Tavares, C. D., & Puigserver, P. (2016). Targeting hepatic glucose metabolism in the treatment of type 2 diabetes. *Nature Reviews Drug Discovery*, 15(11), 786–804.

Timson, D. J. (2019). Fructose 1,6-bisphosphatase: Getting the message across. *Bioscience Reports*, 39(3), BSR20190124.

Xu, K., Yin, N., Peng, M., Stamatiades, E. G., Shyu, A., Li, P., Zhang, X., Do, M. H., Wang, Z., Capistrano, K. J., Chou, C., Levine, A. G., Rudensky, A. Y., & Li, M. O. (2021). Glycolysis fuels phosphoinositide 3-kinase signaling to bolster T cell immunity. *Science*, 371(6527), 405–410.

Xu, Y. X., Huang, Y. Y., Song, R. R., Ren, Y. L., Chen, X., Zhang, C., Mao, F., Li, X. K., Zhu, J., Ni, S. S., Wan, J., & Li, J. (2020). Development of disulfide-derived fructose-1,6-bisphosphatase (FBPase) covalent inhibitors for the treatment of type 2 diabetes. *European Journal of Medicinal Chemistry*, 203, 112500.

Chapter 15

Inhibitors of Fructose 1,6-Bisphosphatase from Natural Sources

Diksha Gulati[1,2,*]
Ajmer Singh Grewal[2]
and Balraj Saini[1]
[1]Chitkara College of Pharmacy, Chitkara University, Punjab, India
[2]Guru Gobind Singh College of Pharmacy, Yamuna Nagar, Haryana, India

Abstract

As the global incidence of diabetes continues to rise, there is an urgent need for the development of safer, more effective, and innovative antihyperglycemic agents. A major contributor to hyperglycemia in type 2 diabetes is the increased endogenous glucose production through gluconeogenesis. However, existing drugs do not directly target this pathway. Since gluconeogenesis plays a pivotal role in glucose overproduction, fructose 1,6-bisphosphatase (FBPase) has emerged as a promising target for therapeutic intervention. FBPase inhibitors offer significant potential to address this unmet need by regulating glucose production. This chapter reviews various chemical classes of FBPase inhibitors, examining their mechanisms of action, roles, and therapeutic potential in diabetes management. FBPase inhibitors function by modulating endogenous glucose metabolism, providing a complementary approach to conventional treatments focusing on insulin secretion and sensitivity. Preclinical and clinical studies have demonstrated that these inhibitors effectively regulate glucose metabolism with minimal adverse effects. However, the development of highly selective inhibitors remains a critical challenge. Future research should prioritize the identification of biomarkers to enhance therapy precision and explore the potential of combination therapies with other antidiabetic agents. These advancements could pave the way for more effective and personalized treatment strategies for diabetes.

Keywords: fructose 1,6-bisphosphatase (FBPase) inhibitors, hyperglycemia, gluconeogenesis, type 2 diabetes, anti-diabetic

---

* Corresponding Author's Email: dikshagulatir@gmail.com

In: Receptor-Targeted Therapies in Diabetes Mellitus
Editors: Ajmer Singh Grewal, Neelam Singh, Swati Verma et al.
ISBN: 979-8-89530-587-4

Abbreviations

AICAR	5-Aminoimidazole-4-carboxamide ribonucleotide
AMP	Adenosine monophosphate
CVS	Cardiovascular system
EGP	Endogeneous glucose production
FBPase	Fructose-1, 6-bisphosphatase
G.I.T.	Gastro-intestinal
G6Pase	Glucose-6-phosphatase
T2DM	Type 2 diabetes mellitus
TCA	Tri-carboxylic Acid
WHO	World health organization

Introduction

Diabetes mellitus is a condition characterized by elevated blood glucose levels, which are normally regulated by insulin produced by the pancreatic β-cells. Insulin enables the body to utilize glucose, derived from carbohydrates, as an energy source. Carbohydrates are essential for the proper functioning of the body's cells. After each meal, blood sugar levels rise, triggering the pancreatic β-cells to release insulin, maintaining a balance between high and low glucose levels. Hyperglycemia, or elevated blood glucose levels, occurs when insufficient insulin is produced or released to regulate blood sugar effectively. Diabetes mellitus affects millions of people worldwide, and its increasing prevalence poses significant challenges for medical practitioners in managing the condition (Sharma et al. 2022). Currently, an estimated 537 million people live with diabetes, a number projected to rise to 783 million by 2045. This includes approximately 61 million individuals in Europe, 51 million in the United States, and 24 million in Africa (Shikov et al. 2021). Type 2 diabetes mellitus (T2DM) is a chronic and debilitating metabolic disorder characterized by persistently elevated blood glucose levels. Contributing factors include reduced insulin sensitivity, relative insulin insufficiency, and increased endogenous glucose production (EGP). Prolonged hyperglycemia is associated with various microvascular and macrovascular complications, including cardiovascular diseases, nephropathy, neuropathy, retinopathy, and cataracts (Kaur et al. 2017). These complications are significant contributors to mortality among individuals with diabetes (Vaidya et al. 2015). Currently, most prescribed anti-diabetic medications function by either addressing peripheral insulin insufficiency or stimulating insulin production. However, these treatments often fail to maintain long-term glycemic control due to significant side effects, including hypoglycemia, obesity, pulmonary edema, gastrointestinal issues, and potential cardiovascular complications (Kaur et al. 2017). Consequently, there is an increasing focus on identifying novel molecular targets to improve glycemic control with fewer adverse effects. One such promising target is FBPase, a rate-limiting enzyme in gluconeogenesis responsible for endogenous glucose production, which contributes to hyperglycemia in individuals with diabetes. Inhibiting FBPase activity could help mitigate the effects of elevated blood and tissue glucose levels, offering a novel approach to diabetes management (Sharma et al. 2021). Most anti-diabetic treatments focus on either enhancing insulin production or reducing insulin resistance in peripheral tissues.

However, FBPase has emerged as a distinct and promising target for pharmacological intervention in diseases such as cancer and T2DM (Liu & Zhang, 2018). This chapter examines the various chemical classes of FBPase inhibitors, their functions, mechanisms of action, and potential therapeutic applications in managing diabetes.

Understanding Gluconeogenesis and FBPase

Glucose is a vital fuel source for various tissues, including red blood cells, renal medullary cells, and neurons (Rizza, 2010). The liver plays a pivotal role in maintaining glucose homeostasis, ensuring blood glucose levels remain within a narrow range of 3.9–7.1 mmol/L (Moore et al. 2012). It stores glucose as glycogen, which can be released into the bloodstream through gluconeogenesis or glycogenolysis. During the fed state, insulin secretion suppresses hepatic glucose production, and some of the ingested glucose is stored as glycogen. During short-term fasting, the liver relies on glycogenolysis (Figure 1) to maintain euglycemia, while in prolonged fasting, gluconeogenesis becomes the primary mechanism as glycogen stores become depleted (Ekberg et al. 1999). The complex process of glucose synthesis involves multiple enzymatic stages that are regulated by hormones, dietary intake, stress levels, and substrate concentrations. Gluconeogenesis occurs primarily in hepatocytes and renal cortical cells, counteracting glucose degradation mediated by glycolytic enzymes. Increased hepatic gluconeogenesis, which contributes up to 40% of glucose production, is a critical pathophysiological factor in T2DM (Gastaldelli et al. 2022). In T2DM, gluconeogenesis significantly influences glucose production both during fasting and postprandial states (Petersen et al. 1966). During a hyperinsulinemic-euglycemic clamp, hyperinsulinemia inhibits glycogenolysis but only modestly reduces gluconeogenesis (by approximately 20%) (Gastaldelli et al. 2001). In this procedure, exogenous insulin is administered at supraphysiological levels, while glucose is infused to maintain a specific blood glucose concentration. Chronic hyperglycemia is associated with microvascular complications, such as damage to the retina, kidneys, and nerves, as well as macrovascular complications, including heart attacks and strokes (Cade, 2008). FBPase is regulated by two natural markers, adenosine monophosphate (AMP) and fructose 2,6-bisphosphate. These regulators, including fructose 2,6-bisphosphate, a substrate analogue of FBPase, control the enzyme's homotetrameric structure and activity (Barciszewski et al. 2016). Fructose-1,6-bisphosphatase (FBPase) plays a crucial role in regulating the gluconeogenesis pathway. It catalyzes the conversion of fructose-1,6-bisphosphate to fructose-6-phosphate and inorganic phosphate. Due to its central role in gluconeogenesis, FBPase is an attractive target for therapeutic interventions. Inhibiting FBPase could prevent the oxidation of three-carbon precursors to glucose without interfering with the TCA cycle, glycolysis, or glycogenolysis (Kaur et al. 2017). Additionally, studies have demonstrated that certain FBPase inhibitors effectively reduce blood sugar levels in both animal models and patients with T2DM (Xu et al. 2020), indicating their potential as a novel class of anti-diabetic drugs.

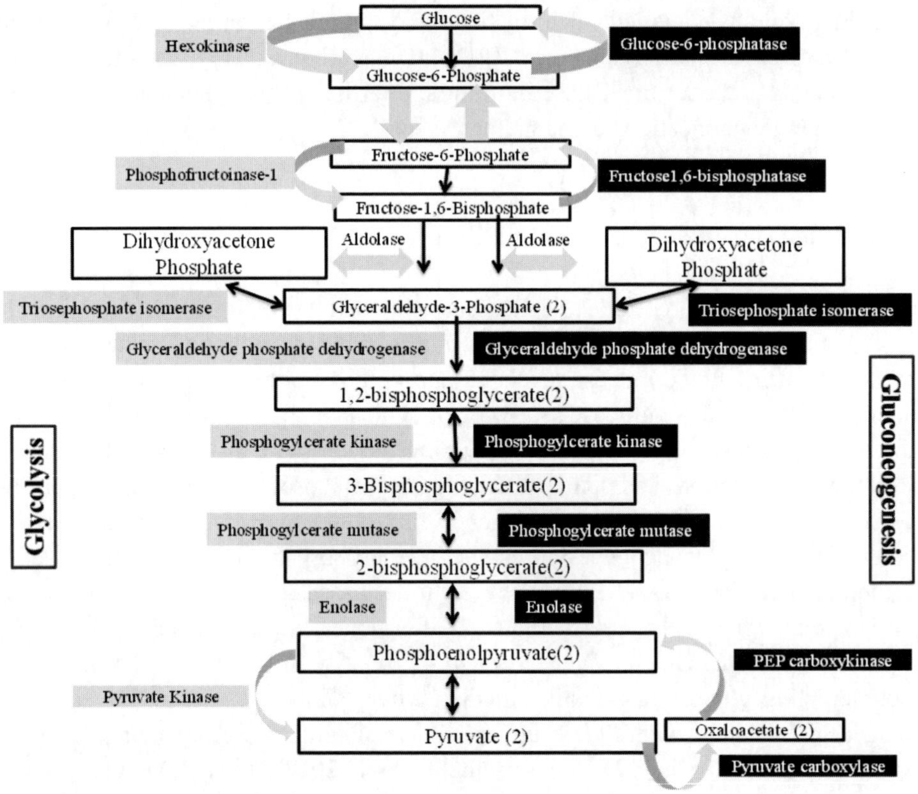

Figure 1. Reactions of gluconeogenesis.

FBPase Inhibitors

FBPase inhibition has gained significant global attention as a novel pharmacological strategy for managing excessive blood sugar levels by preventing hepatic glucose production through gluconeogenesis. FBPase is a desirable drug target due to its pivotal role in the gluconeogenesis pathway. Inhibiting FBPase suppresses glucose production from various substrates without interfering directly with other essential metabolic processes, such as the TCA cycle, glycogenolysis, and glycolysis. Unlike traditional treatments for T2DM, FBPase inhibitors are particularly appealing because they do not induce hypoglycemia. By targeting the primary source of hyperglycemia, these inhibitors have sparked considerable interest for their therapeutic potential (Kaur et al. 2017).

Numerous studies have shown that gluconeogenesis is often elevated in T2DM patients, underscoring the critical role of FBPase in the hyperglycemic state. AICAriboside, also known as 5-aminoimidazole-4-carboxamide ribonucleotide monophosphate (ZMP), has proven to be a valuable tool for studying FBPase inhibition. Its structure closely resembles that of AMP, a physiological allosteric non-competitive inhibitor of FBPase. AICAR can penetrate cell membranes and deliver the inhibitory effect to the enzyme following intracellular phosphorylation, making it an effective research compound for exploring the potential of FBPase-targeted therapies (Vincent et al. 1996). However, recent findings that ZMP also activates AMP-dependent protein kinase (AMPK) have complicated its use as a specific

FBPase inhibitor. Despite this, AICAR continues to be widely used in research to explore the enzyme's role in various processes, including those related to diabetes. For example, it is now understood that one of the key mechanisms behind contraction-induced muscle glucose uptake involves the activation of FBPase (Hayashi et al. 1998; Buhl et al. 2001). AICAR's inhibition of FBPase in liver cells has been shown to significantly reduce gluconeogenesis in a dose-dependent manner in isolated hepatocytes (McCormack et al. 2001). Moreover, animal studies have demonstrated that AICAR treatment lowers plasma glucose levels without increasing blood lactate levels, particularly in diabetic mouse models. Additionally, increases in fructose-1,6-bisphosphate concentrations in liver tissue further support its mode of action. Metabasis Inc. (formerly Gensia Inc.) has pioneered the development of novel FBPase inhibitors using structure-based techniques such as site-directed mutagenesis and X-ray crystallography. These inhibitors target the AMP binding pocket and include AICAR analogues that can enter cells and be phosphorylated. The company has also developed ester prodrugs that could serve as intracellular delivery vehicles for phosphonates (McCormack et al. 2001). As a result, FBPase inhibitors have shown promising efficacy in diabetic animal models, suggesting they could be a viable treatment option for T2DM. Many synthetic FBPase inhibitors with distinctive scaffolds have been discovered through either structure-guided synthesis of AMP mimetics or high-throughput screening of chemical libraries (Proneca et al. 2020). Among these are: (1) non-competitive phosphorus-based inhibitors, which include derivatives of purines, benzimidazoles, thiazoles, and oxazoles; (2) non-competitive inhibitors, which include derivatives of anilinoquinazoline, pseudo-tetrapeptide, and quinolines; and (3) other non-competitive inhibitors, which include derivatives of indoles, benzoxazoles, various N-, O-, and S-containing heterocycles, sulfonyl derivatives, and phytochemicals. Among these, the AMP mimic MB07803 is the only one to have advanced to phase II clinical trials (Mata et al. 2023).

Noncompetitive Inhibitors

Non-competitive inhibitors bind to the AMP site of FBPase, an enzyme crucial for regulating gluconeogenesis. AMP plays a key role in negatively regulating gluconeogenesis by altering the enzyme's conformation from the active R state to the inactive T state. This interaction with the allosteric AMP binding site effectively prevents FBPase from functioning. Consequently, targeting the AMP site of FBPase presents a promising therapeutic approach to reducing elevated glucose levels produced by gluconeogenesis in individuals with T2DM. Additionally, AMP activates AMPK, which is known for its insulin-sensitizing effects, making it an attractive target for T2DM therapy. A variety of compounds, including pharmaceuticals like metformin and thiazolidinediones, can activate AMPK, some of which are already in clinical use for managing T2DM. One such AMP analogue, AICAR monophosphate (ZMP), mimics AMP by directly activating AMPK and enhancing its phosphorylation. This ability to activate AMPK has broadened ZMP's role as a "lead" molecule for investigating other molecular targets implicated in blood glucose regulation, including FBPase, a negative regulator of AMP. ZMP, with an IC50 of 12 ± 1.4 μM, was the first recognized inhibitor of FBPase at the AMP binding site. While its effect on human hepatic FBPase was less potent than AMP (1 ± 0.05 μM), ZMP's *in vivo* inhibition of gluconeogenesis is attributed to its conversion from AICAR and subsequent inhibition of FBPase at the allosteric AMP site (Erion et al. 2005; Song et al. 2002; Bergeron et al. 2001; Coughlan et al. 2014; Young et al. 1996).

Table 1. Natural products with FBPase inhibitory activity

Plant	Active Ingredient	Conclusion	Ref
Ananas comosus L. Merr.	Butane-2,3-diyl diacetate	With few adverse effects, butane-2,3-diyl diacetate is an excellent FBPase inhibitor and a potential DM treatment option.	Hossain et al. 2023
Eclipta prostata, Agave sisalana, Piper aduncum, Curculigo orchioides, Luffa cylindrica, Moringa oleifera, Alium cepa, and Helianthus annuus	Stigmasterol	Stigmasterol exhibits the most encouraging inhibitory effects against FBPase.	Macalalad and Gonzales, 2023
Eryngium cymosum F	Kaempferol-3-O-(2,6-di-O-trans-ρ-coumaryl)-β-d-glucopyranoside	Kaempferol-3-O-(2,6-di-O-trans-ρ-coumaryl)-β-D-glucopyranoside exhibits an inhibitory impact on FBPase.	Romo-Perez et al. 2022
Desmodium caudatum	Prenylquercetin	Desmodium caudatum extract inhibited the activities of FBPase, α-glucosidase, and pancrelipase. It also promoted the consumption of glucose by cells and decreased the amount of lipid present in cells because it contained prenylquercetin and five other flavanoids.	Zhang et al. 2022
Eryngium cymosum F.	Aqueous extract	Aqueous extract of Eryngium cymosum F. showed dual ability to potentially inhibit the activities of FBPase, α-glucosidase, and pancrelipase.	Espinoza-Hernández et al.2021
Eryngium longifolium and Alsophila firma	Caffeic acid, chlorogenic acid, rosmarinic acid, isoflavones in Eryngium longifolium, flavanones or dihydroflavonols in Alsophila firma	Through the inhibition of FBPase and G6Pase, both plants had a notable hypoglycemic effect. In order to rule out alternative action pathways that might combine to create the reported hypoglycemic impact, more research is required.	Andrade-Cetto et al. 2021
Costus spicatus	Cyclohexane, 1,1'-(2-methyl-1,3 propanediyl)	Cyclohexane, 1,1'-(2-methyl-1,3 propanediyl) were found to be multiple inhibitors of PEPCK, α-amylase, β-glucosidase, and FBPase.	Olabisi et al. 2021
Sulawesi Propolis	Broussoflavonol F and glyasperin A	Broussoflavonol F and glyasperin A, on the other hand, SHOW 100% residue similarity when compared to re-docked positive controls and AMP reference.	Sahlan et al. 2020
Alpinia officinarum	Galangin	Galangin has improved the changes caused by STZ in rats' gluconeogenic and glycolytic enzymes as well as their glucose homeostasis.	Aloud et al. 2020
Hedychium coronarium	Terpenoids	This plant's terpenoid-rich fraction may offer an alternate therapy for diabetes and its consequences. Both blood glucose levels and body weight were maintained by the fraction.	Panigrahy et al.2019
Zizyphus spina-christi	Seed embryo extract	ZSC seed embryo extract may have diverse functions through various pathways to provide hypoglycemic and antihyperglycemic effects.	Al-Awar, 2019
Mulberry leaf	Dried powder	Tricetin, gallic acid, chlorogenic acid, and other drug components present in mulberry leaf powder have the ability to regulate various biological processes.	Ge et al. 2018

Plant	Active Ingredient	Conclusion	Ref
Epinephelus morio	NA	Epinephelus morio is able to limit the glucose load via G-6P by activating the gluconeogenic and glycolytic pathways.	Castillo et al. 2018
Ficus carica	Decoction	Ethyl acetate extract of Ficus carica leaves improved the deranged carbohydrate metabolism enzymes, including G6Pase, FBPase, and hexokinase.	Irudayaraj et al. 2017
Caralluma fimbriata	Hydro alcoholic extract	The extract can prevent changes in liver glycogen and key enzymes involved in the metabolism of carbohydrates caused by a high-fat diet, and restore these levels to almost normal.	Gujjala et al. 2017
NA	Geraniol	Geraniol given orally to diabetic rats dramatically inhibited the actions of gluconeogenic enzymes.	Babukumar et al. 2017
Schefflera kwangsiensis	Schekwangsiensides H-K (1-4)	Schekwangsiensides H-K (1-4) had shown mild inhibitory effects against FBPase1 in *in vitro* experiments.	Wang et al. 2016

Competitive Inhibitors

These inhibitors bind directly to the enzyme's active site. While targeting the substrate-binding site is a common approach in inhibitor design, strong competitive inhibitors that bind to the FBPase active site are rare. This challenge arises from the highly charged nature of the active site and the difficulty in developing carbohydrate-based analogs that can effectively compete with the natural substrate, especially at higher concentrations. These factors have contributed to the limited progress in designing inhibitors that target the active site (Heng, 2009).

Uncompetitive Inhibitors

These inhibitors bind to a novel allosteric site on the FBPase subunit interface. Reports suggest that moderately potent uncompetitive inhibitors target a lipophilic region on this interface. However, there is limited information regarding the pharmacokinetic properties or potential drawbacks of these inhibitors (Shikov et al. 2021).

Natural Products as Fbpase Inhibitors

Herbal remedies have been used for centuries to treat various illnesses, with plants known for their ability to enhance insulin production, reduce glucose absorption in the intestines, or activate molecules involved in insulin-dependent processes, contributing to their anti-hyperglycemic effects. The WHO has highlighted medicinal herbs as a primary healthcare source due to their accessibility, affordability, social acceptability, and the trust people place in them. Advances in drug discovery have led to the identification of several synthetic FBPase inhibitors with unique scaffolds, achieved through structure-guided AMP mimetic design or high-throughput screening of chemical libraries (Proenca et al. 2020). Among these, only MB07803, an AMP mimic, has advanced to phase II clinical trials. The most potent natural inhibitors identified to date are listed in Table 1.

Conclusion

T2DM is a chronic, multifactorial metabolic disorder characterized by insulin deficiency, insulin resistance, and excessive EGP, leading to elevated blood glucose levels during both fasting and postprandial states. The medications commonly used to manage diabetes often come with a range of side effects, making long-term use challenging for patients. As a result, there has been growing interest in the discovery of new chemical entities that offer a safer and more efficient approach to treating T2DM. Hyperglycemia in T2DM is primarily driven by gluconeogenesis, a key biochemical process, with FBPase emerging as a promising molecular target for regulating this pathway. The extensive data available in the literature highlights the potential of FBPase inhibitors as a novel strategy for developing safer and more effective treatments for T2DM.

References

Al-Awar, M. (2019). Anti-diabetic activities of Zizyphus spina-christi seeds embryos extract on general characteristics of diabetes, carbohydrate metabolism enzymes and lipids profile in rats. *Jordan Journal of Pharmaceutical Sciences*, 12(2), 91.

Aloud, A. A., Chinnadurai, V., Chandramohan, G., Alsaif, M. A., & Al-Numair, K. S. (2020). Galangin controls streptozotocin-caused glucose homeostasis and reverses glycolytic and gluconeogenic enzyme changes in rats. *Archives of Physiology and Biochemistry*, 126(2), 101-106.

Andrade-Cetto, A., Espinoza-Hernández, F., Mata-Torres, G., & Escandón-Rivera, S. (2021). Hypoglycemic effect of two mexican medicinal plants. *Plants*, 10(10), 2060.

Babukumar, S., Vinothkumar, V., Sankaranarayanan, C., & Srinivasan, S. (2017). Geraniol, a natural monoterpene, ameliorates hyperglycemia by attenuating the key enzymes of carbohydrate metabolism in streptozotocin-induced diabetic rats. *Pharmaceutical Biology*, 55(1), 1442-1449.

Barciszewski, J., Wisniewski, J., Kolodziejczyk, R., Jaskolski, M., Rakus, D., & Dzugaj, A. (2016). T-to-R switch of muscle fructose-1, 6-bisphosphatase involves fundamental changes of secondary and quaternary structure. *Acta Crystallographica Section D: Structural Biology*, 72(4), 536-550.

Bergeron, R., Previs, S. F., Cline, G. W., Perret, P., Russell III, R. R., Young, L. H., & Shulman, G. I. (2001). Effect of 5-aminoimidazole-4-carboxamide-1-β-D-ribofuranoside infusion on *in vivo* glucose and lipid metabolism in lean and obese Zucker rats. *Diabetes*, 50(5), 1076-1082.

Buhl, E. S., Jessen, N., Schmitz, O., Pedersen, S. B., Pedersen, O., Holman, G. D., & Lund, S. (2001). Chronic treatment with 5-aminoimidazole-4-carboxamide-1-β-d-ribofuranoside increases insulin-stimulated glucose uptake and GLUT4 translocation in rat skeletal muscles in a fiber type—specific manner. *Diabetes*, 50(1), 12-17.

Cade, W. T. (2008). Diabetes-related microvascular and macrovascular diseases in the physical therapy setting. *Physical Therapy*, 88(11), 1322-1335.

Castillo, A., Alvarez, A., Cuzon, G., Suárez, J., & Gaxiola, G. (2018). Glycemic response after glucose oral administration of wild juvenile red grouper Epinephelus morio fed two different diets. *Fish Physiology and Biochemistry*, 44, 219-226.

Coughlan, K. A., Valentine, R. J., Ruderman, N. B., & Saha, A. K. (2014). AMPK activation: a therapeutic target for type 2 diabetes? *Diabetes, Metabolic Syndrome and Obesity: Targets and Therapy*, 7, 241-253.

Ekberg, K., Landau, B. R., Wajngot, A., Chandramouli, V., Efendic, S., Brunengraber, H., & Wahren, J. (1999). Contributions by kidney and liver to glucose production in the postabsorptive state and after 60 h of fasting. *Diabetes*, 48(2), 292-298.

Erion, M. D., van Poelje, P. D., Dang, Q., Kasibhatla, S. R., Potter, S. C., Reddy, M. R., Reddy, K. R., Jiang, T., & Lipscomb, W. N. (2005). MB06322 (CS-917): A potent and selective inhibitor of fructose 1, 6-bisphosphatase for controlling gluconeogenesis in type 2 diabetes. *Proceedings of the National Academy of Sciences*, 102(22), 7970-7975.

Espinoza-Hernández, F., Andrade-Cetto, A., Escandón-Rivera, S., Mata-Torres, G., & Mata, R. (2021). Contribution of fasting and postprandial glucose-lowering mechanisms to the acute hypoglycemic effect of traditionally used Eryngium cymosum F. Delaroche. *Journal of Ethnopharmacology*, 279, 114339.

Femi-Olabisi, F. J., Ishola, A. A., Faokunla, O., Agboola, A. O., & Babalola, B. A. (2021). Evaluation of the inhibitory potentials of selected compounds from Costus spicatus (Jacq.) rhizome towards enzymes associated with insulin resistance in polycystic ovarian syndrome: an in silico study. *Journal of Genetic Engineering and Biotechnology*, 19, 1-9.

Gastaldelli, A., Baldi, S., Pettiti, M., Toschi, E., Camastra, S., Natali, A., Landau, B. R., & Ferrannini, E. (2000). Influence of obesity and type 2 diabetes on gluconeogenesis and glucose output in humans: a quantitative study. *Diabetes*, 49(8), 1367-1373.

Gastaldelli, A., Toschi, E., Pettiti, M., Frascerra, S., Quiñones-Galvan, A., Sironi, A. M., Natali, A., & Ferrannini, E. (2001). Effect of physiological hyperinsulinemia on gluconeogenesis in nondiabetic subjects and in type 2 diabetic patients. *Diabetes*, 50(8), 1807-1812.

Ge, Q., Chen, L., Tang, M., Zhang, S., Liu, L., Gao, L., Ma, S., Kong, M., Yao, Q., Feng, F., & Chen, K. (2018). Analysis of mulberry leaf components in the treatment of diabetes using network pharmacology. *European Journal of Pharmacology*, 833, 50-62.

Gujjala, S., Putakala, M., Nukala, S., Bangeppagari, M., Rajendran, R., & Desireddy, S. (2017). Modulatory effects of Caralluma fimbriata extract against high-fat diet induced abnormalities in carbohydrate metabolism in Wistar rats. *Biomedicine & Pharmacotherapy*, 92, 1062-1072.

Hayashi, T., Hirshman, M. F., Kurth, E. J., Winder, W. W., & Goodyear, L. J. (1998). Evidence for 5′ AMP-activated protein kinase mediation of the effect of muscle contraction on glucose transport. *Diabetes*, 47(8), 1369-1373.

Heng, S. (2009). *The Design, Synthesis and Characterization of Enzyme Inhibitors*. Doctoral dissertation, Boston College. Graduate School of Arts and Sciences.

Hossain, M. S., Roney, M., Bin Mohd Yunus, M. Y., & Shariffuddin, J. H. (2024). Virtual screening, molecular docking, molecular dynamics, and MM-GBSA approaches identify prospective fructose-1,6-bisphosphatase inhibitors from pineapple for diabetes management. *Journal of Biomolecular Structure & Dynamics*, 42(24), 13619–13634.

Kaur, R., Dahiya, L., & Kumar, M. (2017). Fructose-1, 6-bisphosphatase inhibitors: a new valid approach for management of type 2 diabetes mellitus. European Journal of Medicinal Chemistry, 141, 473-505.

Liu, G. M., & Zhang, Y. M. (2018). Targeting FBPase is an emerging novel approach for cancer therapy. *Cancer Cell International*, 18(1), 36.

Macalalad, M. A. B., & Gonzales III, A. A. (2023). In silico screening and identification of antidiabetic inhibitors sourced from phytochemicals of Philippine plants against four protein targets of diabetes (PTP1B, DPP-4, SGLT-2, and FBPase). *Molecules*, 28(14), 5301.

Mata, R., Flores-Bocanegra, L., Ovalle-Magallanes, B., & Figueroa, M. (2023). Natural products from plants targeting key enzymes for the future development of antidiabetic agents. *Natural Product Reports*, 40(7), 1198-1249.

McCormack, J. G., Westergaard, N., Kristiansen, M., Brand, C. L., & Lau, J. (2001). Pharmacological approaches to inhibit endogenous glucose production as a means of anti-diabetic therapy. *Current Pharmaceutical Design*, 7(14), 1451-1474.

Moore, M. C., Coate, K. C., Winnick, J. J., An, Z., & Cherrington, A. D. (2012). Regulation of hepatic glucose uptake and storage *in vivo*. *Advances in Nutrition*, 3(3), 286-294.

Panigrahy, S. K., Kumar, A., & Bhatt, R. (2020). *In vitro* and *in vivo* anti-diabetic activity of fractions obtained from the unexplored hedychium coronarium rhizome. *Proceedings of the National Academy of Sciences, India Section B: Biological Sciences*, 90, 605-614.

Petersen, K. F., Price, T. H. O. M. A. S., Cline, G. W., Rothman, D. L., & Shulman, G. I. (1996). Contribution of net hepatic glycogenolysis to glucose production during the early postprandial period. *American Journal of Physiology-Endocrinology and Metabolism*, 270(1), E186-E191.

Proença, C., Oliveira, A., Freitas, M., Ribeiro, D., Sousa, J. L. C., Ramos, M. J., Silva, A. M. S., Fernandes, P. A., & Fernandes, E. (2020). Structural specificity of flavonoids in the inhibition of human fructose 1,6-bisphosphatase. *Journal of Natural Products*, 83(5), 1541–1552.

Rizza, R. A. (2010). Pathogenesis of fasting and postprandial hyperglycemia in type 2 diabetes: implications for therapy. *Diabetes*, 59(11), 2697-2707.

Romo-Pérez, A., Escandón-Rivera, S. M., Miranda, L. D., & Andrade-Cetto, A. (2022). Phytochemical study of Eryngium cymosum F. Delaroche and the inhibitory capacity of its main compounds on two glucose-producing pathway enzymes. *Plants*, 11(7), 992.

Sahlan, M., Al Faris, M. N. H., Aditama, R., Lischer, K., Khayrani, A. C., & Pratami, D. K. (2020). Molecular docking of south Sulawesi propolis against fructose 1, 6-bisphosphatase as a type 2 diabetes mellitus drug. *International Journal of Technology*, 11(5), 910-920.

Sharma, P., Singh, S., Thakur, V., Sharma, N., & Grewal, A. S. (2021). Novel and emerging therapeutic drug targets for management of type 2 diabetes mellitus. *Obesity Medicine*, 23, 100329.

Sharma, P., Singh, S., Sharma, N., Singla, D., Guarve, K., & Grewal, A. S. (2022). Targeting human Glucokinase for the treatment of type 2 diabetes: an overview of allosteric Glucokinase activators. *Journal of Diabetes & Metabolic Disorders*, 21(1), 1129-1137.

Shikov, A. N., Narkevich, I. A., Akamova, A. V., Nemyatykh, O. D., Flisyuk, E. V., Luzhanin, V. G., Povydysh, M. N., Mikhailova, I. V., & Pozharitskaya, O. N. (2021). Medical species used in Russia for the management of diabetes and related disorders. *Frontiers in pharmacology*, 12, 697411.

Song, X. M., Fiedler, M., Galuska, D., Ryder, J. W., Fernström, M., Chibalin, A. V., Wallberg-Henriksson, H., & Zierath, J. R. (2002). 5-Aminoimidazole-4-carboxamide ribonucleoside treatment improves glucose homeostasis in insulin-resistant diabetic (ob/ob) mice. *Diabetologia*, 45, 56-65.

Irudayaraj, S. S., Christudas, S., Antony, S., Duraipandiyan, V., Naif Abdullah, A. D., & Ignacimuthu, S. (2017). Protective effects of Ficus carica leaves on glucose and lipids levels, carbohydrate metabolism enzymes and β-cells in type 2 diabetic rats. *Pharmaceutical Biology*, 55(1), 1074-1081.

Vaidya, V., Gangan, N., & Sheehan, J. (2015). Impact of cardiovascular complications among patients with Type 2 diabetes mellitus: a systematic review. *Expert Review of Pharmacoeconomics & Outcomes Research*, 15(3), 487-497.

Vincent, M. F., Erion, M. D., Gruber, H. E., & Van den Berghe, G. (1996). Hypoglycaemic effect of AICAriboside in mice. *Diabetologia*, 39(10), 1148-1155.

Wang, Y., Liu, Y.-F., Zhang, C.-L., Liang, D., Luo, H., Hao, Z.-Y., Chen, R.-Y., & Yu, D.-Q. (2016). Four new triterpenoid saponins isolated from Schefflera kwangsiensis and their inhibitory activities against FBPase1. *Phytochemistry Letters*, 15, 204-209.

Xu, Y. X., Huang, Y. Y., Song, R. R., Ren, Y. L., Chen, X., Zhang, C., Mao, F., Li, X. K., Zhu, J., Ni, S. S., Wan, J., & Li, J. (2020). Development of disulfide-derived fructose-1, 6-bisphosphatase (FBPase) covalent inhibitors for the treatment of type 2 diabetes. *European Journal of Medicinal Chemistry*, 203, 112500.

Young, M. E., Radda, G. K., & Leighton, B. (1996). Activation of glycogen phosphorylase and glycogenolysis in rat skeletal muscle by AICAR—an activator of AMP-activated protein kinase. *FEBS letters*, 382(1-2), 43-47.

Zhang, Y., Zhang, X., Xiao, Z., Zhang, X., & Sun, H. (2022). Hypoglycemic and hypolipidemic dual activities of extracts and flavonoids from Desmodium caudatum and an efficient synthesis of the most potent 8-prenylquercetin. *Fitoterapia*, 156, 105083.

Chapter 16

Targeting Neurotransmitter Receptors: New Avenues in Diabetes Treatment

Radha Kumari
and Hemlata Nimesh*
Amity Institute of Pharmacy, Amity University, Noida, Uttar Pradesh, India

Abstract

Neurotransmitters are signaling molecules released by neurons that regulate nervous system activity. They include peptides, monoamines, amino acids, and purines. The blood-brain barrier (BBB) regulates neurotransmitter transmission between the central nervous system (CNS) and the peripheral nervous system to maintain brain function. The pancreatic islet, due to its extensive innervation and vascularization, functions as a miniature organ capable of responding to CNS-derived neurotransmitters through both sympathetic and parasympathetic neurons. Additionally, peripheral neurotransmitters, which can be generated in the CNS, are also produced within the islets. These neurotransmitters regulate insulin production to maintain glucose homeostasis through both glucose-dependent and glucose-independent mechanisms. Upon binding to specific membrane receptors, these signaling molecules either stimulate or inhibit hormone release. Dysfunction in islet neurotransmitter receptors is linked to the development of type 2 diabetes (T2D) and β-cell impairment. This chapter explores the role of neurotransmitters and their receptors in the islets, their involvement in T2D pathogenesis, and their potential therapeutic applications for T2D and other metabolic disorders.

Keywords: glucose homeostasis, diabetes, neurotransmitter receptor, pancreatic islets, neurotransmitters, type 2 diabetes

Abbreviations

5-HT	5-Hydroxytryptamine (serotonin)
5-HT1D	Serotonin receptor 1D

* Corresponding Author's Email: hnimesh@amity.edu; hemlatanimesh@gmail.com

In: Receptor-Targeted Therapies in Diabetes Mellitus
Editors: Ajmer Singh Grewal, Neelam Singh, Swati Verma et al.
ISBN: 979-8-89530-587-4

5-HT2B	Serotonin receptor 2B
5-HT3R	Serotonin receptor 3
AADC	Aromatic-L-amino acid decarboxylase
AMPA	α-amino-3-hydroxy-5-methyl-4-isoxazole propionate
BDLG	Basal blood glucose level
cAMP	Cyclic adenosine monophosphate
ChAT	Choline acetyltransferase
DXM	Dextromethorphan
EC	Enterochromaffin
GAD	Glutamate decarboxylase
GSIS	Glucose-stimulated insulin secretion
HDC:	Histidine decarboxylase
M-type receptors	
(mAChRs)	Muscarinic acetylcholine receptors
nAChRs	Nicotinic acetylcholine receptors
NMDA	N-methyl-D-aspartate
NOD	Non-obese diabetic
ROS	Reactive oxygen species
SS	Somatostatin
STAT3	Signal transducer and activator of transcription 3
TPH	Tryptophan hydroxylase
vAChT	Vesicular acetylcholine transporter
VGLUT2	Vesicular glutamate transporter 2
VMAT	Vesicular monoamine transporter

Introduction

Neurotransmitters are signaling chemicals secreted by neurons that bind to various receptors in the central nervous system (CNS), facilitating communication and maintaining proper function between different brain regions. Several neurotransmitters and their receptors, essential for regulating glucose homeostasis, are found in the pancreatic islets. These neurotransmitters can either stimulate or inhibit the synthesis of insulin (β cells), glucagon (α cells), or somatostatin (δ cells) by binding to their respective receptors in the islets. The impact on blood glucose levels is largely determined by the quantity and placement of these neurotransmitter receptors within the islets. These receptors can be either ligand-gated or G-protein-coupled. Malfunctioning neurotransmitter receptors in the islets are associated with the development of T2D and β-cell dysfunction. Targeting specific transmitter systems holds significant promise for the management and prevention of T2D and other metabolic disorders. The pancreatic islets play a critical role in glucose homeostasis. The β cells, the body's sole source of insulin, lower blood glucose levels. When β cells malfunction, insulin secretion is impaired, leading to hyperglycemia and diabetes. Glucose transporters facilitate glucose uptake into the cells when blood glucose levels exceed the Km of the transporters on the β-cell membrane, which is the concentration at which the enzyme's maximum rate of reaction is half. This process leads to membrane depolarization, electrical activity, and the opening of voltage-dependent Ca^{2+}

channels (VDCCs), increasing intracellular Ca^{2+} concentration ($[Ca^{2+}]i$) and initiating insulin granule exocytosis. ATP is produced through glucose metabolism, which is essential for this process (Rorsman & Braun, 2013). Other islet cells also contribute to glucose homeostasis. In response to hypoglycemia, α cells release glucagon to elevate blood sugar, while δ cells release somatostatin to inhibit both insulin and glucagon secretion (Schwartz et al. 2013). Neurotransmitters, including amino acids, monoamines, peptides, and purines, regulate the activity of the nervous system (Sheffler et al. 2020). The blood-brain barrier (BBB) restricts the transfer of neurotransmitters from the CNS to the peripheral nervous system (PNS) to preserve normal brain function. Figure 1 illustrates the diverse molecular structures involved in neurotransmission. Neurotransmitter receptors can be classified into two main types: ionotropic and metabotropic receptors (Ferré et al. 2007). Ionotropic receptors influence cell activity by altering the membrane potential and are associated with ligand-gated ion channels. Metabotropic receptors, primarily G-protein coupled receptors (GPCRs), rely on intracellular second messengers to modulate ion channels or activate signaling cascades, leading to the release of calcium from cells (Pan et al. 2022). The pancreatic islets are vital for glucose regulation, and proper communication between the islets and other organs is essential for maintaining glucose homeostasis (Schwartz et al. 2013).

This chapter explores neurotransmitters' roles in islets and T2D development and their potential therapeutic applications for metabolic disorders.

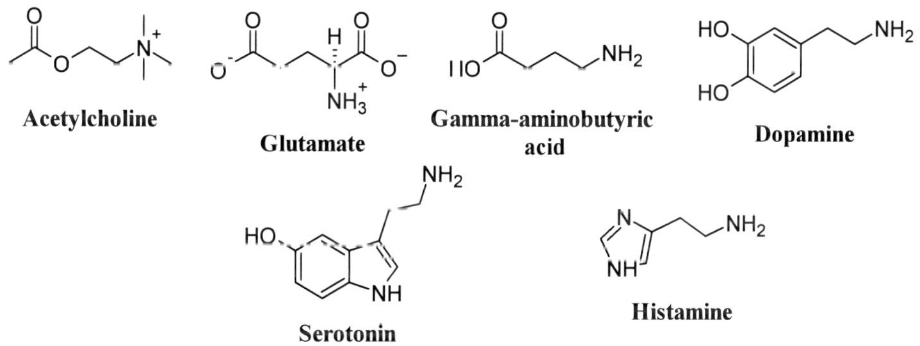

Figure 1. Structure of various neurotransmitters involved in diabetes.

Neurotransmitters and Their Receptors

Monoamines

Monoamine neurotransmitters (MNTs), including serotonin, norepinephrine, dopamine, and histamine, are widely distributed in the central and peripheral nervous systems (Walther et al. 2011). These neurotransmitters are regulated by monoamine transporters, such as vesicular monoamine transporters, norepinephrine transporters, and dopamine transporters, which absorb MNTs to mitigate their effects, or by breakdown through monoamine oxidase (MAO). Dysregulation of MNTs plays a significant role in the development of various mental illnesses (Ng et al. 2015).

Serotonin

In the brain and intestines, tryptophan is converted to 5-hydroxytryptamine (5-HT, serotonin) by tryptophan hydroxylase (TPH) and aromatic L-amino acid decarboxylase (AADC). All 5-HT receptors are GPCRs, except for the 5-HT3R, a ligand-gated ion channel (Freeby et al. 2012). The expression of the 5-HT2B receptor increases during mid-gestation, promoting β-cell proliferation and increasing β-cell mass, while the expression of the 5-HT1D receptor increases later in gestation to reduce β-cell mass (Rorsman & Braun, 2013). The main enzymes, TPH and AADC, in β-cells, produce 5-HT, which is loaded onto vesicles by vesicular monoamine transporters (VMATs) for release alongside insulin, glycine, and GABA (Bird et al. 1980; Kim et al. 2010). Activation of 5-HT3R increases insulin secretion and glucose sensitivity, while 5-HT2BR activity promotes β-cell proliferation. Additionally, 5-HT stimulates insulin secretion in β-cells by serotonylating GTPase (Paulmann et al. 2009). Certain 5-HT receptors, such as 5-HT1FR and 5-HT5AR, are expressed in α cells, and 5-HT1DR is expressed in δ cells, where they inhibit the release of somatostatin (SS) and glucagon (Bennet et al. 2015; Almaça et al. 2016). While δ cells can produce 5-HT, β cells are the primary source, and their paracrine signals suppress glucagon release. A reduction in 5-HT1FR expression on α cells in type 2 diabetes patients may contribute to hyperglycemia (Gromada et al. 2018). Figure 2 illustrates this pathway, highlighting TPH's central role in serotonin production and its physiological effects.

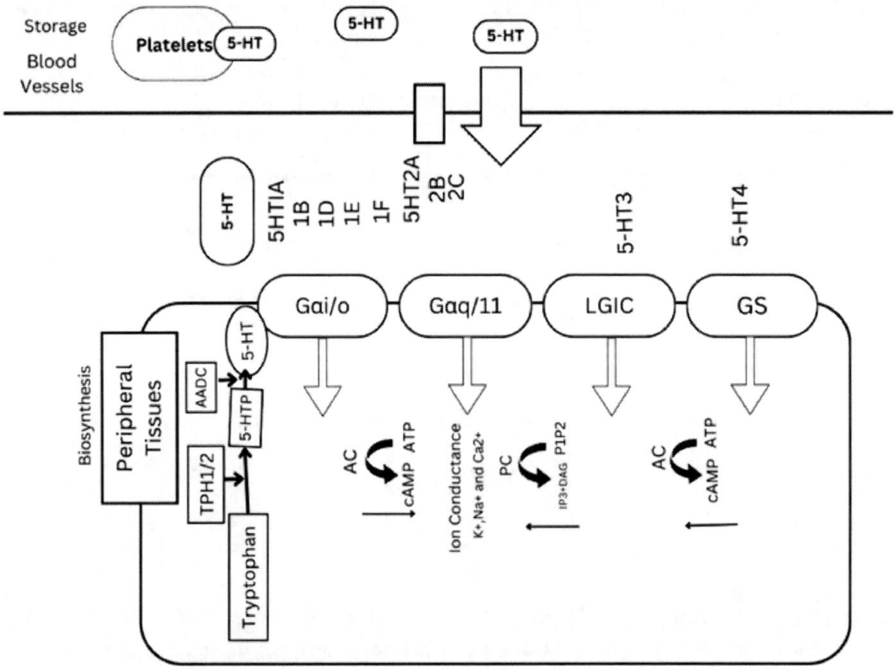

Figure 2. A model of peripheral tissue 5-HT metabolism begins with TPH synthesizing 5-HTP. Serotonin release is regulated by the autonomic nervous system and stored in platelets, with the serotonin transporter (SERT) mediating its release. Most 5-HT receptors are GPCRs, influencing biochemical signaling via the cAMP pathway.

Catecholamines

Dopamine, epinephrine, and norepinephrine are catecholamines (CAs) produced in the central and peripheral nervous systems from phenylalanine or tyrosine (Rubí & Maechler, 2010). Enzymes involved in CA synthesis and specific transporters are present in the α and β cells of both human and rodent islets, suggesting that these cells may be potential sources of CAs. GPCRs are the receptors for CAs (Aslanoglou et al. 2021), and depending on the Gs or Gi/o subunits they interact with, CAs either excite or inhibit cellular activity. Excitatory receptors like α1, β1, β2, β3 adrenergic receptors, and D1 and D5 dopamine receptors increase cAMP levels (Chen et al. 2014), whereas inhibitory receptors like D2, D3, D4 dopamine receptors and α2 adrenergic receptors decrease cAMP levels (Beaulieu & Gainetdinov, 2011). Dopamine transporters (DAT) are found in β cells, using VMAT2 to absorb dopamine and store it in vesicles. Dopamine acts on adrenergic and dopamine receptors when β cells depolarize and release insulin, inhibiting insulin release as part of a negative feedback loop (Rubí et al. 2005). α cells also produce and release dopamine and norepinephrine, interacting with adrenergic β1 receptors to initiate glucagon production. Paracrine, autocrine, and nerve-derived signals in islets may explain part of the increased risk of T2D under chronic stress (Aslanoglou et al. 2021). Blood norepinephrine levels are higher in T2D patients, slowing insulin production and reducing β-cell reactivity to adrenergic signals (Walters et al. 1997; Ortiz-Alonso et al. 1991). High peripheral insulin levels, indicating insulin resistance, prevent CAs from being reabsorbed, continuously activating adrenergic receptors on α and β cells, which disrupts glucose homeostasis and accelerates T2D development (Figlewicz et al. 1993).

Histamine

Histidine decarboxylase (HDC) converts histidine into histamine, which is stored in basophils and mast cells in an inactive form (Munroe et al. 1978). Histamine exerts its effects via histamine receptors (HRs), including H1-4, which activate ion ligand-gated channels. H1R, through Gq/11 coupling, induces cell stimulation and calcium influx. In contrast, H2R and H3R are inhibitory, binding to Gs and Gi/o subunits, respectively (Tanimoto et al. 2004; Nakamura et al. 2013). HDC is expressed in islet α and β cells, with higher expression observed in malignancies, while mast cells and basophils are the primary sources of histamine in islets. Human and rodent β cells express H1R, H2R, and H3R (Nagata et al. 2019). Histamine generally inhibits β-cell growth and insulin release. A first-generation antihistamine, trimeprazine, partially activates H1R, promoting β-cell growth in mice (Kuznetsova et al. 2016). Cetirizine, an H1R antagonist, improves glucose tolerance in mice on a high-fat diet, but does not affect diabetes development in NOD mice (Anvari et al. 2014). Selective H3R agonists reduce insulin synthesis and cell proliferation in MIN6 cells, whereas JNJ-5207852, a selective H3R inverse agonist, enhances insulin secretion and may stimulate β-cell proliferation (Nakamura et al. 2013). Both H2R agonists and antagonists can inhibit insulin secretion, with species-specific differences in receptor sites (Nagata et al. 2019; Nakamura et al. 2013). H3R, expressed in α cells, can inhibit glucagon synthesis. JNJ-39758979, a selective H4R antagonist, reduces diabetic nephropathy progression, likely due to decreased tissue inflammation, though direct evidence of H4R expression in islets is lacking (Pini et al. 2018). Elevated histaminergic activity in T2D is linked to increased reactive oxygen species (ROS) due to hyperglycemia, which accelerates vascular injury and heightens cardiovascular disease risk. In type 1 diabetes (T1D), histamine production from mast cell infiltration in islets worsens immune-mediated damage and β-cell death. H2R antagonists, commonly used for peptic ulcers, are associated with a lower prevalence of non-alcoholic fatty liver disease (NAFLD) in men, likely due to their antioxidant and anti-inflammatory effects (Shen & Liangpunsakul, 2016). However, prolonged use of H2R antagonists may increase the risk of T2D, suggesting potential adverse effects in diabetic patients (Yuan et al. 2021).

Amino Acids

Gamma-Aminobutyric Acid (GABA)

In GABAergic neurons, GABA, the most significant inhibitory neurotransmitter in the mammalian CNS, is synthesized from glutamate by the enzyme glutamate decarboxylase (GAD). The density of GABA and GABA receptors in the pancreatic islets is comparable to that in the central nervous system (Okada et al. 1976). GABA receptors include GABA-A, a ligand-gated ion channel, and GABA-B, a member of the GPCR family. GABA-A activation leads to chloride influx, which prevents depolarization and reduces target cell excitability. GABA-B exerts inhibitory effects by coupling with Gi/o proteins, inhibiting cAMP synthesis. In the pancreatic islets, β cells secrete GABA along with insulin, and GABA acts as an autocrine signal to bind to GABA-A receptors on β cells, reducing insulin release (Reetz et al. 1991). Furthermore, GABA receptor activation has been shown to increase β-cell proliferation. In α cells, the paracrine signal from GABA binding to GABA-A receptors prevents glucagon secretion and cell division (Feng et al. 2017). When glucose levels are insufficient to trigger action potentials in β cell membranes, GABA-A receptor activation gently depolarizes β cells by altering the chloride potential, stimulating the release of both insulin and GABA (Braun et al. 2010). However, when glucose levels exceed a certain threshold, GABA acts to prevent excessive insulin release (Dong et al. 2006). The GABA-B receptor agonist reduces insulin release at high glucose concentrations (25 mmol/L), and both GABA-B receptor 1 and 2 mRNAs have been identified in islets from rats, humans, and MIN6 cells (Rachdi et al. 2020). Reduced GABA content is associated with β-cell dysfunction and diminished insulin content in islets from individuals and animals with type 2 diabetes (T2D) (Menegaz et al. 2019). GAD autoantibodies are essential for diagnosing autoimmune diabetes (Regnell & Lernmark, 2017). Additionally, GABA influences T cells and other innate immune cells, modulating the immune response by inhibiting NF-κB activation and protecting β cells from inflammation.

Glutamate

Glutamate, a nonessential amino acid, serves as the primary excitatory neurotransmitter in the central nervous system. In pancreatic islets, glutamate is primarily produced in α cells, with minimal contribution from blood vessels (Zhou et al. 2014). Once synthesized, vesicular glutamate transporter 2 (VGLUT2) packages glutamate into secretory granules, where it is co-released with glucagon in response to low glucose levels (Tapiero et al. 2002). Both glycine and glutamate activate NMDA receptors, which play a critical role in regulating intracellular calcium and sodium balance (Huang et al. 2017). Fast excitatory synaptic transmission in the islets is mediated by non-NMDA receptors, such as kainate receptors and α-amino-3-hydroxy-

5-methyl-4-isoxazole propionate (AMPA) receptors (Marquard et al. 2015). Ionotropic and metabotropic glutamate receptors regulate islet function and glucose homeostasis. Ionotropic NMDA receptors on β cells facilitate calcium influx and transient insulin secretion; however, prolonged activation can impair glucose-stimulated insulin secretion (GSIS) and lead to excitotoxicity, ultimately resulting in β-cell death. Conversely, inhibition of NMDA receptors has been shown to enhance GSIS and improve glucose tolerance (Marquard et al. 2015; Otter & Lammert, 2016). Non-NMDA receptors, including AMPA and kainate receptors, contribute to excitatory synaptic transmission and the regulation of glucagon secretion, forming feedback loops that influence islet hormone release (Cabrera et al. 2008). Metabotropic glutamate receptors (mGluRs), classified into groups I, II, and III, play crucial roles in islet function by modulating insulin and glucagon secretion. For instance, mGluR4 and mGluR8 in α and PP cells inhibit insulin and glucagon release, while mGluR5 interacts with NMDA receptors to optimize insulin secretion (Storto et al. 2006). Elevated plasma glutamate levels are associated with chronic conditions such as obesity, diabetes, and oxidative stress, contributing to excitotoxicity and inflammation (Gaggini et al. 2017). Targeting glutamate receptors, particularly using NMDA receptor antagonists, holds promise for treating T2D. Agents such as dextromethorphan (DXM) and its derivative Lam39M have been shown to improve insulin secretion, enhance glycemic control, and protect islet cells from apoptosis (Welters et al. 2017).

Acetylcholine

In human islets, acetylcholine (ACh) is primarily derived from both neurons and α cells, whereas in rodents, it predominantly originates from cholinergic nerve terminals (Rodriguez-Diaz et al. 2011). Within α cells, ACh is stored in separate vesicles from glucagon by the vesicular acetylcholine transporter (vAChT), enabling its independent release. In rodents, α cells are located at the periphery of the islets, facilitating paracrine ACh signaling to neighboring cells. However, in humans, α cells are dispersed throughout the islets (Duttaroy et al. 2004b). The enzyme choline acetyltransferase (ChAT) catalyzes the conversion of choline and acetyl-coenzyme A into ACh, which is stored in cholinergic neurons in both the central and peripheral autonomic nervous systems via vAChT. Cholinergic receptors are classified into muscarinic (mAChRs) and nicotinic (nAChRs) receptors. Muscarinic receptors, which are G-protein-coupled receptors (GPCRs), mediate excitatory or inhibitory responses through interactions with either Gi/o (M2, M4) or Gq/11 (M1, M3, M5) subunits. In contrast, nicotinic receptors are ligand-gated ion channels composed of multiple subunits (Rodriguez-Diaz, Abdulreda, et al. 2011). The primary subunits of nicotinic acetylcholine receptors (nAChRs) in rodents are α7 and β2, whereas in human islets, they are α5 and β2 (Klee et al. 2016). Nicotine, a well-known risk factor for type 2 diabetes (T2D), functions as a natural agonist of nAChRs (Pan et al. 2015). Interestingly, long-term low-dose nicotine administration in db/db mice has been shown to enhance insulin sensitivity and improve glucose metabolism. Activation of nAChRs can stimulate insulin secretion, increase β-cell mass, and protect β-cells from cytokine-induced toxicity. In α5nAChR-deficient mice, increased nicotine intake has ambiguous effects on glucose homeostasis (Fowler et al. 2011). Conversely, deletion of the α7-nAChR results in insulin resistance and impaired glucose tolerance (Wang et al. 2011). Moreover, selective α7-nAChR agonists, such as PUN-282987, demonstrate beneficial effects via the STAT3 pathway, enhancing insulin sensitivity and reducing inflammation in mouse liver, adipose tissue, and muscle. (Xu et al. 2012).

Conclusion

Neurotransmitters, including peptides, monoamines, amino acids, and purines, are essential signaling molecules released by neurons to regulate nervous system activity. These molecules can cross the blood-brain barrier (BBB) and interact with both the central and peripheral nervous systems, including the pancreatic islets, which play a crucial role in glucose homeostasis. Neurotransmitters such as serotonin, catecholamines, and histamine modulate the secretion of insulin and glucagon in response to glucose levels. For instance, serotonin influences β-cell proliferation and insulin secretion, while catecholamines and histamine affect β-cell function and glucose regulation, both of which are critical in the development of T2D. Dysregulation of neurotransmitter receptors in islets is linked to β-cell dysfunction and the progression of T2D. The receptors for these neurotransmitters, including both ionotropic and metabotropic types, play significant roles in islet hormone release and glucose regulation. Research into specific neurotransmitter pathways offers promising opportunities for managing and treating T2D, underscoring the complex interactions between neurotransmitters and islet function.

References

Almaça, J., Molina, J., Menegaz, D., Pronin, A. N., Tamayo, A., Slepak, V., Berggren, P. O., & Caicedo, A. (2016). Human Beta Cells Produce and Release Serotonin to Inhibit Glucagon Secretion from Alpha Cells. *Cell Reports*, 17(12), 3281–3291.

Anvari, E., Wang, X., Sandler, S., & Welsh, N. (2014). The H1-receptor antagonist cetirizine ameliorates high-fat diet-induced glucose intolerance in male C57BL/6 mice, but not diabetes outcome in female non-obese diabetic (NOD) mice. *Upsala Journal of Medical Sciences*, 120(1), 40–46.

Aslanoglou, D., Bertera, S., Sánchez-Soto, M., Benjamin Free, R., Lee, J., Zong, W., Xue, X., Shrestha, S., Brissova, M., Logan, R. W., Wollheim, C. B., Trucco, M., Yechoor, V. K., Sibley, D. R., Bottino, R., & Freyberg, Z. (2021). Dopamine regulates pancreatic glucagon and insulin secretion via adrenergic and dopaminergic receptors. *Translational Psychiatry*, 11(1), 59.

Beaulieu, J. M., & Gainetdinov, R. R. (2011). The Physiology, Signaling, and Pharmacology of Dopamine Receptors. *Pharmacological Reviews*, 63(1), 182–217.

Bennet, H., Balhuizen, A., Medina, A., Dekker Nitert, M., Ottosson Laakso, E., Essén, S., Spégel, P., Storm, P., Krus, U., Wierup, N., & Fex, M. (2015). Altered serotonin (5-HT) 1D and 2A receptor expression may contribute to defective insulin and glucagon secretion in human type 2 diabetes. *Peptides*, 71, 113–120.

Bird, J. L., Wright, E. E., & Feldman, J. M. (1980). Pancreatic Islets: A Tissue Rich in Serotonin. *Diabetes*, 29(4), 304–308.

Braun, M., Ramracheya, R., Bengtsson, M., Clark, A., Walker, J. N., Johnson, P. R., & Rorsman, P. (2010). γ-Aminobutyric Acid (GABA) Is an Autocrine Excitatory Transmitter in Human Pancreatic β -Cells. *Diabetes*, 59(7), 1694–1701.

Cabrera, O., Jacques-Silva, M. C., Speier, S., Yang, S. N., Köhler, M., Fachado, A., Vieira, E., Zierath, J. R., Kibbey, R., Berman, D. M., Kenyon, N. S., Ricordi, C., Caicedo, A., & Berggren, P. O. (2008). Glutamate Is a Positive Autocrine Signal for Glucagon Release. *Cell Metabolism*, 7(6), 545–554.

Dong, H., Kumar, M., Zhang, Y., Gyulkhandanyan, A., Xiang, Y. Y., Ye, B., Perrella, J., Hyder, A., Zhang, N., Wheeler, M., Lu, W. Y., & Wang, Q. (2006). Gamma-aminobutyric acid up- and downregulates insulin secretion from beta cells in concert with changes in glucose concentration. *Diabetologia*, 49(4), 697–705.

Duncan, A., Heyer, M. P., Ishikawa, M., Caligiuri, S. P. B., Liu, X., Chen, Z., Micioni Di Bonaventura, M. V., Elayouby, K. S., Ables, J. L., Howe, W. M., Bali, P., Fillinger, C., Williams, M., O'Connor, R. M., Wang, Z., Lu, Q., Kamenecka, T. M., Ma'ayan, A., O'Neill, H. C., & Ibanez-Tallon, I. (2019). Habenular TCF7L2 links nicotine addiction to diabetes. *Nature*, 574(7778), 372–377.

Duttaroy, A., Zimliki, C. L., Gautam, D., Cui, Y., Mears, D., & Wess, J. (2004). Muscarinic Stimulation of Pancreatic Insulin and Glucagon Release Is Abolished in M3 Muscarinic Acetylcholine Receptor-Deficient Mice. *Diabetes*, 53(7), 1714–1720.

Feng, A. L., Xiang, Y. Y., Gui, L., Kaltsidis, G., Feng, Q., & Lu, W. Y. (2017). Paracrine GABA and insulin regulate pancreatic alpha cell proliferation in a mouse model of type 1 diabetes. *Diabetologia*, 60(6), 1033–1042.

Ferré, S., Ciruela, F., Woods, A. S., Lluis, C., & Franco, R. (2007). Functional relevance of neurotransmitter receptor heteromers in the central nervous system. *Trends in Neurosciences*, 30(9), 440–446.

Figlewicz, D. P., Bentson, K., & Ocrant, I. (1993). The effect of insulin on norepinephrine uptake by PC12 cells. *Brain Research Bulletin*, 32(4), 425–431.

Fowler, C. D., Lu, Q., Johnson, P. M., Marks, M. J., & Kenny, P. J. (2011). Habenular α5 nicotinic receptor subunit signalling controls nicotine intake. *Nature*, 471(7340), 597–601.

Freeby, M., Ichise, M., & Harris, P. E. (2012). Vesicular monoamine transporter, type 2 (vmat2) expression as it compares to insulin and pancreatic polypeptide in the head, body and tail of the human pancreas. *Islets*, 4(6), 393–397.

Gaggini, M., Carli, F., Rosso, C., Buzzigoli, E., Marietti, M., Della Latta, V., Ciociaro, D., Abate, M. L., Gambino, R., Cassader, M., Bugianesi, E., & Gastaldelli, A. (2018). Altered amino acid concentrations in NAFLD: Impact of obesity and insulin resistance. *Hepatology*, 67(1), 145–158.

Gromada, J., Chabosseau, P., & Rutter, G. A. (2018). The α-cell in diabetes mellitus. *Nature Reviews Endocrinology*, 14(12), 694–704.

Hauge-Evans, A. C., Reers, C., Kerby, A., Franklin, Z. J., Amisten, S., King, A., Hassan, Z., Vilches-Flores, A., Zayd Tippu, Persaud, S. J., & Jones, P. B. (2014). Effect of hyperglycaemia on muscarinic M3 receptor expression and secretory sensitivity to cholinergic receptor activation in islets. *Diabetes, Obesity & Metabolism*, 16(10), 947–956.

Hauser, A. S., Attwood, M. M., Rask-Andersen, M., Schiöth, H. B., & Gloriam, D. E. (2017). Trends in GPCR drug discovery: new agents, targets and indications. *Nature Reviews. Drug Discovery*, 16(12), 829–842.

Huang, X. T., Li, C., Peng, X. P., Guo, J., Yue, S. J., Liu, W., Zhao, F. Y., Han, J. Z., Huang, Y. H., Yang, L., Cheng, Q. M., Zhou, Z. G., Chen, C., Feng, D. D., & Luo, Z. Q. (2017). An excessive increase in glutamate contributes to glucose-toxicity in β-cells via activation of pancreatic NMDA receptors in rodent diabetes. *Scientific Reports*, 7, Article 44120.

Kim, H., Toyofuku, Y., Lynn, F. C., Chak, E., Uchida, T., Mizukami, H., Fujitani, Y., Kawamori, R., Miyatsuka, T., Kosaka, Y., Yang, K., Honig, G., van der Hart, M., Kishimoto, N., Wang, J., Yagihashi, S., Tecott, L. H., Watada, H., & German, M. S. (2010). Serotonin regulates pancreatic beta cell mass during pregnancy. *Nature Medicine*, 16(7), 804–808.

Klee, P., Bosco, D., Guérardel, A., Somm, E., Toulotte, A., Maechler, P., & Schwitzgebel, V. M. (2016). Activation of Nicotinic Acetylcholine Receptors Decreases Apoptosis in Human and Female Murine Pancreatic Islets. *Endocrinology*, 157(10), 3800–3808.

Kuznetsova, A., Yu, Y., Hollister-Lock, J., Opare-Addo, L., Rozzo, A., Sadagurski, M., Norquay, L., Reed, J. E., El Khattabi, I., Bonner-Weir, S., Weir, G. C., Sharma, A., & White, M. F. (2016). Trimeprazine increases IRS2 in human islets and promotes pancreatic β cell growth and function in mice. *JCI Insight*, 1(3), e80749.

Marquard, J., Otter, S., Welters, A., Stirban, A., Fischer, A., Eglinger, J., Herebian, D., Kletke, O., Skelin Klemen, M., Stožer, A., Wnendt, S., Piemonti, L., Köhler, M., Ferrer, J., Thorens, B., Schliess, F., Slak Rupnik, M., Heise, T., Berggren, P. O., Klöcker, N., Meissner, T., Mayatepek, E., Eberhard, D., Kragl, M., & Lammert, E. (2015). Characterization of pancreatic NMDA receptors as possible drug targets for diabetes treatment. *Nature Medicine*, 21(4), 363–372.

Menegaz, D., Hagan, D. W., Almaça, J., Cianciaruso, C., Rodriguez-Diaz, R., Molina, J., Dolan, R. M., Becker, M. W., Schwalie, P. C., Nano, R., Lebreton, F., Kang, C., Sah, R., Gaisano, H. Y., Berggren, P. O., Baekkeskov, S., Caicedo, A., & Phelps, E. A. (2019). Mechanism and effects of pulsatile GABA secretion from cytosolic pools in the human beta cell. *Nature Metabolism*, 1(11), 1110–1126.

Molina, J., Rodriguez-Diaz, R., Fachado, A., Jacques-Silva, M. C., Berggren, P.-O., & Caicedo, A. (2014). Control of Insulin Secretion by Cholinergic Signaling in the Human Pancreatic Islet. *Diabetes*, 63(8), 2714–2726.

Munroe, W. A., Lewis, C. A., & Dunlap, R. B. (1978). Kinetics of sulfhydryl group modification of thymidylate synthetase: a proposal for activation of catalytic cysteinly residues. *Biochemical and Biophysical Research Communications*, 80(2), 355–360.

Nagata, M., Yokooji, T., Nakai, T., Miura, Y., Tomita, T., Taogoshi, T., Sugimoto, Y., & Matsuo, H. (2019). Blockade of multiple monoamines receptors reduce insulin secretion from pancreatic β-cells. *Scientific Reports*, 9(1), 16438.

Nakamura, T., Yoshikawa, T., Noguchi, N., Sugawara, A., Kasajima, A., Sasano, H., & Yanai, K. (2013). The expression and function of histamine H3receptors in pancreatic beta cells. *British Journal of Pharmacology*, 171(1), 171–185.

Ng, J., Papandreou, A., Heales, S. J., & Kurian, M. A. (2015). Monoamine neurotransmitter disorders—clinical advances and future perspectives. *Nature Reviews Neurology*, 11(10), 567–584.

Okada, Y., Taniguchi, H., & Schimada, C. (1976). High Concentration of GABA and High Glutamate Decarboxylase Activity in Rat Pancreatic Islets and Human Insulinoma. *Science*, 194(4265), 620–622.

Ortiz-Alonso, F. J., Herman, W. H., Zobel, D. L., Perry, T. J., Smith, M. J., & Halter, J. B. (1991). Effect of epinephrine on pancreatic beta-cell and alpha-cell function in patients with NIDDM. *Diabetes*, 40(9), 1194–1202.

Otter, S., & Lammert, E. (2016). Exciting Times for Pancreatic Islets: Glutamate Signaling in Endocrine Cells. *Trends in Endocrinology & Metabolism*, 27(3), 177–188.

Pan, A., Wang, Y., Talaei, M., Hu, F. B., & Wu, T. (2015). Relation of active, passive, and quitting smoking with incident type 2 diabetes: a systematic review and meta-analysis. *The Lancet Diabetes & Endocrinology*, 3(12), 958–967.

Pan, X., Tao, S., & Tong, N. (2022). Potential therapeutic targeting neurotransmitter receptors in diabetes. *Frontiers in Endocrinology*, 13, 884549.

Chen, Y., Hong, F., Chen, H., Fan, R. F., Zhang, X. L., Zhang, Y., & Zhu, J. X. (2014). Distinctive expression and cellular distribution of dopamine receptors in the pancreatic islets of rats. *Cell and Tissue Research*, 357(3), 597–606.

Paulmann, N., Grohmann, M., Voigt, J. P., Bert, B., Vowinckel, J., Bader, M., Skelin, M., Jevšek, M., Fink, H., Rupnik, M., & Walther, D. J. (2009). Intracellular Serotonin Modulates Insulin Secretion from Pancreatic β-Cells by Protein Serotonylation. *PLoS Biology*, 7(10), e1000229.

Pini, A., Grange, C., Veglia, E., Argenziano, M., Cavalli, R., Guasti, D., Calosi, L., Ghè, C., Solarino, R., Thurmond, R. L., Camussi, G., Chazot, P. L., & Rosa, A. C. (2018). Histamine H4 receptor antagonism prevents the progression of diabetic nephropathy in male DBA2/J mice. *Pharmacological Research*, 128, 18–28.

Pini, A., Obara, I., Battell, E., Chazot, P. L., & Rosa, A. C. (2016). Histamine in diabetes: Is it time to reconsider? *Pharmacological Research*, 111, 316–324.

Rachdi, L., Maugein, A., Pechberty, S., Armanet, M., Hamroune, J., Ravassard, P., Marullo, S., Albagli, O., & Scharfmann, R. (2020). Regulated expression and function of the GABAB receptor in human pancreatic beta cell line and islets. *Scientific Reports*, 10(1), 13469.

Reetz, A., Solimena, M., Matteoli, M., Folli, F., Takei, K., & De Camilli, P. (1991). GABA and pancreatic beta-cells: colocalization of glutamic acid decarboxylase (GAD) and GABA with synaptic-like microvesicles suggests their role in GABA storage and secretion. *The EMBO Journal*, 10(5), 1275–1284.

Regnell, S. E., & Lernmark, Å. (2017). Early prediction of autoimmune (type 1) diabetes. *Diabetologia*, 60(8), 1370–1381.

Rodriguez-Diaz, R., Abdulreda, Midhat H., Formoso, Alexander L., Gans, I., Ricordi, C., Berggren, P. O., & Caicedo, A. (2011). Innervation Patterns of Autonomic Axons in the Human Endocrine Pancreas. *Cell Metabolism*, 14(1), 45–54.

Rodriguez-Diaz, R., Dando, R., Jacques-Silva, M. C., Fachado, A., Molina, J., Abdulreda, M. H., Ricordi, C., Roper, S. D., Berggren, P. O., & Caicedo, A. (2011). Alpha cells secrete acetylcholine as a non-neuronal paracrine signal priming beta cell function in humans. *Nature Medicine*, 17(7), 888–892.

Rorsman, P., & Braun, M. (2013). Regulation of Insulin Secretion in Human Pancreatic Islets. *Annual Review of Physiology*, 75(1), 155–179.

Rubí, B., & Maechler, P. (2010). Minireview: new roles for peripheral dopamine on metabolic control and tumor growth: let's seek the balance. *Endocrinology*, 151(12), 5570–5581.

Rubí, B., Ljubicic, S., Pournourmohammadi, S., Carobbio, S., Armanet, M., Bartley, C., & Maechler, P. (2005). Dopamine D2-like Receptors Are Expressed in Pancreatic Beta Cells and Mediate Inhibition of Insulin Secretion. *Journal of Biological Chemistry*, 280(44), 36824–36832.

Scholz, O., Otter, S., Welters, A., Wörmeyer, L., Dolenšek, J., Skelin Klemen, M., Pohorec, V., Eberhard, D., Mrugala, J., Hamacher, A., Koch, A., Sanz, M., Hoffmann, T., Hogeback, J., Herebian, D., Klöcker, N., Piechot, A., Mayatepek, E., Meissner, T., Stožer, A., & Lammert, E. (2021). Peripherally active dextromethorphan derivatives lower blood glucose levels by targeting pancreatic islets. *Cell Chemical Biology*, 28(10), 1474–1488.

Schwartz, M. W., Seeley, R. J., Tschöp, M. H., Woods, S. C., Morton, G. J., Myers, M. G., & D'Alessio, D. (2013). Cooperation between brain and islet in glucose homeostasis and diabetes. *Nature*, 503(7474), 59–66.

Sheffler, Z. M., Reddy, V., & Pillarisetty, L. S. (2020). *Physiology, Neurotransmitters*. PubMed; StatPearls Publishing.

Shen, H., & Liangpunsakul, S. (2016). Histamine H2-receptor antagonist use is associated with lower prevalence of nonalcoholic fatty liver disease. *Journal of Clinical Gastroenterology*, 50(7), 596–601.

Storto, M., Capobianco, L., Battaglia, G., Molinaro, G., Gradini, R., Riozzi, B., Di Mambro, A., Mitchell, K. J., Bruno, V., Vairetti, M. P., Rutter, G. A., & Nicoletti, F. (2006). Insulin secretion is controlled by mGlu5 metabotropic glutamate receptors. *Molecular pharmacology*, 69(4), 1234–1241.

Tang, S., Luc Baeyens, Shen, C., Peng, S. J., Chien, H., Scheel, D., Chamberlain, C. E., & German, M. S. (2017). Human pancreatic neuro-insular network in health and fatty infiltration. *Diabetologia*, 61(1), 168–181.

Tanimoto, A., Matsuki, Y., Tomita, T., Takakazu Sasaguri, Shohei Shimajiri, & Yasuyuki Sasaguri. (2004). Histidine decarboxylase expression in pancreatic endocrine cells and related tumors. *Pathology International*, 54(6), 408–412.

Tapiero, H., Mathé, G., Couvreur, P., & Tew, K. D. (2002). II. Glutamine and glutamate. *Biomedicine & Pharmacotherapy*, 56(9), 446–457.

Walters, J. M., Ward, G. M., Barton, J., Arackal, R., Boston, R. C., Best, J. D., & Alford, F. P. (1997). The effect of norepinephrine on insulin secretion and glucose effectiveness in non—insulin-dependent diabetes. *Metabolism*, 46(12), 1448–1453.

Walther, D. J., Stahlberg, S., & Vowinckel, J. (2011). Novel roles for biogenic monoamines: from monoamines in transglutaminase-mediated post-translational protein modification to monoaminylation deregulation diseases. *FEBS Journal*, 278(24), 4740–4755.

Welters, A., Kluppel, C., Mrugala, J., Wormeyer, L., Meissner, T., Mayatepek, E., Heiss, C., Eberhard, D., & Lammert, E. (2017). NMDAR antagonists for the treatment of diabetes mellitus-Current status and future directions. *Diabetes, obesity & metabolism*, 19(Suppl 1), 95–106.

Xu, T. Y., Guo, L. L., Wang, P., Song, J., Le, Y. Y., Viollet, B., & Miao, C. Y. (2012). Chronic Exposure to Nicotine Enhances Insulin Sensitivity through α7 Nicotinic Acetylcholine Receptor-STAT3 Pathway. *PLoS ONE*, 7(12), e51217.

Yuan, J., He, Q., Nguyen, L. H., Wong, M. C. S., Huang, J., Yu, Y., Xia, B., Tang, Y., He, Y., & Zhang, C. (2021). Regular use of proton pump inhibitors and risk of type 2 diabetes: results from three prospective cohort studies. *Gut*, 70(6), 1070–1077.

Zhou, Y., Waanders, L. F., Holmseth, S., Guo, C., Berger, U. V., Li, Y., Lehre, A. C., Lehre, K. P., & Danbolt, N. C. (2014). Proteome analysis and conditional deletion of the EAAT2 glutamate transporter provide evidence against a role of EAAT2 in pancreatic insulin secretion in mice. *The Journal of biological chemistry*, 289(3), 1329–1344.

Chapter 17

Targeting G Protein-Coupled Receptors in Type 2 Diabetes: From Molecular Mechanisms to Therapeutic Innovation

Aniruddha Sen*
Department of Biochemistry, All India Institute of Medical Sciences, Gorakhpur, Uttar Pradesh, India

Abstract

G protein-coupled receptors (GPCRs) are crucial in regulating glucose homeostasis and insulin secretion, making them key therapeutic targets for type 2 diabetes mellitus (T2DM). This chapter highlights important receptors, including the free fatty acid receptor 1 (FFAR1/GPR40) and the glucagon-like peptide-1 receptor (GLP-1R), and explores the molecular mechanisms underlying GPCR function in glucose metabolism. These receptors are central to the pathogenesis of T2DM, influencing appetite, insulin secretion, and inflammation. We review recent advancements in GPCR-targeted therapies, such as small molecule modulators and GLP-1 receptor agonists, which have demonstrated efficacy in enhancing glycemic control and promoting weight loss. Additionally, we examine the clinical implications, safety concerns, and future potential of these treatments, with a focus on challenges related to receptor selectivity, drug resistance, and adverse effects.

Keywords: G protein-coupled receptors (GPCRs), type 2 diabetes, glucose homeostasis, insulin sensitivity, GLP-1 receptor, β-cell dysfunction

Abbreviations

AI	Artificial Intelligence
cAMP	Cyclic Adenosine Monophosphate
CB1	Cannabinoid Receptor 1
CNS	Central Nervous System
DAG	Diacylglycerol

* Corresponding Author's Email: aniruddhasen7122@gmail.com

In: Receptor-Targeted Therapies in Diabetes Mellitus
Editors: Ajmer Singh Grewal, Neelam Singh, Swati Verma et al.
ISBN: 979-8-89530-587-4

FDA	Food and Drug Administration
FFAR1/ GPR40	Free Fatty Acid Receptor 1
GI	Gastrointestinal
GLP-1R	Glucagon-Like Peptide-1 Receptor
GPCR	G Protein-Coupled Receptor
GPR119	G Protein-Coupled Receptor 119
GPR120	G Protein-Coupled Receptor 120
GRK	GPCR Kinase
GSIS	Glucose-Stimulated Insulin Secretion
HbA1c	Hemoglobin A1c (Glycated Hemoglobin)
HTS	High-Throughput Screening
IP3	Inositol Trisphosphate
T2DM	Type 2 Diabetes Mellitus

Introduction

Type 2 diabetes mellitus (T2DM) is a chronic metabolic disorder marked by insulin resistance and progressive dysfunction of pancreatic beta cells, ultimately leading to hyperglycemia. T2DM is among the most pressing global health issues, contributing significantly to morbidity and mortality worldwide. The condition results from a combination of genetic and environmental factors that impair insulin action and secretion, leading to a gradual onset of insulin resistance and diminished cellular responsiveness to insulin. Over time, cells require higher insulin doses to absorb glucose from the bloodstream (Goyal et al. 2024). Initially, pancreatic beta cells compensate by producing more insulin; however, this adaptive response eventually fails, leading to insufficient insulin release and persistent hyperglycemia. T2DM affects multiple organs, including the liver, muscle, and adipose tissue. Insulin resistance in the liver increases glucose production, while impaired glucose uptake in muscle tissue raises blood glucose levels. Dysfunctional adipose tissue, with altered adipokine secretion, worsens insulin resistance and promotes inflammation in T2DM patients (Padhi et al. 2020). Receptors that regulate glucose metabolism play crucial roles in the pathophysiology and treatment of T2DM. In particular, G protein-coupled receptors (GPCRs) are essential in managing glucose homeostasis and insulin secretion. As cell surface receptors, GPCRs respond to external signals by triggering intracellular pathways that regulate cellular growth, metabolism, and differentiation. Specific GPCRs, such as the free fatty acid receptor 1 (FFAR1/GPR40) and glucagon-like peptide-1 receptor (GLP-1R), are particularly important in T2DM. FFAR1/GPR40, activated by long-chain fatty acids, enhances glucose-stimulated insulin secretion to better control postprandial glucose levels. GLP-1R, activated by the incretin hormone GLP-1, promotes insulin secretion, inhibits glucagon release, and induces satiety, helping to maintain blood glucose levels within a normal range (DeFronzo et al. 2015; Westman, 2021). Given their role in glucose metabolism, GPCRs hold significant therapeutic potential as drug targets in T2DM. GPCR-targeted therapies can enhance insulin secretion and sensitivity while regulating appetite, addressing multiple facets of T2DM simultaneously. Pharmacological advancements have led to the development of GPCR-targeted drugs, including GLP-1 receptor agonists, which improve glycemic control and support weight loss in T2DM patients by mimicking endogenous GLP-1 action (Bellou et al. 2018). Small-molecule modulators that selectively activate or inhibit GPCRs are also under investigation, offering promising options for personalized diabetes treatment and better patient outcomes. These advancements highlight the transformative potential of GPCR-targeted therapies in T2DM management (Artasensi et al. 2020). This chapter aims to provide insights into the therapeutic potential of targeting GPCRs in T2DM, addressing current advancements and future directions for improving disease management and patient outcomes.

G-Protein Coupled Receptors in Glucose Homeostasis

Structure and Function of GPCRs

GPCRs form a large family of cell surface receptors that respond to extracellular signals by activating specific intracellular signaling pathways. Structurally, GPCRs share a common architecture featuring seven transmembrane helices, with an extracellular N-terminus and an intracellular C-terminus. Upon ligand binding, GPCRs undergo conformational changes that enable the activation of associated G-proteins, which relay signals to downstream effectors, triggering cellular responses (Varney & Benovic, 2024). The versatility of GPCRs arises from their ability to interact with a range of ligands, including hormones, neurotransmitters, and metabolites. These interactions initiate multiple signaling pathways, such as the cyclic adenosine monophosphate (cAMP) and phosphatidylinositol pathways, and activate various kinases that regulate cellular responses (Zhang et al. 2017). In glucose homeostasis, GPCRs significantly influence insulin secretion, glucose uptake, and metabolic balance, playing a crucial role in maintaining normal blood glucose levels.

Key GPCRs Involved in Glucose Metabolism

Free Fatty Acid Receptor 1 (FFAR1/GPR40)

FFAR1, also known as GPR40, is a GPCR that responds to long-chain free fatty acids by binding with these ligands, thereby enhancing glucose-stimulated insulin secretion (GSIS). Upon activation, FFAR1 increases intracellular calcium levels, which then stimulate insulin release, aiding in postprandial glucose regulation (Regard et al. 2007). FFAR1 agonists hold therapeutic potential by promoting insulin release without causing hypoglycemia, a common and uncomfortable side effect of many antidiabetic medications. Clinical trials have shown encouraging results for FFAR1 agonists as potential treatments for T2DM (Dallatana et al. 2023).

Glucagon-Like Peptide-1 Receptor (GLP-1R)

GLP-1R is another crucial GPCR involved in glucose metabolism, activated by the incretin hormone GLP-1 and expressed in pancreatic beta cells, the central nervous system, and the gastrointestinal tract. Activation of GLP-1R by its ligand enhances insulin secretion through glucose-dependent mechanisms, inhibits glucagon release, and slows gastric emptying, all contributing to improved glycemic control (Wong et al. 2023). Due to their effectiveness in lowering blood glucose levels and promoting weight loss, GLP-1R agonists have become essential treatments for T2DM. By replicating GLP-1's natural actions, these agents provide notable benefits with a favorable safety profile (Zhang et al. 2024).

Signaling Pathways Mediated by GPCRs in T2DM

GPCRs are vital in regulating glucose homeostasis by activating signaling pathways through ligand binding and G protein coupling, which then modulate various downstream effectors, including adenylyl cyclase, phospholipase C, and ion channels. This cascade influences insulin secretion, glucose uptake, and metabolic balance (Souza et al. 2021). For instance, FFAR1 activation engages Gq proteins that stimulate phospholipase C, producing inositol trisphosphate (IP3) and diacylglycerol (DAG), which increase intracellular calcium and promote insulin secretion (Johnson et al. 2017). Additionally, GLP-1R activation involves Gs protein coupling, leading to adenylyl cyclase activation and elevated cAMP levels, which enhance insulin gene transcription and secretion, contributing to better glucose regulation (Tao & Liang, 2014; Röthe et al. 2019). Table 1 summarizes the roles and therapeutic potential of key GPCRs in glucose metabolism, alongside the pathways they mediate in T2DM management.

Table 1. Key GPCRs and their role in glucose metabolism: targets and pathways

GPCR	Ligand	Primary Target Tissues	Mechanism of Action	Therapeutic Potential
FFAR1/GPR40	Long-chain free fatty acids	Pancreatic beta cells, liver, muscle	Enhances GSIS via increased intracellular calcium	FFAR1 agonists may improve postprandial glucose regulation without inducing hypoglycemia
GLP-1R	GLP-1	Pancreatic beta cells, CNS, GI tract	Enhances insulin secretion, inhibits glucagon release, slows gastric emptying	GLP-1R agonists lower blood glucose and promote weight loss in T2DM patients
GPR119	Lipid derivatives, incretin hormones	Pancreatic beta cells, intestines	Stimulates insulin secretion, inhibits glucagon release	Promising in improving glycemic control and enhancing insulin sensitivity
Cannabinoid receptor 1 (CB1)	Endocannabinoids	CNS, adipose tissue, liver, muscle	Modulates appetite, glucose metabolism, and insulin sensitivity	Potential target for obesity and metabolic syndrome treatment
GPR40	Fatty acids	Pancreatic beta cells, liver	Enhances insulin secretion by increasing calcium levels	GPR40 agonists are under investigation for improving insulin secretion in T2DM
GPR120	Long-chain polyunsaturated fatty acids	Adipose tissue, liver, muscle	Enhances insulin sensitivity, reduces inflammation	Target for improving insulin sensitivity and reducing metabolic inflammation in T2DM

GPCR-Targeted Therapies For T2DM

GPCR-targeted therapies have emerged as promising options for the treatment of T2DM because of their significant role in regulating glucose metabolism and insulin secretion. Advances in pharmacology have led to the development of various GPCR modulators that specifically target these receptors, increasing their therapeutic potential.

Pharmacological Advances in GPCR Modulators

GLP-1 Receptor Agonists

GLP-1 receptor agonists have emerged as one of the most significant advancements in GPCR-targeted therapies for T2DM. These agonists mimic the action of the endogenous incretin hormone GLP-1, which is crucial for regulating glucose homeostasis. GLP-1 activation boosts glucose-dependent insulin secretion, suppresses glucagon release, and slows gastric emptying, leading to reduced postprandial glucose spikes (Wendell et al. 2020). GLP-1R agonists, including exenatide, liraglutide, and semaglutide, have demonstrated substantial success in lowering HbA1c (glycated hemoglobin) levels, promoting weight loss, and providing cardiovascular benefits, making them indispensable in T2DM management (Dallatana et al. 2023).

Small Molecule Modulators

In addition to GLP-1 receptor agonists, small-molecule modulators of GPCRs have gained significant attention as potential treatments for T2DM. These modulators can function as agonists, antagonists, or allosteric modulators, offering a versatile approach to regulating GPCR activity. One such example is FFAR1 (GPR40) agonists, which enhance insulin secretion by binding to the GPR40 receptor on pancreatic beta cells when glucose enters. Other receptors involved in energy balance and metabolism, such as CB1 or GPR119, also play key roles in improving glycemic control and promoting weight loss (Obot et al. 2021; Gao & Jockers, 2021).

Mechanisms of Action of GPCR-Targeted Drugs

GPCR-targeted drugs work by modulating specific signaling pathways that regulate glucose metabolism and insulin secretion through the activation of their respective ligands. Upon ligand binding, GPCRs undergo conformational changes, leading to G protein binding/activation, which in turn activates or inhibits downstream signaling molecules such as adenylyl cyclase, phospholipase C, or various kinases to induce physiological responses (Varney & Benovic, 2024). For instance, GLP-1R agonists stimulate GLP-1Rs on pancreatic beta cells, promoting the production of cAMP, which enhances gene transcription and exocytosis to increase insulin secretion. Similarly, FFAR1 agonists activate Gq proteins, which in turn stimulate phospholipase C to generate IP3 and DAG; these second messengers increase intracellular calcium levels, facilitating insulin release (Lee et al. 2018).

Clinical Efficacy and Safety of GPCR-Targeted Therapies

Clinical studies have demonstrated the efficacy and safety of GPCR-targeted therapies in treating T2DM. GLP-1R agonists, in particular, have proven highly effective at lowering HbA1c levels and body weight while maintaining a favorable safety profile. These agents not only improve glycemic control but also offer cardiovascular benefits by reducing major adverse cardiovascular events (Deepak et al. 2021). Both liraglutide and semaglutide exemplify this dual benefit by addressing both glycemic control and cardiovascular outcomes simultaneously (Ghislain & Poitout, 2021). Small-molecule modulators like FFAR1 agonists have shown promising results in clinical trials, improving insulin secretion and glycemic control without inducing hypoglycemia, which is a major concern with many other antidiabetic drugs

(Laeremans et al. 2022). However, challenges remain, including drug resistance and potential side effects such as gastrointestinal discomfort associated with GLP-1 receptor agonists.

Current GPCR-Targeted Drugs on the Market

Overview of Approved GPCR-Targeted Drugs

GPCR-targeted drugs for treating T2DM have advanced significantly in recent years, earning regulatory approval and demonstrating remarkable clinical benefits. GLP-1R agonists, in particular, have revolutionized the management of T2DM. Drugs such as exenatide, liraglutide, lixisenatide, albiglutide, and dulaglutide are widely adopted by regulatory agencies. These medications mimic GLP-1's action, reducing glucagon release, slowing gastric emptying, increasing satiety, and improving glycemic control and weight loss (As et al. 2017). Zhang et al. (2024) highlighted the rapid efficacy of these agents in managing glycemia and promoting weight loss (Zhang et al. 2024). In addition to GLP-1R agonists, drugs targeting free fatty acid receptor 1 (FFAR1/GPR40), like fasiglifam/TAK-875, have shown promise in increasing insulin secretion to improve glucose regulation (Addis et al. 2024). However, liver toxicity issues led to the discontinuation of TAK-875, prompting ongoing research into safer alternatives (Piper et al. 2022).

Case Studies and Clinical Trials

Efficacy in Enhancing Insulin Secretion

GPCR-targeted drugs, particularly GLP-1R agonists, have been extensively studied in clinical trials for their ability to enhance insulin secretion, with significant improvements in beta-cell function and glucose-dependent insulin release. In a T2DM patient study, liraglutide demonstrated a significant enhancement in both insulin secretion and beta-cell function compared to a placebo (Yuan et al. 2024). Similarly, exenatide treatment led to sustained improvements in insulin secretion and glucose control over a 52-week period (Yang et al. 2021). Clinical trials involving FFAR1 agonists have also shown promising results. Fasiglifam, in particular, demonstrated efficacy in increasing insulin secretion and reducing HbA1c levels compared to a placebo in one randomized controlled trial, suggesting its potential as an alternative therapy for T2DM. However, further research is needed to develop safer FFAR1 agonists to minimize the adverse effects observed in earlier trials (Jamaluddin & Gorvin, 2023).

Impact on Insulin Sensitivity

GPCR-targeted therapies not only enhance insulin secretion but also improve insulin sensitivity, a crucial factor in the management of T2DM. GLP-1R agonists, for example, have been shown to increase insulin sensitivity by reducing glucotoxicity and lipotoxicity, which are major contributors to insulin resistance. One such therapy, dulaglutide, has demonstrated significant improvements in both insulin sensitivity and body weight reduction in T2DM patients (Reimann & Gribble, 2016). Additionally, GPCR modulators, such as GPR119 agonists, which stimulate insulin secretion and inhibit glucagon release, have been shown to enhance insulin sensitivity and overall glycemic control (Gao & Jockers, 2021). These findings underscore the potential of GPCR-targeted therapies to offer comprehensive benefits for managing both insulin secretion and sensitivity in T2DM patients.

Challenges in GPCR-Based Drug Development

Specificity and Selectivity of GPCR Targeting

One of the primary challenges in GPCR drug development is achieving high specificity and selectivity. GPCRs constitute a large and diverse family of receptors found in various tissues, where they perform critical physiological roles. Due to their widespread expression, targeting a specific GPCR without affecting others can be difficult, often resulting in off-target effects and unintended side effects (Yuan et al. 2024). The challenge of receptor specificity is further compounded by the conserved nature of GPCR ligand-binding sites. However, advances in structure-based drug design and the development of high-resolution GPCR structures have facilitated the creation of more selective ligands. One promising approach is the use of allosteric modulators, which target sites distinct from the orthosteric binding sites. This method allows for more precise modulation of receptor activity, thereby enhancing selectivity. Despite their potential, the identification and optimization of allosteric modulators remain complex and resource-intensive (Laeremans et al. 2022; Shen et al. 2024).

Potential Adverse Effects

GPCR-targeted therapies, while effective, may lead to various adverse side effects due to the wide range of physiological functions these receptors regulate. For example, while GLP-1R agonists are highly effective in improving glycemic control and promoting weight loss, they are associated with common side effects such as nausea, vomiting, and diarrhea, which should be carefully considered when selecting these agents for treatment (Gao & Jockers, 2021). Additionally, prolonged activation or inhibition of GPCRs can result in compensatory mechanisms, including receptor desensitization, which can complicate therapeutic outcomes over time. Achieving an optimal balance between therapeutic efficacy and safety is crucial; as such, comprehensive preclinical and clinical evaluations must be conducted before these drugs are approved for use in the general population (Yang et al. 2021).

Development of Drug Resistance

Drug resistance remains a major challenge in the development of GPCR-targeted therapies, particularly for chronic conditions like T2DM, where long-term medication usage is often necessary. Repeated or excessive stimulation of GPCRs can lead to receptor desensitization, internalization, and downregulation, which reduces the drug's efficacy over time (Willard et al. 2020). This process is largely driven by GPCR kinases (GRKs), which phosphorylate the receptors, binding arrestin proteins to block further G protein activation and promote receptor internalization (Usman et al. 2020). To overcome this, strategies such as the development of biased agonists which preferentially activate beneficial signaling pathways over desensitization pathways are being explored (Cao et al. 2024).

Innovative Approaches in GPCR-Targeted Therapies

Advances in Drug Discovery Techniques

GPCR-targeted therapies have seen significant progress in recent years, largely driven by advances in drug discovery techniques such as structural biology, computational modeling, and high-throughput screening (HTS) (Table 2). Notably, innovations like cryo-electron microscopy (cryo-EM) and X-ray crystallography have enabled high-resolution structural elucidation of GPCRs, revealing intricate details about receptor conformation and potential binding sites. These advancements have laid the groundwork for rational drug design, allowing for the creation of more selective and potent GPCR modulators (Deepak et al. 2021). Structure-based drug design has become a cornerstone of GPCR-targeted therapy development. Advances in computational techniques, including molecular docking and simulations, have further facilitated the identification of potential drug candidates. Virtual screening of compound libraries, aided by these techniques, has increased the probability of discovering new, effective GPCR modulators. HTS has also revolutionized drug discovery in the GPCR space. The integration of automation and machine learning algorithms into HTS processes has optimized screening efficiency, improving hit rates and accelerating the overall drug discovery pipeline. This combination of techniques represents a powerful approach to developing the next generation of GPCR-targeted therapies.

Personalized Medicine and GPCR Modulation

Personalized medicine has become increasingly important for the management of T2DM, with GPCR modulation playing a central role in this approach. T2DM patients exhibit considerable variability in GPCR expression and function, which influences the efficacy and safety of treatments. Thus, tailoring therapeutic strategies to individual characteristics is essential for optimizing clinical outcomes. Genetic analyses have revealed that genetic variations in GPCR genes can significantly affect the response to drugs, emphasizing the importance of personalized treatment strategies (Rehman et al. 2024). Pharmacogenomics, the study of genetic variations that impact drug responses, enables the selection of GPCR-targeted therapies based on an individual's genetic profile (Kolar et al. 2017). For instance, understanding gene polymorphisms allows for the identification of specific agonists or antagonists that are most likely to be effective, reducing the likelihood of adverse side effects and improving overall treatment outcomes. Moreover, advancements in biomarker discovery have led to the identification of molecular signatures related to GPCR signaling pathways, providing valuable tools for monitoring therapeutic responses.

Table 2. Advances in drug discovery techniques for GPCR-targeted therapies

Technique	Description	Impact on GPCR Drug Discovery
Cryo-EM	Provides high-resolution structural details of GPCRs, enabling precise mapping of receptor conformations and binding sites	Facilitates structure-based drug design by allowing researchers to visualize receptor–ligand interactions at atomic resolution
X-ray Crystallography	Elucidates 3D structures of GPCRs, offering insight into receptor architecture and potential drug binding sites	Enables the identification of specific receptor conformations and guides rational drug design to improve selectivity
Structure-Based Drug Design	Uses detailed structural information to design ligands that fit specific binding pockets within GPCRs	Improves the specificity of GPCR-targeted therapies, reducing off-target effects and enhancing therapeutic efficacy
Computational Modeling & Simulations	Employs molecular docking and simulations to predict interactions between GPCRs and potential drug candidates	Accelerates virtual screening of compound libraries, increasing the efficiency of identifying lead compounds
High-Throughput Screening (HTS)	Tests thousands of compounds quickly to identify those with the desired biological activity on GPCR targets	Increases the speed of identifying active compounds and optimizes hit rates, especially when combined with automation and AI
Machine Learning & Automation	Utilizes AI algorithms to analyze data from HTS and predict receptor–ligand interactions	Enhances the accuracy of drug discovery and optimizes the screening process, reducing the time and cost of drug development

These biomarkers enable clinicians to adjust therapies dynamically, ensuring that patients receive the most effective and safest treatments available (Tian et al. 2022). Integrating biomarkers into personalized medicine can enhance the management of T2DM and other metabolic disorders by offering targeted therapies that are customized to the individual's unique genetic makeup and disease profile (Atanes & Persaud, 2020).

Future Prospects and Research Directions

Newer targeted therapies for treating T2DM that focus on GPCRs are poised to drive significant advancements in the field. Ongoing research, combined with technological breakthroughs, is pushing the boundaries of GPCR modulation. A promising approach involves the development of biased agonists, which specifically activate certain signaling pathways within GPCRs while avoiding others. This selective activation could enhance therapeutic effects and minimize undesirable side effects, providing a more targeted and precise approach to GPCR regulation (Sloop et al. 2018). Another exciting avenue is the exploration of allosteric modulators. Unlike conventional orthosteric ligands that bind directly to the main active sites of GPCRs, allosteric modulators interact with receptors at distinct sites, offering a new layer of control over receptor activity. This approach could increase the specificity of receptor activation, reducing the likelihood of desensitization and resistance, thus providing a more sustainable therapeutic effect. Furthermore, the integration of artificial intelligence (AI) and machine learning is expected to revolutionize GPCR drug discovery. AI-powered algorithms can rapidly analyze large-scale databases, predict interactions between drugs and receptors, and optimize lead compounds with unprecedented speed and accuracy. This data-driven approach will likely accelerate the development of novel GPCR-targeted therapeutics, improving both their precision and efficiency (Laeremans et al. 2022). These innovative strategies hold great promise for advancing the future of T2DM treatment, offering more effective and personalized therapies for patients.

Conclusion

GPCRs have emerged as pivotal regulators of glucose metabolism, insulin secretion, and energy balance, positioning them as promising targets for novel T2DM therapies. GLP-1R agonists, in particular, have already transformed T2DM management by improving glycemic control and promoting weight loss, with proven efficacy and safety in clinical practice. However, the development of GPCR-targeted therapies faces challenges, including receptor specificity, drug resistance, and potential adverse effects. Recent advancements in structural biology, high-throughput screening, and computational modeling have played a crucial role in overcoming these challenges, enabling more precise drug design and personalized treatment approaches. The future of GPCR-targeted therapies in T2DM is promising, with ongoing research exploring innovative strategies such as allosteric modulators, biased agonists, and the integration of machine learning in drug discovery. These breakthroughs are set to enhance therapeutic efficacy, minimize side effects, and offer personalized treatment options based on individual genetic profiles. As research continues to progress, GPCR-based therapies are poised to further revolutionize T2DM treatment, improving patient outcomes and quality of life.

References

Addis, P., Bali, U., Baron, F., Campbell, A., Harborne, S., Jagger, L., Milne, G., Pearce, M., Rosethorne, E. M., Satchell, R., Swift, D., Young, B., & Unitt, J. F. (2024). Key aspects of modern GPCR drug discovery. *SLAS Discovery: Advancing Life Sciences R & D*, 29(1), 1–22.

Artasensi, A., Pedretti, A., Vistoli, G., & Fumagalli, L. (2020). Type 2 Diabetes Mellitus: A Review of Multi-Target Drugs. *Molecules*, 25(8), Article 8.

As, H., Mm, A., M, R.-A., Hb, S., & De, G. (2017). Trends in GPCR drug discovery: new agents, targets and indications. *Nature Reviews. Drug Discovery*, 16(12), 829–842.

Atanes, P., & Persaud, S. J. (2020). Chapter 18—GPCR targets in type 2 diabetes. In B. Jastrzebska & P. S.-H. Park (Eds.), *GPCRs* (pp. 367–391). Academic Press.

Bellou, V., Belbasis, L., Tzoulaki, I., & Evangelou, E. (2018). Risk factors for type 2 diabetes mellitus: An exposure-wide umbrella review of meta-analyses. *PloS One*, 13(3), e0194127.

Cao, D., Zhang, P., & Wang, S. (2024). Advances in structure-based drug design: The potential for precision therapeutics in psychiatric disorders. *Neuron*, 112(4), 526–538.

Dallatana, A., Cremonesi, L., Trombetta, M., Fracasso, G., Nocini, R., Giacomello, L., & Innamorati, G. (2023). G Protein-Coupled Receptors and the Rise of Type 2 Diabetes in Children. *Biomedicines*, 11(6), 1576.

Deepak, R. N. V. K., Verma, R. K., Hartono, Y. D., Yew, W. S., & Fan, H. (2021). Recent Advances in Structure, Function, and Pharmacology of Class A Lipid GPCRs: Opportunities and Challenges for Drug Discovery. *Pharmaceuticals*, 15(1), 12.

DeFronzo, R. A., Ferrannini, E., Groop, L., Henry, R. R., Herman, W. H., Holst, J. J., Hu, F. B., Kahn, C. R., Raz, I., Shulman, G. I., Simonson, D. C., Testa, M. A., & Weiss, R. (2015). Type 2 diabetes mellitus. *Nature Reviews Disease Primers*, 1(1), 1–22.

Gao, W., & Jockers, R. (2021). Pharmacogenomics of GPCR genes in type 2 diabetes and obesity. *Current Opinion in Endocrine and Metabolic Research*, 16, 128–135.

Ghislain, J., & Poitout, V. (2021). Targeting lipid GPCRs to treat type 2 diabetes mellitus—Progress and challenges. *Nature Reviews. Endocrinology*, 17(3), 162–175.

Goyal, R., Singhal, M., & Jialal, I. (2024). *Type 2 Diabetes*. StatPearls Publishing.

Jamaluddin, A., & Gorvin, C. M. (2023). Rising Stars: Targeting G protein-coupled receptors to regulate energy homeostasis. *Journal of Molecular Endocrinology*, 70(4), e230014.

Johnson, R. J., Applegarth, J., Bennett, S., Caskey, S., Coatney, C., Corsbie, K., Cotter, A., Cotter, D., Coulis, A., Hansen, H., Hart, W., Koehler, C., Koelper, A., Kuhlman, S., Mitchell, C., Moskal, B., Murfield, O., Paton, A., Schemenauer, D., Stankavich, B., Taylor, C., Waibel, B., & Williams, L. D. (2017). Proteopedia entry: G-protein coupled receptors. *Multimedia in Biochemistry and Molecular Biology Education*, 45(3), 277–278.

Kolar, G. R., Grote, S. M., & Yosten, G. L. C. (2017). Targeting orphan G protein-coupled receptors for the treatment of diabetes and its complications: C-peptide and GPR146. *Journal of Internal Medicine*, 281(1), 25–40.

Laeremans, T., Sands, Z. A., Claes, P., De Blieck, A., De Cesco, S., Triest, S., Busch, A., Felix, D., Kumar, A., Jaakola, V. P., & Menet, C. (2022). Accelerating GPCR drug discovery with conformation-stabilizing VHHs. *Frontiers in Molecular Biosciences*, 9, 863099.

Lee, Y., Basith, S., & Choi, S. (2018). Recent advances in structure-based drug design targeting class A G protein-coupled receptors utilizing crystal structures and computational simulations. *Journal of Medicinal Chemistry*, 61(1), 1–46.

Obot, D. N., Udom, G. J., Udoh, A. E., Onyeukwu, N. J., Olusola, A. J., Udoh, I. M., Umana, I. K., Yemitan, O. K., & Okokon, J. E. (2021). Advances in the molecular understanding of G protein-coupled receptors and their future therapeutic opportunities. *Future Journal of Pharmaceutical Sciences*, 7(1), 194.

Padhi, S., Nayak, A. K., & Behera, A. (2020). Type II diabetes mellitus: A review on recent drug based therapeutics. *Biomedicine & Pharmacotherapy*, 131, 110708.

Piper, N. B. C., Whitfield, E. A., Stewart, G. D., Xu, X., & Furness, S. G. B. (2022). Targeting appetite and satiety in diabetes and obesity, via G protein-coupled receptors. *Biochemical Pharmacology*, 202, 115115.

Regard, J. B., Kataoka, H., Cano, D. A., Camerer, E., Yin, L., Zheng, Y.-W., Scanlan, T. S., Hebrok, M., & Coughlin, S. R. (2007). Probing cell type-specific functions of Gi *in vivo* identifies GPCR regulators of insulin secretion. *The Journal of Clinical Investigation*, 117(12), 4034–4043.

Rehman, S., Rahimi, N., & Dimri, M. (2024). *Biochemistry, G Protein Coupled Receptors*. StatPearls Publishing.

Reimann, F., & Gribble, F. M. (2016). G protein-coupled receptors as new therapeutic targets for type 2 diabetes. *Diabetologia*, 59(2), 229–233.

Röthe, J., Thor, D., Winkler, J., Knierim, A. B., Binder, C., Huth, S., Kraft, R., Rothemund, S., Schöneberg, T., & Prömel, S. (2019). Involvement of the Adhesion GPCRs Latrophilins in the Regulation of Insulin Release. *Cell Reports*, 26(6), 1573-1584.e5.

Shen, S., Liao, Q., Gu, L., Zhu, Y., Liu, Y., Zhang, X., Zhang, J., Shi, Q., Sun, Y., Wang, J., & Lin, L. (2024). G protein-coupled receptor-biased signaling: Potential drug discovery to facilitate treatment of metabolic diseases. *Acta Materia Medica*, 3, 31–45.

Sloop, K. W., Emmerson, P. J., Statnick, M. A., & Willard, F. S. (2018). The current state of GPCR-based drug discovery to treat metabolic disease. *British Journal of Pharmacology*, 175(21), 4060–4071.

Souza, C., Sun, X., & Oh, D. (2021). Metabolic Functions of G Protein-Coupled Receptors and β-Arrestin-Mediated Signaling Pathways in the Pathophysiology of Type 2 Diabetes and Obesity. *Frontiers in Endocrinology*, 12, 715877.

Tao, Y. X., & Liang, X. F. (2014). G protein-coupled receptors as regulators of glucose homeostasis and therapeutic targets for diabetes mellitus. *Progress in Molecular Biology and Translational Science*, 121, 1–21.

Tian, H., Zhang, T., Qin, S., Huang, Z., Zhou, L., Shi, J., Nice, E. C., Xie, N., Huang, C., & Shen, Z. (2022). Enhancing the therapeutic efficacy of nanoparticles for cancer treatment using versatile targeted strategies. *Journal of Hematology & Oncology*, 15(1), 132.

Usman, S., Khawer, M., Rafique, S., Naz, Z., & Saleem, K. (2020). The current status of anti-GPCR drugs against different cancers. *Journal of Pharmaceutical Analysis*, 10(6), 517–521.

Varney, M. J., & Benovic, J. L. (2024). The Role of G Protein–Coupled Receptors and Receptor Kinases in Pancreatic β-Cell Function and Diabetes. *Pharmacological Reviews*, 76(2), 267–299.

Wendell, S. G., Fan, H., & Zhang, C. (2020). G Protein-Coupled Receptors in Asthma Therapy: Pharmacology and Drug Action. *Pharmacological Reviews*, 72(1), 1–49.

Westman, E. C. (2021). Type 2 Diabetes Mellitus: A Pathophysiologic Perspective. *Frontiers in Nutrition*, 8, 707371.

Willard, F. S., Ho, J. D., & Sloop, K. W. (2020). Discovery and pharmacology of the covalent GLP-1 receptor (GLP-1R) allosteric modulator BETP: A novel tool to probe GLP-1R pharmacology. *Advances in Pharmacology*, 88, 173–191.

Wong, T. S., Gao, W., Chen, G., Qiu, C., He, G., Ye, F., Wu, Z., Zeng, Z., & Du, Y. (2023). Cryo-EM structure of orphan G protein-coupled receptor GPR21. *MedComm*, 4(1), e205.

Yang, D., Zhou, Q., Labroska, V., Qin, S., Darbalaei, S., Wu, Y., Yuliantie, E., Xie, L., Tao, H., Cheng, J., Liu, Q., Zhao, S., Shui, W., Jiang, Y., & Wang, M. W. (2021). G protein-coupled receptors: Structure- and function-based drug discovery. *Signal Transduction and Targeted Therapy*, 6(1), 7.

Yuan, W., Shi, X., & Lee, L. T. O. (2024). RNA therapeutics in targeting G protein-coupled receptors: Recent advances and challenges. Molecular Therapy. *Nucleic Acids*, 35(2), 102195.

Zhang, C., Wang, Y., Kimura, T., & Al-Mrabeh, A. H. (2024). Editorial: The role of GPCRs in obesity. *Frontiers in Endocrinology*, 15, 1404969.

Zhang, H., Qiao, A., Yang, D., Yang, L., Dai, A., de Graaf, C., Reedtz-Runge, S., Dharmarajan, V., Zhang, H., Han, G. W., Grant, T. D., Sierra, R. G., Weierstall, U., Nelson, G., Liu, W., Wu, Y., Ma, L., Cai, X., Lin, G., Wu, X., Geng, Z., Dong, Y., Song, G., Griffin, P. R., Lau, J., Cherezov, V., Yang, H., Hanson, M. A., Stevens, R. C., Zhao, Q., Jiang, H., Wang, M. W., & Wu, B. (2017). Structure of the full-length glucagon class B G-protein-coupled receptor. *Nature*, 546(7657), 259–264.

Zhang, M., Chen, T., Lu, X., Lan, X., Chen, Z., & Lu, S. (2024). G protein-coupled receptors (GPCRs): Advances in structures, mechanisms, and drug discovery. *Signal Transduction and Targeted Therapy*, 9(1), 1–43.

Chapter 18

The Role of GAD65 in Early Detection of Latent Autoimmune Diabetes in Adults (LADA)

Lima Patowary[1,2]
and Trideep Saikia[1,2,*]
[1]School of Pharmaceutical Sciences, Girijananda Chowdhury University, Guwahati, Assam, India
[2]Department of Pharmaceutical Sciences, Dibrugarh University, Dibrugarh, Assam, India

Abstract

A crucial autoantigen, glutamic acid decarboxylase 65 (GAD65), triggers the production of autoantibodies (GADA), which are key biomarkers for identifying latent autoimmune diabetes in adults (LADA). The presence of these autoantibodies in LADA suggests an autoimmune pathogenesis, with an inverse relationship between GADA levels and C-peptide levels, which serve as indicators of insulin production. The distinct mobility regions within the GAD65 molecule, which overlap with the region containing important antigenic epitopes, suggest that the C-terminal region of GAD65 may be particularly flexible, potentially playing a key role. In diabetic patients, GADA epitope-specific assays could improve the specificity of clinical diagnostics. This chapter covers the pathophysiology of LADA, its role in the autoimmune response, and the biochemical characteristics of GAD65. It also discusses the significance of GAD65 autoantibodies in diagnostic methods, early detection, and clinical management.

Keywords: Latent autoimmune diabetes in adults (LADA), glutamic acid decarboxylase 65 (GAD65), autoantibodies, early detection, clinical management

Abbreviations

APC	Antigen-presenting cells
CVD	Cardiovascular diseases
ELISA	Enzyme-linked immunosorbent assays
GABA	Gamma aminobutyric acid

* Corresponding Author's Email: trideep.saikia3@gmail.com

In: Receptor-Targeted Therapies in Diabetes Mellitus
Editors: Ajmer Singh Grewal, Neelam Singh, Swati Verma et al.
ISBN: 979-8-89530-587-4

GAD65	65 kDa glutamic acid decarboxylase
GADA	Glutamic acid decarboxylase antibodies
HLA	Human leukocyte antigen
IA-2A	Insulinoma-associated antigen-2 autoantibodies
IAA	Insulin autoantibody
ICA	Islet cell antibodies
LADA	Latent autoimmune diabetes in adults
RIA	Radio immune assay
T1DM	Type 1 diabetes mellitus
T2DM	Type 2 diabetes mellitus
ZnT8A	Zinc transporter-8 autoantibodies

Introduction

Latent autoimmune diabetes in adults (LADA) is a unique form of diabetes that combines characteristics of both type 1 diabetes mellitus (T1DM) and type 2 diabetes mellitus (T2DM). First described by Tuomi et al. (1993), the term LADA was used to identify a subgroup of patients with T2DM-like features but who also display immune markers typical of T1DM. Often referred to as "type 1.5 diabetes," LADA accounts for approximately 2% to 12% of all adult diabetes cases (Hu et al. 2022; Zhu et al. 2020). Studies have reported that 4% to 14% of patients initially diagnosed with T2DM are later found to have LADA based on autoantibody testing performed at various centers globally (Mishra et al. 2018; Pozzilli & Pieralice, 2018). Diagnosing LADA generally relies on three main criteria: adult onset of the disease (typically after age 30), the presence of at least one islet autoantibody indicating autoimmune activity, and no need for insulin treatment for at least six months after diagnosis. However, the specific application of these criteria can vary; while adult onset is typically required, the age threshold (either 30 or 35 years) is still debated. The delayed insulin dependency that differentiates LADA from adult-onset T1DM often includes an initial period of six to twelve months without insulin therapy, although this guideline is somewhat flexible and may be adjusted based on the physician's judgment (Brophy et al. 2008). Fasting C-peptide levels are useful in indicating ongoing insulin production and a "latent" onset of the condition (Rasouli et al. 2016; Takeda et al. 2002). The most widely accepted criterion is the detection of autoantibodies that indicate autoimmune activity, setting LADA apart from T2DM (Fourlanos et al. 2005). The standard diagnostic approach for LADA involves testing for islet autoantibodies, such as glutamic acid decarboxylase antibodies (GADA), insulin autoantibody (IAA), zinc transporter-8 autoantibodies (ZnT8A), and insulinoma-associated antigen-2 autoantibodies (IA-2A). Most LADA patients are GADA-positive, as GADA is a major autoantigen in β-cell-specific autoimmunity (Cernea et al. 2009; Fourlanos et al. 2005). Cross-sectional studies have linked GADA titer to the phenotypic variability of LADA patients (Mohan's, 2023). GADA affinity can vary up to 10,000-fold among GADA-positive LADA patients and is associated with the subsequent need for insulin therapy, inversely correlating with β-cell function (Krause et al. 2014). The clinical importance of developing early diabetes biomarkers is well-supported by previous research. For example, a rapid lateral flow immunoassay for tyrosine-phosphatase-like protein IA-2 (IA-2As) and GAD65 autoantibodies using an electrochemiluminescence assay has shown high sensitivity and specificity for early T1DM diagnosis, facilitating early intervention (Kikkas et al. 2014; Miao et al. 2013). Additionally, a radio-binding assay with radiolabeled GAD65(96–585) has proven highly sensitive in identifying individuals at high risk for T1DM (Wuragil et al. 2022). Similar to T1DM, autoimmunity appears to be the initial pathogenic mechanism in LADA (Insel et al. 2015). T1DM is a chronic autoimmune disorder characterized by reduced insulin production due to the destruction of pancreatic β-cells, accompanied by the presence of multiple islet autoantibodies. In contrast, LADA primarily presents with GADA positivity. Recent studies highlight the role of 65 kDa glutamic acid decarboxylase (GAD65) in the pathogenesis of T1DM (Hampe et al. 2013; Towns et al. 2011). Elevated levels of GAD65 in asymptomatic diabetic patients may indicate early disease onset (Lenmark & Larsson, 2013; Zampetti et al. 2014). GAD65 may serve as a marker for reduced β-cell function in early T1DM (Ludvigsson et al. 2012). Compared to other markers, GAD antibodies are more effective in tracking disease progression, as they share similar properties with GAD65 (Towns et al. 2011). Therefore, GAD65 holds potential as a serological biomarker for detecting pre-diabetic conditions and could be a promising target for clinical diagnostic development (Zampetti et al. 2014). This chapter examines the pathophysiology of LADA, the biochemical properties of GAD65, its role in the autoimmune response, and various diagnostic approaches, emphasizing the significance of GAD65 autoantibodies in early detection and clinical management. Additionally, it reviews recent research, advances in detection technologies, and potential therapeutic targets related to GAD65, with the aim of improving early diagnosis and treatment outcomes for LADA.

Pathophysiology

T1DM, T2DM, and LADA are often grouped under elderly-onset diabetes without precise distinctions (Table 1). However, identifying specific forms of diabetes can be aided by examining pathogenic factors such as insulin resistance, β-cell function, and immunological activity (Ravikumar et al. 2023). Similar to T1DM, LADA is marked by the presence of autoantibodies, indicating an autoimmune mechanism. Although the pathophysiology of LADA is not fully understood, studies suggest it is primarily driven by cell-mediated immunity (Brooks-Worrell et al. 1999; Signore et al. 2015). *In vitro* research on LADA patients has demonstrated that peripheral blood mononuclear cells (PBMCs) can inhibit insulin secretion in human islets, highlighting the role of cell-mediated autoimmunity in LADA (Brooks-Worrell et al. 1999). Research from Japan on pancreatic biopsies from LADA patients found that T-cell infiltration is a primary characteristic of insulitis, providing strong evidence for a cellular immune-driven onset in LADA (Shimada et al. 1999). Additionally, a reduction in regulatory T cells and functional irregularities in these cells are believed to contribute to LADA's autoimmunity (Li et al. 2011). Recent research increasingly suggests that innate immunity directly influences autoimmune diabetes mellitus (Wang et al. 2015). LADA and T1DM share certain immunological markers, including pancreatic β-cell-specific autoantibodies, similar profiles of proinflammatory cytokines at both cellular and systemic levels, and persistent alterations in some immune cell phenotypes (Hu et al. 2022). However, individuals with LADA generally exhibit higher levels of C-peptide, an indicator of insulin production, and often do not require insulin immediately after diagnosis. This suggests a milder autoimmune process and a slower progression of β-cell loss (Carlsson et al. 2000; Hernandez et al. 2015). Unlike T2DM, patients with LADA produce less insulin, which eventually leads to a quicker dependence on insulin therapy (Hernandez et al. 2015; Zampetti et al. 2014). This gradual progression distinguishes LADA from both T1DM and T2DM, highlighting the importance of differential diagnosis for optimal treatment.

Turner et al. (1997) analyzed data from the UK Perspective Diabetes Study (UKPDS), which showed that 84% of patients initially diagnosed with T2DM and testing positive for GADA became insulin-dependent within six years, contrasting with only 14% among those without antibodies. This suggests that, similar to T1DM, autoimmunity is a key pathological factor in LADA. Findings from the HUNT Study further revealed that 64% of LADA patients were GADA-positive years before diagnosis (Sørgjerd et al. 2012), a pattern also seen in the Finnish Botnia Study (Lundgren et al. 2010). While LADA patients typically test positive for GADA, T1DM patients often exhibit multiple islet autoantibodies (Regnell & Lernmark, 2017; Tuomi et al. 1999). The European multicenter Action LADA study found that 90% of antibody-positive LADA patients were GADA-positive, with only 10% testing positive for antibodies against zinc transporter 8 (ZnT8A) or insulinoma-associated antigen-2 (IA-2A) (Hawa et al. 2013). Multiple antibodies were present in 24% of Action LADA participants and 10% of LADA patients in the Norwegian HUNT Study (Hawa et al. 2013; Sørgjerd et al. 2012). There is an inverse relationship between GADA levels and C-peptide levels, which measure insulin production, making GADA a valuable marker for the presence and extent of autoimmune activity (Carlsson, 2019). Compared to T1DM patients, LADA patients generally produce more insulin at diagnosis, suggesting that factors beyond autoimmune beta-cell destruction may influence LADA's pathophysiology. Insulin resistance, though less prominent than in T2DM, has been observed in LADA patients and is associated with variations in BMI (Carlsson, 2019; Lundgren et al. 2010). Research from Sweden and Norway suggests that insulin resistance is more common in LADA patients with lower autoimmune activity, as reflected by lower GADA levels, than in those with higher levels of autoimmunity (Ravikumar et al. 2023).

Table 1. Comparison of clinical features between LADA, T1DM and T2DM (Hu et al. 2022; Keshavarz et al. 2022; Ravikumar et al. 2023)

Clinical and Genetic Characteristics	LADA	T1DM	T2DM
Diagnosis Age	Generally, >30-35 years	Mostly in childhood but very rarely in adult	Any
Resistance to insulin	High	Absent	High
β-cell function	Decrease	Loss of function	May be normal or a little increased
Insulin Requirement	Usually after 6 months of diagnosis	Required from the time of diagnosis	Absent or may require years after diagnosis
Body mass index	Normal rarely obese	Normal or might be underweight (<18.5)	>25.0 to >30.0 Overweight or obese
Family history	May or may not present	May or may not present	Frequently present
Risk of complications	High risk of CVD	High risk of CVD	High risk of CVD

Understanding GAD65 as a Biomarker for Lada

GAD is a primary autoantigen in autoimmune diabetes and is considered the most sensitive marker for diagnosing LADA (Cernea et al. 2009). While GAD and GABA are largely associated with GABA-ergic neurons, they are also present in non-neuronal tissues, including the pancreas, where GABA is stored within β-cells in synaptic-like vesicles (Towns & Pietropaolo, 2011; Buddhala et al. 2009). Although the function of GAD in islet β-cells remains unclear, it may influence the paracrine regulation of somatostatin, glucagon, and insulin release (Bu & Tobin, 1994). GAD has two main isoforms, GAD65 and GAD67; differing in molecular weight and subcellular localization. GAD65 is found in synaptic-like vesicles, while GAD67 resides in the cytoplasm of β-cells. Despite GAD67's higher expression in β-cells, only GAD65 is antigenic in T1DM autoimmunity (Buddhala et al. 2009; Fenalti & Buckle, 2010). The C-terminal region of GAD65 is flexible and contains key antigenic epitopes, while the N-terminal region undergoes palmitoylation, which localizes GAD65 to the Golgi and influences its antigenicity (Solimena et al. 1998; Christgau et al. 1992). GAD65's membrane anchoring and release may play critical roles in its autoantigenic function (Towns & Pietropaolo, 2011). Differences in epitope binding further distinguish LADA from T1DM. LADA patients generally have higher levels of GAD65-NAb (N-terminal antibodies) and lower levels of GAD65-CAb (C-terminal antibodies) compared to T1DM patients (Jin et al. 2011; Peng et al. 2023). LADA patients with GAD65-CAb tend to have reduced β-cell function, as evidenced by lower C-peptide levels and increased insulin dependence (Schlosser et al. 2005). In genetically susceptible individuals, the autoimmune response in LADA may spread from the N-terminal to the middle region of GAD65, marking the progression of β-cell decline (Hampe et al. 2002b).

Diagnostic Approaches for Lada

Current Diagnostic Criteria

Diagnosing LADA involves identifying the distinct characteristics that differentiate it from T1DM and T2DM. LADA's slow progression and initial independence from insulin often lead to it being misclassified as T2DM. The primary diagnostic criteria and distinguishing factors for LADA are outlined in Table 2 below.

Combining these criteria with careful attention to the patient's clinical progression and autoantibody presence can confirm a diagnosis of LADA. It's important to note that diagnosis may be challenging and may require ongoing monitoring and testing. Accurate diagnosis is essential for effective LADA management, often involving the earlier initiation of insulin therapy to preserve residual beta-cell function and reduce the risk of long-term complications.

Table 2. List of current diagnostic criteria for the LADA

Diagnostic Criteria	Explanation	Reference
Age of Onset	LADA usually manifests in adults over 30, frequently in the 30- to 50-year-old age range.	Biniek et al. 2023
Positive autoantibodies to islet β cells	An essential feature of autoimmune diabetes is the existence of autoantibodies against islet β cells (e.g., GADA, ICA, IAA, IA-2A, ZnT8A). Pancreatic β cells are attacked by an autoimmune response in LADA.	Yin et al. 2022
Autoantibody Testing	Diagnosis depends on the existence of autoantibodies linked to diabetes. The GADA is the most often tested autoantibody. LADA can be verified by a positive GADA test; research suggests that 83% of LADA cases can be diagnosed by looking for this antibody. Other than GADA, ICA, IAA, and IA-2A are additional autoantibodies that may be tested.	Biniek et al. 2023; Vich-Pérez et al. 2023
Insulin Requirement	The fact that patients do not need insulin therapy for at least six months following diagnosis is a significant diagnostic criterion for LADA. This sets LADA apart from traditional T1DM, where insulin is usually needed right away.	Buzzetti et al. (2020)
C-Peptide Levels	Measurement of C-peptide levels help assess residual β-cell function. Levels less than 0.3 nmol/L suggest severe dysfunction of the β-cell, which calls for a treatment plan akin to that of T1DM. In the "grey area," or levels between 0.3 and 0.7 nmol/L, a combination of approaches might be required. Levels greater than 0.7 nmol/L indicate a T2DM-like treatment strategy with close observation for advancement.	Buzzetti et al. 2020; Pozzilli & Pieralice, 2018
Clinical Features	Compared to typical T2DM patients, patients with LADA may have characteristics like a lower BMI (often <25 kg/m2), a family history of autoimmune diseases, and less obvious insulin resistance.	Pozzilli & Pieralice, 2018
Family History of Autoimmune Diseases and Progressive Nature	The diagnosis of LADA may be supported by a history of autoimmune diseases in the family. In contrast to T2DM, which can be controlled for many years with oral medications, LADA leads to insulin dependence more quickly.	Carlsson et al. 2007

Role of Autoantibodies in Diagnosis

GADA is crucial in diagnosing LADA as the primary marker, detected in approximately 70–80% of cases at diagnosis. Testing for GADA is essential to differentiate autoimmune diabetes, such as T1DM and LADA, from T2DM (Rosário et al. 2007). In a meta-analysis involving 377 diabetic patients, GADA levels were used to identify LADA, dividing participants into 318 with T2DM and 59 with LADA. Compared to T2DM patients, those with LADA showed lower fasting glucose levels, fewer complications, an earlier age of diagnosis, higher insulin use, and a higher estimated Glucose Disposal Rate (eGDR). An eGDR above 9.75 mg/kg/min and age under 40.5 years were strongly linked to LADA, aiding early detection and referral in southeast Mexico (Nolasco-Rosales et al. 2023). Elevated GADA levels in LADA patients can predict the rate of β-cell decline and the eventual need for insulin, with higher titers indicating quicker progression to insulin dependence. Diagnosing LADA involves detecting GADA alongside clinical criteria, such as adult-onset diabetes and no need for insulin for at least six months, distinguishing it from T1DM, which necessitates immediate insulin therapy (Mohan's, 2023). Although GADA testing alone usually suffices to distinguish LADA from T2DM, sensitivity diminishes in older patients. GADA testing thus allows for early intervention and monitoring of β-cell function, which is especially beneficial for LADA patients, who often require earlier insulin therapy than typical T2DM patients (Rosário et al. 2007). ICA, another important marker, is also used to diagnose autoimmune diabetes, including LADA. Although GADA is the most common autoantibody in LADA, ICA testing is useful when GADA results are inconclusive. Around 20–50% of LADA patients present ICA, supporting the autoimmune etiology of diabetes (Zimmet et al. 1994). Detecting ICA alongside GADA and other autoantibodies, such as IA-2A and ZnT8A, enhances diagnostic accuracy, particularly in patients with atypical diabetes symptoms. ICA presence suggests ongoing immune-mediated β-cell destruction, which may lead to earlier insulin dependence. Initiating early insulin therapy in ICA-positive LADA patients may help preserve β-cell function and improve long-term glycemic control (Kawasaki et al. 2023; Rajkumar & Levine, 2023). Other markers such as IAA, IA-2A, and ZnT8A also assist in diagnosing LADA. IAA indicates an autoimmune reaction against insulin and is often one of the earliest markers during an autoimmune attack on β cells, helping distinguish LADA from T2DM, which usually lacks autoimmune markers (Fourlanos et al. 2005; Sutkowska et al. 2021). IA-2A, an antibody targeting a protein involved in insulin secretion, further confirms autoimmune diabetes when present. Though less common than GADA, IA-2A is found in many LADA patients (Bottazzo et al. 2005). ZnT8A, which targets a protein essential for insulin secretion, also signals an autoimmune response, and when combined with other markers such as IA-2A and GADA, improves diagnostic precision for autoimmune diabetes (Yi et al. 2006).

GAD65 and Immune Response

The most widely used and accurate autoantibody marker for LADA diagnosis is GAD65. GAD65 is a crucial biomarker for differentiating LADA from T2DM and other types of diabetes, as it is positive in about 90% of LADA patients. Over the past few years, GAD65's specificity has increased dramatically from 94% to 99%, increasing its dependability in clinical settings. A T1DM like phenotype, which includes a lower BMI and an increased risk of developing insulin dependency, is linked to high GAD65 levels (Towns & Pietropaolo, 2011)

GAD65 Autoantibody Production

GAD65 antibodies are significant in various autoimmune conditions, including LADA. B cells, which are activated in response to the autoimmune process that targets pancreatic β cells, produce GAD65 antibodies. The B cells responsible for secreting these autoantibodies, which can penetrate the blood-brain barrier and impact neurological processes, clonally expand as a result of this activation (Tohid, 2016). T cells are part of the immune response; they identify GAD65 as a target. When it comes to LADA, this immune reaction causes the β cells that produce insulin to be destroyed, which causes hyperglycemia and other symptoms of the disease. Antibodies against GAD65 show that these cells are still being attacked by the immune system (Buzzetti., 2020; Ravikumar et al. 2023).

Interaction with the Immune System

Immune Recognition and Autoantibody Production

Autoantibody generation: One of the main autoantigens in autoimmune diabetes is GAD65, and one of the hallmarks of the autoimmune response is the generation of autoantibodies against GAD65. GADA is often employed as a diagnostic indicator for LADA and T1DM, signifying a continuous immune assault on pancreatic β cells (Gu Urban et al. 2015; Towns & Pietropaolo, 2011).

Mechanism of immune activation: T cells, especially CD4+ T helper cells, along with B cells that produce GADA, play key roles in the immune response to GAD65. These T cells recognize various GAD65 epitopes, triggering autoreactive T cells that contribute to β-cell destruction (Dik et al. 2021).

Cross-Presentation and T-Cell Activation

Antigen presentation: Due to its primary location in the cytoplasm of pancreatic β cells, GAD65 is difficult for the immune system to recognize. Antigen-presenting cells (APCs) have the ability to present GAD65 to CD4+ T cells, which can subsequently grant permission to CD8+ T cells to present GAD65 cross-presentation, thereby initiating a cytotoxic response against β cells (Dik et al. 2021).

Role of HLA molecules: Individuals with particular haplotypes of the human leukocyte antigen (HLA), like HLA-A*02:01, are more prone to autoimmune reactions against GAD65 because these haplotypes are linked to the presentation of peptides derived from GAD65. The severity and onset of autoimmune diabetes may be influenced by this genetic predisposition (Dik et al. 2021).

Gut Microbiome Interaction

Microbial influence on immune response: The gut microbiome may influence the immune system's reaction to GAD65. For instance, the removal of certain gut bacteria that produce

GAD-like proteins could provoke an unintended immune response. In this case, T cells, originally trained to recognize microbial GAD, may mistakenly target GAD65 in pancreatic β cells due to structural similarities between the two (Bedi et al. 2022).

Implications for Disease Progression

Elevated GADA titers are associated with a more rapid decline in β-cell function and an increased likelihood of developing insulin dependency in LADA patients. Studies have shown that over a three-year period, C-peptide levels in LADA patients with high GADA levels (≥180 units/mL) declined more significantly compared to those with low GADA titers (<180 units/mL) or patients with T2DM (Liu et al. 2015). In a multicenter prospective study by Liu et al. it was found that only 42% of LADA patients with initially high GADA titers maintained residual β-cell function (fasting C-peptide >0.2 nmol/L) after three years, compared to 90% of patients with low GADA titers and 97% of patients with type 2 diabetes. This highlights how GADA levels can predict disease progression in LADA patients (Liu et al. 2015). Autoantibodies against GAD65 indicate an ongoing immune response that targets and destroys pancreatic β cells (Towns & Pietropaolo, 2011). In LADA patients with initially high GADA titers (92%), persistent positive GADA at three years was more common compared to those with low GADA titers (26%), suggesting that a prolonged autoimmune response is linked to higher GADA levels. Identifying elevated GADA titers can influence treatment strategies for LADA patients, as they may benefit from more aggressive management to preserve β-cell function and delay insulin dependency. Investigational treatments aimed at controlling the autoimmune response in LADA, such as the GAD-alum vaccination, are currently being explored (Björklund et al. 2022).

Screening for GAD65 for Detection and Predictive Values in Lada

GADA is found using a variety of assays, such as immunofluorescence methods and enzyme-linked immunosorbent assays (ELISA). Recent developments have resulted in the creation of extremely sensitive assays that can identify serum levels of GAD65 at low levels, potentially increasing the accuracy of diagnoses (Zong et al. 2023). More recent techniques concentrate on identifying GAD65-GADA complexes, which could shed light on the ongoing destruction of β-cells and improve knowledge of the autoimmune process. These complexes may function as extra biomarkers to track the course of a disease and its response to treatment (Gu Urban et al. 2015).

ELISA

This widely used technique looks for antibodies in patient serum by coating GAD65 antigens on a plate. The presence of GAD65 antibodies is indicated by a colorimetric change caused by an enzyme-conjugated secondary antibody (Zong et al. 2023).

Radio Immune Assay (RIA)

This method counts the quantity of radiolabeled antibodies attached to the antigen by using GAD65 antigens that have been radiolabeled. Although it offers high sensitivity, handling radioactive materials with caution is necessary (Walikonis & Lennon, 1998).

Immunoprecipitation

In this technique, antibodies in patient samples are identified by their capacity to precipitate the antigen-antibody complex using fluorescent or radiolabeled GAD65 proteins. Because of its complexity, it is not as widely used, despite having a high specificity (Burbelo et al. 2010). List all the predictive values for GAD65 in the diagnosis and progression of LADA are reported in Table 3 (Buzzetti et al. 2020; Hoppu et al. 2004; Towns & Pietropaolo, 2011).

Table 3. List of predictive values of GAD65 in LADA

Predictive Value	Details
Prevalence	GADA is present in approximately 70-80% of LADA patients at diagnosis.
Disease Progression	Higher GADA titers are associated with a more rapid decline in β-cell function and an earlier need for insulin.
Insulin Dependency	Elevated GADA levels predict an increased likelihood of developing insulin dependency sooner compared to those with lower levels.
Differentiation from T2DM	GADA testing helps differentiate LADA from T2DM, which typically lacks autoimmune markers.
Early Intervention	Positive GADA results can prompt earlier initiation of insulin therapy, potentially preserving β-cell function.
Monitoring Disease	GADA levels can be used to monitor the progression of autoimmune destruction and adjust treatment plans accordingly.
Age and eGDR Correlation	GADA is correlated with younger age and higher eGDR values in LADA patients, aiding in early identification and referral.

Importance of Early Diagnosis

Predicting disease progression: The rate at which insulin dependency will progress can be predicted by early detection of GAD65 autoantibodies. β-cell function is more likely to decline in patients with high GADA titers, requiring early insulin therapy (Towns & Pietropaolo, 2011).

Differentiating diabetes types: One important biomarker that helps differentiate T2DM from LADA is GAD65. When patients with T2DM are first diagnosed, identifying GAD65 positivity can result in more tailored treatment plans (Towns & Pietropaolo, 2011).

Guiding treatment decisions: Customized treatment regimens, such as the possibility of early insulin therapy and closer monitoring of glycemic control in GAD65-positive patients, are made possible by the early detection of GAD65 autoantibodies (Pipi et al. 2014).

Understanding autoimmune mechanisms: Finding GAD65 autoantibodies helps medical professionals comprehend the pathophysiology of the disease and the function of β-cell destruction by shedding light on the autoimmune mechanisms underpinning LADA (Wuragil et al. 2022).

Potential for immunotherapy: Immunotherapy strategies, like GAD65-based vaccines, that aim to maintain β-cell function and alter the autoimmune response may become more viable if detected early (Pipi et al. 2014).

Public health implications: An early intervention in at-risk populations may result from public health strategies and screening protocols taking into account the prevalence of GAD65 autoantibodies in older adults (Sangma et al. 2022).

Conclusion

In summary, effective disease management depends on the early detection of LADA by identifying GAD65 autoantibodies. As an autoantigen, GAD65 is essential in the autoimmune process and sets LADA apart from other forms of diabetes. Recognizing GAD65's biochemical characteristics and how it interacts with the immune system improves our capacity to identify and track LADA. Early detection techniques that offer use of GADA screening insightful information about the course of the disease, enabling prompt intervention and customized treatment regimens. All things considered, the addition of GAD65 autoantibody testing greatly increases the precision and efficacy of LADA diagnosis.

References

Bedi, S., Richardson, T. M., Jia, B., Saab, H., Brinkman, F. S. L., & Westley, M. (2022). Similarities between bacterial GAD and human GAD65: Implications in gut mediated autoimmune type 1 diabetes. *PloS one*, 17(2), e0261103.

Biniek, B., Kosiński, M., Żurawska-Kliś, M., Wojtczak, A., & Cypryk, K. (2023). Clinical approach to the differential diagnosis between immune-mediated diabetes and type 2 diabetes in adult patients. *Family Medicine & Primary Care Review*, 25(1), 18–24.

Björklund, A., Hals, I. K., Grill, V., & Ludvigsson, J. (2022). Latent Autoimmune Diabetes in Adults: Background, Safety and Feasibility of an Ongoing Pilot Study with Intra-Lymphatic Injections of GAD-Alum and Oral Vitamin D. *Frontiers in endocrinology*, 13, 926021.

Bottazzo, G. F., Bosi, E., Cull, C. A., Bonifacio, E., Locatelli, M., Zimmet, P., Mackay, I. R., & Holman, R. R. (2005). IA-2 antibody prevalence and risk assessment of early insulin requirement in subjects presenting with type 2 diabetes (UKPDS 71). *Diabetologia*, 48(4), 703–708.

Brooks-Worrell, B. M., Juneja, R., Minokadeh, A., Greenbaum, C. J., & Palmer, J. P. (1999). Cellular immune responses to human islet proteins in antibody-positive type 2 diabetic patients. *Diabetes*, 48(5), 983–988.

Brophy, S., Yderstraede, K., Mauricio, D., Hunter, S., Hawa, M., Pozzilli, P., Schernthaner, G., Schloot, N., Buzzetti, R., Davies, H., Leslie, D., Williams, R., & Action LADA Group. (2008). Time to insulin initiation cannot be used in defining latent autoimmune diabetes in adults. *Diabetes care*, 31(3), 439–441.

Bu, D. F., & Tobin, A. J. (1994). The exon-intron organization of the genes (GAD1 and GAD2) encoding two human glutamate decarboxylases (GAD67 and GAD65) suggests that they derive from a common ancestral GAD. *Genomics*, 21(1), 222-228.

Buddhala, C., Hsu, C. C., & Wu, J. Y. (2009). A novel mechanism for GABA synthesis and packaging into synaptic vesicles. *Neurochemistry International*, 55(1-3), 9-12.

Burbelo, P. D., Hirai, H., Issa, A. T., Kingman, A., Lernmark, A., Ivarsson, S. A., Notkins, A. L., & Iadarola, M. J. (2010). Comparison of radioimmunoprecipitation with luciferase immunoprecipitation for autoantibodies to GAD65 and IA-2beta. *Diabetes Care*, 33(4), 754–756.

Buzzetti, R., Tuomi, T., Mauricio, D., Pietropaolo, M., Zhou, Z., Pozzilli, P., & Leslie, R. D. (2020). Management of Latent Autoimmune Diabetes in Adults: A Consensus Statement from an International Expert Panel. *Diabetes*, 69(10), 2037–2047.

Carlsson, A., Sundkvist, G., Groop, L., & Tuomi, T. (2000). Insulin and glucagon secretion in patients with slowly progressing autoimmune diabetes (LADA). *Journal of Clinical Endocrinology & Metabolism*, 85(1), 76–80.

Carlsson, S. (2019). Etiology and pathogenesis of latent autoimmune diabetes in adults (LADA) compared to type 2 diabetes. *Frontiers in Physiology*, 10, 320.

Carlsson, S., Midthjell, K., & Grill, V. (2007). Influence of Family History of Diabetes on Incidence and Prevalence of Latent Autoimmune Diabetes of the Adult. *Diabetes Care*, 30(12), 3040–3045.

Cernea, S., Buzzetti, R., & Pozzilli, P. (2009). β-cell protection and therapy for latent autoimmune diabetes in adults. *Diabetes care*, 32(Suppl 2), S246.

Christgau, S., Aanstoot, H. J., Schierbeck, H., Begley, K., Tullin, S., Hejnaes, K., & Baekkeskov, S. (1992). Membrane anchoring of the autoantigen GAD65 to microvesicles in pancreatic beta-cells by palmitoylation in the NH2-terminal domain. *The Journal of Cell Biology*, 118(2), 309–320.

Dik, A., Widman, G., Schulte-Mecklenbeck, A., Witt, J. A., Pitsch, J., Golombeck, K. S., Wagner, J., Gallus, M., Strippel, C., Hansen, N., Mönig, C., Räuber, S., Wiendl, H., Elger, C. E., Surges, R., Meuth, S. G., Helmstaedter, C., Gross, C. C., Becker, A. J., & Melzer, N. (2021). Impact of T cells on neurodegeneration in anti-GAD65 limbic encephalitis. *Annals of clinical and translational neurology*, 8(12), 2289–2301.

Falorni, A., Gambelunghe, G., Forini, F., Kassi, G., Cosentino, A., Candeloro, P., Bolli, G. B., Brunetti, P., & Calcinaro, F. (2000). Autoantibody recognition of COOH-terminal epitopes of GAD65 marks the risk for insulin requirement in adult-onset diabetes mellitus. *The Journal of Clinical Endocrinology & Metabolism*, 85(1), 309-316.

Fenalti, G., & Buckle, A. M. (2010). Structural biology of the GAD autoantigen. *Autoimmunity Reviews*, 9(3), 148-152.

Gu Urban, G. J., Friedman, M., Ren, P., Törn, C., Fex, M., Hampe, C. S., Lernmark, Å., Landegren, U., & Kamali-Moghaddam, M. (2015). Elevated Serum GAD65 and GAD65-GADA Immune Complexes in Stiff Person Syndrome. *Scientific Reports*, 5, 11196.

Hampe, C. S., Hammerle, L. P., Bekris, L., Örtqvist, E., Persson, B., & Lernmark, Å. (2002a). Stable GAD65 autoantibody epitope patterns in type 1 diabetes children five years after onset. *Journal of Autoimmunity*, 18(1), 49-53.

Hampe, C. S., Kockum, I., Landin-Olsson, M., & Törn, C. (2002b). GAD65 antibody epitope patterns of type 1.5 diabetic patients are consistent with slow-onset autoimmune diabetes. *Diabetes Care*, 25(8), 1481.

Hampe, C. S., Maitland, M. E., Gilliam, L. K., Phan, T. H., Sweet, I. R., Radtke, J. R., Bota, V., Ransom, B. R., & Hirsch, I. B. (2013). High titers of autoantibodies to glutamate decarboxylase in type 1 diabetes patients: epitope analysis and inhibition of enzyme activity. *Endocrine Practice*, 19(4), 663-668.

Hawa, M. I., Kolb, H., Schloot, N., Beyan, H., Paschou, S. A., Buzzetti, R., Mauricio, D., De Leiva, A., Yderstræde, K., Beck-Nielsen, H., Tuomilehto, J., Sarti, C., Thivolet, C., Hadden, D., Hunter, S., Schernthaner, G., Scherbaum, W. A., Williams, R., Brophy, S., Pozzilli, P., & Leslie, R. D.; Action LADA consortium. (2013). Adult-onset autoimmune diabetes in Europe is prevalent with a broad clinical phenotype: Action LADA 7. *Diabetes Care*, 36(4), 908–913.

Hernandez, M., Mollo, A., Marsal, J. R., Esquerda, A., Capel, I., Puig-Domingo, M., Pozzilli, P., de Leiva, A., Mauricio, D., & Action LADA Consortium. (2015). Insulin secretion in patients with latent autoimmune diabetes (LADA): half way between type 1 and type 2 diabetes: action LADA 9. *BMC Endocrine Disorders*, 15, 1-6.

Hoppu, S., Ronkainen, M. S., Kulmala, P., Akerblom, H. K., Knip, M., & Childhood Diabetes in Finland Study Group (2004). GAD65 antibody isotypes and epitope recognition during the prediabetic process in siblings of children with type I diabetes. *Clinical and Experimental Immunology*, 136(1), 120–128.

Hu, J., Zhang, R., Zou, H., Xie, L., Zhou, Z., & Xiao, Y. (2022). Latent autoimmune diabetes in adults (LADA): from immunopathogenesis to Immunotherapy. *Frontiers in Endocrinology*, 13, 917169.

Insel, R. A., Dunne, J. L., Atkinson, M. A., Chiang, J. L., Dabelea, D., Gottlieb, P. A., Greenbaum, C. J., Herold, K. C., Krischer, J. P., Lernmark, Å., Ratner, R. E., Rewers, M. J., Schatz, D. A., Skyler, J. S., Sosenko, J. M., & Ziegler, A. G. (2015). Staging presymptomatic type 1 diabetes: A scientific statement of JDRF, the Endocrine Society, and the American Diabetes Association. *Diabetes Care*, 38(10), 1964–1974.

Jin, P., Huang, G., Lin, J., Luo, S., & Zhou, Z. (2011). Epitope analysis of GAD65 autoantibodies in adult-onset type 1 diabetes and latent autoimmune diabetes in adults with thyroid autoimmunity. *Acta diabetologica*, 48, 149-155.

Kawasaki E. (2023). Anti-Islet Autoantibodies in Type 1 Diabetes. *International journal of molecular sciences*, 24(12), 10012.

Keshavarzi, E., Noveiry, B. B., & Rezaei, N. (2022). The relationship between GAD65 autoantibody and the risk of T1DM onset. *Journal of Diabetes & Metabolic Disorders*, 21(2), 1935-1942.

Kikkas, I., Mallone, R., Larger, E., Volland, H., & Morel, N. (2014). A rapid lateral flow immunoassay for the detection of tyrosine phosphatase-like protein IA-2 autoantibodies in human serum. *PLoS One*, 9(7), e103088.

Krause, S., Landherr, U., Agardh, C. D., Hausmann, S., Link, K., Hansen, J. M., Lynch, K. F., Powell, M., Furmaniak, J., Rees-Smith, B., Bonifacio, E., Ziegler, A. G., Lernmark, A., & Achenbach, P. (2014). GAD autoantibody affinity in adult patients with latent autoimmune diabetes, the study participants of a GAD65 vaccination trial. *Diabetes Care*, 37(6), 1675-1680.

Li, Y., Zhao, M., Hou, C., Liang, G., Yang, L., Tan, Y., Wang, Z., Yin, H., Zhou, Z., & Lu, Q. (2011). Abnormal DNA methylation in CD4+ T cells from people with latent autoimmune diabetes in adults. *Diabetes research and clinical practice*, 94(2), 242-248.

Liu, L., Li, X., Xiang, Y., Huang, G., Lin, J., Yang, L., Zhao, Y., Yang, Z., Hou, C., Li, Y., Liu, J., Zhu, D., Leslie, R. D., Wang, X., Zhou, Z., & LADA China Study Group (2015). Latent autoimmune diabetes in adults with low-titer GAD antibodies: similar disease progression with type 2 diabetes: a nationwide, multicenter prospective study (LADA China Study 3). *Diabetes care*, 38(1), 16–21.

Ludvigsson, J., Krisky, D., Casas, R., Battelino, T., Castaño, L., Greening, J., Kordonouri, O., Otonkoski, T., Pozzilli, P., Robert, J. J., Veeze, H. J., Palmer, J., Samuelsson, U., Elding Larsson, H., Åman, J., Kärdell, G., Neiderud Helsingborg, J., Lundström, G., Albinsson, E., Carlsson, A., Nordvall, M., Fors, H., Arvidsson, C. G., Edvardson, S., Hanås, R., Larsson, K., Rathsman, B., Forsgren, H., Desaix, H., Forsander, G., Nilsson, N. Ö., Åkesson, C. G., Keskinen, P., Veijola, R., Talvitie, T., Raile, K., Kapellen, T., Burger, W., Neu, A., Engelsberger, I., Heidtmann, B., Bechtold, S., Leslie, D., Chiarelli, F., Cicognani, A., Chiumello, G., Cerutti, F., Zuccotti, G. V., Gomez Gila, A., Rica, I., Barrio, R., Clemente, M., López Garcia, M. J., Rodriguez, M., Gonzalez, I., Lopez, J. P., Oyarzabal, M., Reeser, H. M., Nuboer, R., Stouthart, P., Bratina, N., Bratanic, N., de Kerdanet, M., Weill, J., Ser, N., Barat, P., Bertrand, A. M., Carel, J. C., Reynaud, R., Coutant, R., & Baron, S. (2012). GAD65 antigen therapy in recently diagnosed type 1 diabetes mellitus. *New England Journal of Medicine*, 366(5), 433–442.

Lundgren, V. M., Isomaa, B., Lyssenko, V., Laurila, E., Korhonen, P., Groop, L. C., Tuomi, T., & Botnia Study Group (2010). GAD antibody positivity predicts type 2 diabetes in an adult population. *Diabetes*, 59(2), 416–422.

Miao, D., Guyer, K. M., Dong, F., Jiang, L., Steck, A. K., Rewers, M., Eisenbarth, G. S., & Yu, L. (2013). GAD65 autoantibodies detected by electrochemiluminescence assay identify high risk for type 1 diabetes. *Diabetes*, 62(12), 4174-4178.

Mishra, R., Hodge, K. M., Cousminer, D. L., Leslie, R. D., & Grant, S. F. (2018). A global perspective of latent autoimmune diabetes in adults. *Trends in Endocrinology & Metabolism*, 29(9), 638-650.

Mohan's, D. (2023). *Latent Autoimmune Diabetes of Adults (LADA)*. Dr Mohan's Diabetes Center in Chennai. https://drmohans.com/lada/

Nolasco-Rosales, G. A., Ramírez-González, D., Rodríguez-Sánchez, E., Ávila-Fernandez, Á., Villar-Juarez, G. E., González-Castro, T. B., Tovilla-Zárate, C. A., Guzmán-Priego, C. G., Genis-Mendoza, A. D., Ble-Castillo, J. L., Marín-Medina, A., & Juárez-Rojop, I. E. (2023). Identification and phenotypic characterization of patients with LADA in a population of southeast Mexico. *Scientific reports*, 13(1), 7029.

Peng, Y., Li, X., Xiang, Y., Yan, X., Zhou, H., Tang, X., Cheng, J., Niu, X., Liu, J., Ji, Q., Ji, L., Huang, G., & Zhou, Z. (2022). GAD65 antibody epitopes and genetic background in latent autoimmune diabetes in youth (LADY). *Frontiers in Immunology*, 13, 836952.

Pipi, E., Marketou, M., & Tsirogianni, A. (2014). Distinct clinical and laboratory characteristics of latent autoimmune diabetes in adults in relation to type 1 and type 2 diabetes mellitus. *World journal of diabetes*, 5(4), 505–510.

Pozzilli, P., & Pieralice, S. (2018). Latent Autoimmune Diabetes in Adults: Current Status and New Horizons. *Endocrinology and metabolism*, 33(2), 147–159.

Rajkumar, V., & Levine, S. N. (2023). *Latent Autoimmune Diabetes*. StatPearls Publishing. Treasure Island (FL).

Ravikumar, V., Ahmed, A., & Anjankar, A. (2023). A Review on Latent Autoimmune Diabetes in Adults. *Cureus*, 15(10), e47915.

Rosário, P. W. S., Reis, J. S., Fagundes, T. A., Calsolari, M. R., Amim, R., Silva, S. C., & Purisch, S. (2007). Latent autoimmune diabetes in adults (LADA): usefulness of anti-GAD antibody titers and benefit of early insulinization. *Arquivos Brasileiros de Endocrinologia & Metabologia*, 51, 52-58.

Sangma, H., Singh, A., Srivastava, A., & Misra, V. (2022). Prevalence of Latent Autoimmune Diabetes in Adult Based on the Presence of GAD 65 Antibodies in North-Eastern Uttar Pradesh, India. *Annals of the National Academy of Medical Sciences*, 58(01), 017–021.

Schlosser, M., Banga, J. P., Madec, A. M., Binder, K. A., Strebelow, M., Rjasanowski, I., Wassmuth, R., Gilliam, L. K., Luo, D., & Hampe, C. S. (2005). Dynamic changes of GAD65 autoantibody epitope specificities in individuals at risk of developing type 1 diabetes. *Diabetologia*, 48(5), 922–930.

Shimada, A., Imazu, Y., Morinaga, S., Funae, O., Kasuga, A., Atsumi, Y., & Matsuoka, K. (1999). T-cell insulitis found in anti-GAD65+ diabetes with residual beta-cell function. A case report. *Diabetes care*, 22(4), 615-617.

Signore, A., Capriotti, G., Chianelli, M., Bonanno, E., Galli, F., Catalano, C., Quintero, A. M., De Toma, G., Manfrini, S., Pozzilli, P., & Action LADA Group. (2015). Detection of insulitis by pancreatic scintigraphy with 99mTc-labeled IL-2 and MRI in patients with LADA (Action LADA 10). *Diabetes Care*, 38(4), 652-658.

Solimena, M. (1998). Vesicular autoantigens of type 1 diabetes. *Diabetes/Metabolism Research and Reviews*, 14(3), 227–240.

Sørgjerd, E. P., Skorpen, F., Kvaløy, K., Midthjell, K., & Grill, V. (2012). Time dynamics of autoantibodies are coupled to phenotypes and add to the heterogeneity of autoimmune diabetes in adults: The HUNT study. *Diabetologia*, 55(5), 1310–1318.

Sutkowska, E., Ostrowska, M., & Sutkowska, M. (2021). Insulin Autoimmune Syndrome as Part of Pre-Clinical LADA. *Diabetes, Metabolic Syndrome and Obesity*, 14, 1557-1561.

Sørgjerd, E. P., Skorpen, F., Kvaløy, K., Midthjell, K., & Grill, V. (2012). Time dynamics of autoantibodies are coupled to phenotypes and add to the heterogeneity of autoimmune diabetes in adults: The HUNT study. Diabetologia, 55(5), 1310–1318. Clinical, autoimmune, and genetic characteristics of adult-onset diabetic patients with GAD autoantibodies in Japan (Ehime Study). *Diabetes care*, 25(6), 995-1001.

Tohid, H. (2016). Anti-glutamic acid decarboxylase antibody positive neurological syndromes. *Neurosciences*, 21(3), 215–222.

Towns, R., & Pietropaolo, M. (2011). GAD65 autoantibodies and its role as biomarker of Type 1 diabetes and Latent Autoimmune Diabetes in Adults (LADA). *Drugs of the Future*, 36(11), 847.

Tuomi, T., Carlsson, A., Li, H., Isomaa, B., Miettinen, A., Nilsson, A., Nissén, M., Ehrnström, B. O., Forsén, B., Snickars, B., Lahti, K., Forsblom, C., Saloranta, C., Taskinen, M. R., & Groop, L. C. (1999). Clinical and genetic characteristics of type 2 diabetes with and without GAD antibodies. *Diabetes*, 48, 150-157.

Tuomi, T., Groop, L. C., Zimmet, P. Z., Rowley, M. J., Knowles, W., & Mackay, I. R. (1993). Antibodies to glutamic acid decarboxylase reveal latent autoimmune diabetes mellitus in adults with a non—insulin-dependent onset of disease. *Diabetes*, 42(2), 359-362.

Turner, R., Stratton, I., Horton, V., Manley, S., Zimmet, P., Mackay, I. R., Shattock, M., Bottazzo, G. F., & Holman, R. (1997). UKPDS 25: autoantibodies to islet-cell cytoplasm and glutamic acid decarboxylase for prediction of insulin requirement in type 2 diabetes. *The Lancet*, 350(9087), 1288-1293.

Vich-Pérez, P., Abánades-Herranz, J. C., Mora-Navarro, G., Carrasco-Sayalero, Á. M., Salinero-Fort, M. Á., Sevilla-Machuca, I., Sanz-Pascual, M., Álvarez Hernández-Cañizares, C., & De Burgos-Lunar, C. (2023). Development and validation of a clinical score for identifying patients with high risk of latent autoimmune adult diabetes (LADA): The LADA primary care-protocol study. *PLOS ONE*, 18(2), e0281657.

Walikonis, J. E., & Lennon, V. A. (1998). Radioimmunoassay for glutamic acid decarboxylase (GAD65) autoantibodies as a diagnostic aid for stiff-man syndrome and a correlate of susceptibility to type 1 diabetes mellitus. *Mayo Clinic proceedings*, 73(12), 1161–1166.

Wang, Y., Yuan, W., Guo, H., & Jiang, Y. (2015). High frequency of activated NKp46+ natural killer cells in patients with new diagnosed of latent autoimmune diabetes in adults. *Autoimmunity*, 48(4), 267-273.

Aulanni'am, A., Wuragil, D. K., Susanto, H., Herawati, A., Nugroho, Y. M., Laili Fajri, W. N., Putri, P. F., Susiati, S., Trijoyo Purnomo, J. D., Taufiq, A., & Soeatmadji, D. W. (2021). The early detection of type 1 diabetes mellitus and latent autoimmune diabetes in adults (LADA) through rapid test reverse-flow immunochromatography for glutamic acid decarboxylase 65 kDa (GAD65). *Heliyon*, 8(1), e08695.

Yi, B., Huang, G., & Zhou, Z. (2016). Different role of zinc transporter 8 between type 1 diabetes mellitus and type 2 diabetes mellitus. *Journal of Diabetes Investigation*, 7(4), 459–465.

Yin, W., Luo, S., Xiao, Z., Zhang, Z., Liu, B., & Zhou, Z. (2022). Latent autoimmune diabetes in adults: a focus on β-cell protection and therapy. *Frontiers in endocrinology*, 13, 959011.

Zampetti, S., Campagna, G., Tiberti, C., Songini, M., Arpi, M. L., De Simone, G., Cossu, E., Cocco, L., Osborn, J., Bosi, E., Giorgino, F., Spoletini, M., Buzzetti, R., & NIRAD Study Group (2014). High GADA titer increases the risk of insulin requirement in LADA patients: a 7-year follow-up (NIRAD study 7). *European journal of endocrinology*, 171(6), 697-704.

Zimmet, P. Z., Tuomi, T., Mackay, I. R., Rowley, M. J., Knowles, W., Cohen, M., & Lang, D. A. (1994). Latent autoimmune diabetes mellitus in adults (LADA): the role of antibodies to glutamic acid decarboxylase in diagnosis and prediction of insulin dependency. *Diabetic Medicine*, 11(3), 299–303.

Zong, S., Vinke, A. M., Du, P., Hoffmann, C., Mané-Damas, M., Molenaar, P. C., Damoiseaux, J. G. M. C., Losen, M., Rouhl, R. P. W., & Martinez-Martinez, P. (2023). Anti-GAD65 autoantibody levels measured by ELISA and alternative types of immunoassays in relation to neuropsychiatric diseases versus diabetes mellitus type 1. *Frontiers in Neurology*, 14, 1111063.

Chapter 19

Navigating Diabetes Mellitus: Alpha-Glucosidase Inhibitors as Therapeutic Allies

Suman Baishnab
Ajmal Tariq Hussain*
Shrishti Shandily
and Pallavi Malik
Amity Institute of Pharmacy, Amity University Uttar Pradesh, Lucknow Campus, India

Abstract

Alpha-glucosidase inhibitors (AGIs) are a class of drugs used to manage type 2 diabetes mellitus. They work by slowing the absorption of glucose into the bloodstream, helping to control blood sugar levels after meals. AGIs are often used in combination with other anti-diabetic medications, such as metformin, due to their moderate effect on blood sugar regulation. Whether used alone or in combination with other oral hypoglycemic agents and insulin, AGIs help achieve glycemic control, although they may cause mild, transient gastrointestinal side effects. Acarbose inhibits the enzyme by competing with polysaccharides and oligosaccharides at the active site, while miglitol competes with disaccharides. Both acarbose and voglibose are minimally absorbed in their original forms, resulting in low systemic bioavailability, which is therapeutically beneficial. Less than 2% of orally administered acarbose enters the bloodstream. AGIs have been shown to improve postprandial hyperglycemia, a key contributor to cardiovascular diseases. These medications should not be used in patients with known hypersensitivity to the drug or its components, diabetic ketoacidosis, colonic ulceration, partial intestinal obstruction, or those with a tendency for intestinal blockage.

Keywords: alpha-glucosidase, alpha-glucosidase inhibitors, miglitol, diabetes mellitus, voglibose, type 2 diabetes mellitus

* Corresponding Author's Email: ajmaltariq413@gmail.com

In: Receptor-Targeted Therapies in Diabetes Mellitus
Editors: Ajmer Singh Grewal, Neelam Singh, Swati Verma et al.
ISBN: 979-8-89530-587-4

Abbreviations

ACE	Angiotensin Converting Enzyme
AGI	Alpha Glucosidase Inhibitors
ARB	Angiotensin Receptor Blockers
BCDS	Beijing Community Diabetes Study
BMI	Body Mass Index
DALY	Daily Adjusted Life Years
DNJ	1-deoxynojirimycin
DPP4	Dipeptidyl Peptidase 4
FDA	Food & Drugs Administration
FPG	Fasting Plasma Glucose
GLP1	Glucagon-like Peptide 1
HbA1C	Glycosylated Haemoglobin
HDL	High Density Lipoproteins
IGT	Impaired Glucose Tolerance
LDL	Low Density Lipoproteins
OGTT	Oral Glucose Tolerance Test
OHA	Oral Hypoglycaemic Agents
PPG	Post Prandial Glucose
PPI	Post Prandial Insulin
RCT	Randomized Controlled Trials
RYGB	Roux-en-Y Gastric Bypass Surgery
SGLT2	Sodium Glucose Cotransporter 2
T2DM	Type 2 Diabetes Mellitus
UKPDS	United Kingdom Prospective Diabetes Study

Introduction

High blood sugar levels, resulting from abnormalities in insulin production, action, or both, characterize a set of metabolic diseases collectively called diabetes. Chronic hyperglycemia associated with diabetes can harm, malfunction, and eventually cause failure in several organs, including the kidneys, heart, blood vessels, nerves, and eyes. Insulin insufficiency is caused by autoimmune destruction of pancreatic β-cells and resistance to the action of insulin, both of which contribute to the development of diabetes. Diabetes patients exhibit anomalies in the metabolism of proteins, lipids, and carbohydrates due to insufficient insulin activity in target tissues. This deficiency is primarily caused by a decreased tissue response to insulin and insufficient insulin synthesis. It can be difficult to determine whether abnormal insulin action or insufficient insulin secretion is the primary cause of hyperglycemia, as these anomalies often coexist. Severe hyperglycemia can lead to weight loss, increased appetite, thirst, frequent urination, and impaired vision. In addition to slowing growth, chronic hyperglycemia may increase susceptibility to infections. Uncontrolled diabetes can result in nonketotic hyperosmolar syndrome or hyperglycemia with ketoacidosis, both of which are acute and potentially fatal conditions. Diabetes can lead to peripheral neuropathy, increasing the risk of foot ulcers, amputations, and Charcot's joints; retinopathy, which may cause vision loss; nephropathy, which can lead to renal failure; and autonomic neuropathy, which can cause symptoms in the gastrointestinal, genitourinary, cardiovascular systems, and sexual function. Diabetes also increases the risk of peripheral arterial disease, cerebrovascular disease, and atherosclerotic cardiovascular disease. Hypertension and abnormalities in lipoprotein metabolism are common in individuals with diabetes (Metzger et al. 2010). Diabetes mellitus includes type 1 diabetes, an autoimmune disease that destroys insulin-producing beta cells (Atkinson et al. 2014); type 2 diabetes (T2DM), often associated with lifestyle factors such as poor diet and inactivity (Chatterjee et al. 2017); prediabetes, in which blood glucose levels are elevated but not yet classified as T2DM (Tabák et al. 2012); and gestational diabetes, which occurs during pregnancy and increases the risk of developing future T2DM (Metzger et al. 2010).

Prevalence and Impact on Global Health

The incidence of diabetes has surged globally, with adult cases increasing from 4.7% to 8.5%, raising the affected population from 108 million in 1980 to 476 million in 2017. In 2017, diabetes contributed to 1.4 million deaths worldwide, significantly affecting low- and middle-income countries. The highest prevalence is found in the Eastern Mediterranean, parts of Asia and Africa, and regions such as the Western Pacific and Southeast Asia (Arokiasamy et al. 2021). A comprehensive study across 195 countries revealed a marked increase in diabetes cases since 1990, recording 22.9 million new incidences, 476 million cases, 1.37 million deaths, and 67.9 million disability-adjusted life years (DALYs) in 2017, with projections of 26 million incidences, 570.9 million cases, 1.59 million deaths, and 79.3 million DALYs for 2025. While T1DM-related mortality and DALYs have decreased, T2DM trends align with total diabetes statistics, influenced heavily by high BMI and lifestyle factors (Lin et al. 2020). The International Diabetes Federation reported that in 2015, 415 million individuals aged 20–79 had diabetes, a number expected to rise to 642 million by 2040. Additionally, 318 million people exhibit elevated blood sugar levels below the T2DM threshold, which significantly impacts life expectancy and mortality (Ogurtsova et al. 2017).

Overview of Treatment Approaches

The primary goals of diabetes treatment are to alleviate symptoms, prevent complications, and maintain healthy blood glucose levels. This includes reducing symptoms such as excessive thirst and fatigue, as well as preventing long-term complications like cardiovascular disease, kidney disease, nerve damage, eye disorders, and foot problems. Achieving these goals requires lifestyle modifications, medication, self-monitoring of blood glucose, and regular screenings. By focusing on these objectives, healthcare providers and patients can effectively manage diabetes, improve health outcomes, and enhance quality of life. The following are the approaches to diabetes treatment:

Lifestyle Modifications

- *Dietary changes:* Eating a balanced diet with appropriate portions of carbohydrates, proteins, and fats is essential for effective diabetes management. Focusing on low-glycemic index foods, which are absorbed more gradually and lead to smaller blood sugar spikes, helps in controlling blood glucose levels. Maintaining a healthy weight through diet can further enhance insulin sensitivity and lower the risk of complications (Evert et al. 2019).
- *Physical activity:* Regular exercise, including aerobic and strength training, improves insulin sensitivity, lowers blood glucose levels, and reduces cardiovascular risks. The American Diabetes Association recommends at least 150 minutes of moderate-intensity exercise per week for most adults with diabetes (Colberg et al. 2016).
- *Smoking cessation:* Smoking is a major risk factor for complications such as cardiovascular disease, kidney disease, and neuropathy. Quitting smoking can significantly enhance health outcomes for individuals with diabetes (Yeh et al. 2010).

Pharmacological Treatments

- *Oral medications:* Metformin is the first oral medication typically prescribed for T2DM, as it reduces glucose production in the liver and enhances insulin sensitivity. Other oral medications, such as sulfonylureas, DPP-4 inhibitors, and GLP-1 agonists, help lower blood glucose through various mechanisms. Combination therapy using multiple oral medications is often employed to achieve improved glucose control (American Diabetes Association, 2021).
- *Insulin therapy:* Insulin is the primary treatment for T1DM and is also often required for T2DM patients who cannot manage their blood glucose levels with oral medications alone. Different insulin types, delivery methods, and regimens (e.g., basal-bolus, premixed) are used to optimize therapy and minimize the risk of hypoglycemia (Home et al. 2014).
- *Other treatments:* In certain cases, bariatric surgery may be considered for individuals with T2DM and obesity, as it can improve blood glucose control and reduce the need for medications. Pancreatic islet cell transplantation is an experimental treatment for T1DM, that aims to restore natural insulin production (Affinati et al. 2019).

Monitoring and Evaluation

- *Blood glucose monitoring:* Regular self-monitoring of blood glucose levels, via fingerstick tests or continuous glucose monitoring, is essential for adjusting treatment and achieving optimal blood glucose control (Janapala et al. 2019).
- *Glycosylated hemoglobin (HbA1c) testing:* HbA1c measures average blood glucose levels over the past 2-3 months and is used to assess long-term diabetes management. The American Diabetes Association recommends an HbA1c target of less than 7% for

most individuals, with personalized goals based on factors such as age, diabetes duration, and risk of hypoglycemia (Sherwani et al. 2016).

- *Screening for complications:* Regular screenings for diabetes-related complications, including retinopathy, nephropathy, neuropathy, and cardiovascular disease, are crucial for early detection and effective management (Beck et al. 2017).

Understanding Alpha-Glucosidase Inhibitors

By postponing the breakdown and absorption of complex carbs, alpha-glucosidase inhibitors (AGIs) are antihyperglycemic medications that reduce blood sugar levels. These are enzymes on the brush border of enterocytes that break oligosaccharides into monosaccharides, and they do so in a competitive manner. Their main function is to slow the rise in plasma glucose after meals. These inhibitors lower postprandial plasma glucose by 40 to 50 mg/dL and HbA1c by 0.5% to 1.0% in individuals with non-insulin-dependent diabetes mellitus (Lebovitz 1997). Acarbose is the most well-studied and commonly used AGI. It works as a competitive and reversible inhibitor of intestinal alpha-glucosidases, which delays the digestion and absorption of carbohydrates, helping to control blood glucose levels (DiNicolantonio et al. 2015). Miglitol is another AGI that functions similarly to acarbose. Like acarbose, it is a competitive and reversible inhibitor of intestinal alpha-glucosidases (Akmal et al. 2024). Voglibose is an AGI primarily used in Asia, including Japan and China. It inhibits alpha-glucosidase activity in the small intestine, thereby delaying the digestion and absorption of carbohydrates (Göke et al. 1995).

Mechanism of Action

Enzymes called α-glucosidase, which hydrolyse non-absorbable oligosaccharides and polysaccharides into absorbable monosaccharides, are competitively inhibited by the pseudo-carbohydrates acarbose, voglibose, and miglitol, which are found in the brush border of enterocytes. Among these drugs, acarbose is the most utilized. *Actinoplanes utahensis* is a microbe that undergoes fermentation to produce this pseudo tetrasaccharide, which has a nitrogen bond between the first and second glucose units (Puls, 1996). This natural tetrasaccharide alteration has significance due to its stability and strong affinity for the brush border α-glucosidases of the small intestine. After sucrase, maltase, and dextranase, acarbose is the most potent inhibitor of glucoamylase. Inhibiting α-amylase is another function it has; however, it does not affect β-glucosidases like lactase (Derosa and Maffioli, 2012).

Pharmacokinetics and Pharmacodynamics of Alpha-Glucosidase Inhibitors

Acarbose

- *Absorption:* Unaltered acarbose is absorbed in very small amounts, less than 2% in humans and rats after oral administration, and approximately 4% in dogs. However, the absorption of drug-related radioactivity is higher, likely due to the breakdown of intestinal contents into more absorbable metabolites, primarily in the colon (Ahr et al. 1989).

- *Distribution:* In rats, acarbose is rapidly and unevenly distributed throughout organs and tissues, primarily in the extracellular space. Due to fast renal excretion, acarbose is highly concentrated in the kidneys and urine. It crosses the placental barrier more slowly than maternal plasma and only slightly penetrates the blood-brain barrier. Radioactive material from acarbose accumulates in the kidneys, liver, and adrenal glands after repeated doses, gradually disappearing after about half a day. Nursing rats also release acarbose-related radioactivity into their milk (Ahr et al. 1989).
- *Metabolism:* Digestive enzymes and intestinal bacteria break down glucose and 4-methyl pyrogallol from the original carbohydrate, which are then further metabolized. The body utilizes the amino acids resulting from the breakdown of ring B (Krause and Ahr, 1996).
- *Excretion:* Acarbose remains unchanged and is almost entirely eliminated through the urine. The non-absorbed portions are excreted in the feces, with only a small amount eliminated through the bile system, indicating minimal enterohepatic circulation (Krause and Ahr, 1996).

Miglitol

- *Absorption:* In rats and dogs, miglitol is rapidly and fully absorbed at doses below 5 mg/kg. However, human absorption is incomplete, even at lower doses. Similar to glucose absorption, the process involves both extracellular diffusion and transcellular transport (Krause and Ahr, 1996).
- *Distribution:* Miglitol is primarily located in the extracellular space and is distributed rapidly and unevenly. It does not easily penetrate the brain but is found in significant amounts in the kidneys and urine. During breastfeeding, miglitol is gradually transferred into milk after passing through the placental barrier (Ahr et al. 1997).
- *Metabolism:* In humans, dogs, and rodents, miglitol is eliminated intact through the urine (Krause and Ahr, 1996).
- *Excretion:* The kidneys eliminate miglitol almost completely and rapidly. When administered at modest dosages, miglitol has only been detected in trace amounts in the stool of rats and dogs (Scott and Spencer, 2000).

Voglibose

- *Absorption*: Following oral administration, voglibose is absorbed slowly and poorly, with plasma concentrations often undetectable at therapeutic doses (Kaku, 2014). Only a small percentage of voglibose is absorbed, approximately 5.9% in rats and 2.7% in dogs. At higher doses, absorption is modestly reduced (Krause and Ahr, 1996).
- *Distribution*: Following absorption, voglibose is distributed across various organs and tissues, but its systemic availability is limited. Maximum concentrations are reached within an hour after oral administration, with the highest levels found in the kidneys and intestinal wall. The blood-brain barrier and erythrocyte membranes are somewhat

impermeable to voglibose. In rats and humans, approximately 15% of voglibose binds to plasma proteins (Krause and Ahr, 1996).

- *Metabolism*: The metabolism of voglibose is minimal. Ninety percent of the radioactivity exhaled by rats and dogs following oral administration corresponds directly to the drug, with no observable metabolites detected.
- *Excretion*: Although exact information on excretion is not provided, it is expected that voglibose would be eliminated largely unaltered, similar to acarbose (Krause and Ahr, 1996).

Adverse Effects and Tolerability

Acarbose offers benefits, but its side effects limit its use in healthy individuals. A study tested low-dose acarbose (50 mg) before high-carbohydrate meals in healthy subjects to assess its effectiveness and tolerability. The results showed that acarbose significantly reduced glucose levels, particularly at the beginning, 15 minutes after, and at peak levels, as measured with continuous glucose monitors. However, most participants experienced mild symptoms such as nausea, bloating, gas, and stomach discomfort. Despite these side effects, 50 mg of acarbose before meals was well-tolerated and effectively reduced glucose increases by more than 17% (Isman et al. 2023). Miglitol's effectiveness and tolerability were assessed in a randomized, double-blind, placebo-controlled study involving 105 Chinese patients with T2DM who were not responding to diet and sulfonylureas. Patients received either placebo or miglitol for 24 weeks. Compared to a placebo, miglitol significantly reduced HbA1c and postprandial glucose levels. Both groups had similar rates of diarrhea, hypoglycemia, and abdominal pain. Miglitol is considered a useful adjuvant medication in these patients, improving metabolic control and being well-tolerated (Hsieh et al. 2011). A review and meta-analysis of clinical studies on voglibose found that it did not significantly affect fasting blood sugar, insulin, body weight, BMI, adiponectin, triglycerides, total cholesterol, or HDL cholesterol. However, it was shown to significantly lower HbA1c and increase LDL cholesterol levels in patients with type 2 diabetes (Nowrouzi-Sohrabi et al. 2020).

Dosage and Administration

Oral administration of AGIs typically occurs three times a day, with the first dose taken at the start of a major meal. Treatment often begins with a lower dose, such as 25 mg of acarbose, 0.2 mg of miglitol, and voglibose, which is gradually increased over time. Dosage adjustments should be made every four to eight weeks based on the patient's HbA1c, postprandial glucose (PPG), and drug tolerance (Hedrington and Davis, 2019). For adults, the maximum doses are up to 100 mg of acarbose and miglitol, and 0.6 mg of voglibose, taken three times daily. These drugs can be used safely and effectively in both younger and older adults (Göke et al. 1995).

Future Directions and Emerging Research

Recent research has highlighted AGIs as effective and safer treatments for T2DM compared to other hypoglycemics, with both synthetic and natural AGIs showing good selectivity and high binding affinity (Agrawal et al. 2022). Despite their promise, microbial production of AGIs, such as 1-deoxynojirimycin (DNJ), remains limited, necessitating improvements through fermentation and metabolic strategies. Bioactive substances like flavonoids, polyphenols, and alkaloids found in fruits, vegetables, dairy products, and grains are utilized in the production of hypoglycemic products, with fermentation enhancing their nutritional content and bioactivity (Ren et al. 2023). A review identified eight plant molecules procyanidin A2, alaternin, taxumariene F, akebonoic acid, morusin, rhaponticin, mulberrofuran K, and psoralidin as having high alpha-glucosidase inhibitory efficacy, with some also improving insulin signaling. These molecules show potential for diabetes therapy, but further clinical research is needed to assess their mechanisms and safety (Dirir et al. 2022). AGIs such as acarbose have also been shown to treat hypoglycemia following Roux-en-Y gastric bypass (RYGB) surgery. Acarbose, taken 15 minutes before meals, prevented hypoglycemia in all eight RYGB patients studied, significantly raising their lowest plasma glucose levels, likely by reducing early GLP-1 release and the hyperinsulinemic response (Salehi et al. 2018; Valderas et al. 2012). In a recent evaluation, AGI therapy successfully treated postprandial hypoglycemia in four RYGB patients, with three experiencing long-term symptom relief, suggesting AGIs as a primary treatment for post-Roux-en-Y hypoglycemia (Frankhouser et al. 2013). Furthermore, the Beijing Community Diabetes Study (BCDS) showed that long-term acarbose use in T2DM patients resulted in a 50% reduction in the relative risk of myocardial infarction and a 52% reduction in all-cause mortality after ten years, indicating that acarbose, as part of a multimodal therapeutic approach, can improve cardiovascular outcomes in T2DM patients (Zhang et al. 2021).

Conclusion

AGIs are drugs that reduce the gut's ability to absorb carbohydrates. Examples include acarbose, miglitol, and voglibose. These drugs lower blood glucose levels, both fasting and postprandially, as well as HbA1c levels, compared to a placebo. They also slightly reduce postprandial insulin levels and BMI. However, evidence does not indicate significant effects on diabetes-related morbidity or mortality. AGIs may cause gastrointestinal side effects, such as flatulence, diarrhea, and stomach pain, which can be managed by starting with lower doses. Future research should focus on comparing AGIs with other diabetic drugs, investigating combination treatments, assessing their impact on impaired glucose tolerance, confirming potential cardiovascular benefits, and developing new formulations to improve tolerability. AGIs remain useful in managing T2DM, particularly in treating postprandial hyperglycemia, but further studies are needed to optimize their use and enhance patient outcomes.

References

Affinati, A. H., Esfandiari, N. H., Oral, E. A., & Kraftson, A. T. (2019). Bariatric surgery in the treatment of type 2 diabetes. *Current Diabetes Reports*, 19(12), 156.

Agrawal, N., Sharma, M., Singh, S., & Goyal, A. (2022). Recent advances of α-glucosidase inhibitors: A comprehensive review. *Current Topics in Medicinal Chemistry*, 22(25), 2069–2086.

Ahr, H. J., Boberg, M., Krause, H. P., Maul, W., Müller, F. O., Ploschke, H. J., Weber, H., & Wünsche, C. (1989). Pharmacokinetics of acarbose. Part I: Absorption, concentration in plasma, metabolism and excretion after single administration of [14C]acarbose to rats, dogs, and man. *Arzneimittelforschung*, 39(10), 1254-1260.

Akmal, M., Patel, P., & Wadhwa, R. (2024). *Alpha Glucosidase Inhibitors*. StatPearls Publishing.

Arokiasamy, P., Salvi, S., & Selvamani, Y. (2021). Global burden of diabetes mellitus. In *Handbook of Global Health* (pp. 1–44). Springer.

American Diabetes Association. (2021). 9. Pharmacologic approaches to glycemic treatment: Standards of medical care in diabetes-2021. *Diabetes Care*, 44(Suppl 1), S111–S124.

Atkinson, M. A., Eisenbarth, G. S., & Michels, A. W. (2014). Type 1 diabetes. *The Lancet*, 383(9911), 69–82.

Beck, R. W., Riddlesworth, T. D., Ruedy, K., Ahmann, A., Haller, S., Kruger, D., McGill, J. B., Polonsky, W., Price, D., Aronoff, S., Aronson, R., Toschi, E., Kollman, C., Bergenstal, R., & DIAMOND Study Group. (2017). Continuous glucose monitoring versus usual care in patients with type 2 diabetes receiving multiple daily insulin injections: A randomized trial. *Annals of Internal Medicine*, 167(6), 365–374.

Chatterjee, S., Khunti, K., & Davies, M. J. (2017). Type 2 diabetes. The Lancet, 389(10085), 2239–2251.

Colberg, S. R., Sigal, R. J., Yardley, J. E., Riddell, M. C., Dunstan, D. W., Dempsey, P. C., Horton, E. S., Castorino, K., & Tate, D. F. (2016). Physical activity/exercise and diabetes: A position statement of the American Diabetes Association. *Diabetes Care*, 39(11), 2065.

Derosa, G., & Maffioli, P. (2012). α-Glucosidase inhibitors and their use in clinical practice. *Archives of Medical Science: AMS*, 8(5), 899.

DiNicolantonio, J. J., Bhutani, J., & O'Keefe, J. H. (2015). Acarbose: Safe and effective for lowering postprandial hyperglycaemia and improving cardiovascular outcomes. *Open Heart*, 2(1), e000327.

Dirir, A. M., Daou, M., Yousef, A. F., & Yousef, L. F. (2022). A review of alpha-glucosidase inhibitors from plants as potential candidates for the treatment of type-2 diabetes. *Phytochemistry Reviews*, 21(4), 1049–1079.

Evert, A. B., Dennison, M., Gardner, C. D., Garvey, W. T., Lau, K. H. K., MacLeod, J., Mitri, J., Pereira, R F., Rawlings, K., Robinson, S., Saslow, L., Uelmen, S., Urbanski, P. B., & Yancy, W. S., Jr (2019). Nutrition therapy for adults with diabetes or prediabetes: a consensus report. *Diabetes Care*, 42(5), 731–754.

Frankhouser, S. Y., Ahmad, A. N., Perilli, G. A., Quintana, B. J., & Vengrove, M. A. (2013). Post-gastric-bypass hypoglycemia successfully treated with alpha-glucosidase inhibitor therapy. *Endocrine Practice*, 19(3), 511–514.

Göke, B., Fuder, H., Wieckhorst, G., Theiss, U., Stridde, E., Littke, T., Kleist, P., Arnold, R., & Lücker, P. W. (1995). Voglibose (AO-128) is an efficient alpha-glucosidase inhibitor and mobilizes the endogenous GLP-1 reserve. *Digestion*, 56(6), 493–501.

Hedrington, M. S., & Davis, S. N. (2019). Considerations when using alpha-glucosidase inhibitors in the treatment of type 2 diabetes. *Expert Opinion on Pharmacotherapy*, 20(18), 2229–2235.

Home, P., Riddle, M., Cefalu, W. T., Bailey, C. J., Bretzel, R. G., Del Prato, S., Leroith, D., Schernthaner, G., van Gaal, L., & Raz, I. (2014). Insulin therapy in people with type 2 diabetes: opportunities and challenges? *Diabetes Care*, 37(6), 1499–1508.

Hsieh, S.-H., Shih, K.-C., Chou, C.-W., & Chu, C.-H. (2011). Evaluation of the efficacy and tolerability of miglitol in Chinese patients with type 2 diabetes mellitus inadequately controlled by diet and sulfonylureas. *Acta Diabetologica*, 48(1), 71–77.

Isman, A., Nyquist, A., Moel, M., Zhang, X., & Zalzala, S. (2023). The efficacy and tolerability of intermittent prandial acarbose to reduce glucose spikes in healthy individuals. *Translational Medicine of Aging*, 7, 12–19.

Janapala, R. N., Jayaraj, J. S., Fathima, N., Kashif, T., Usman, N., Dasari, A., Jahan, N., & Sachmechi, I. (2019). Continuous Glucose Monitoring Versus Self-monitoring of Blood Glucose in Type 2 Diabetes Mellitus: A Systematic Review with Meta-analysis. *Cureus*, 11(9), e5634.

Kaku, K. (2014). Efficacy of voglibose in type 2 diabetes. *Expert Opinion on Pharmacotherapy*, 15(8), 1181–1190.

Krause, H. P., & Ahr, H. J. (1996). Pharmacokinetics and metabolism of glucosidase inhibitors. In *Oral Antidiabetics* (pp. 541–555). Springer.

Lebovitz, H. E. (1997). Alpha-glucosidase inhibitors. *Endocrinology and Metabolism Clinics of North America*, 26(3), 539–551.

Lin, X., Xu, Y., Pan, X., Xu, J., Ding, Y., Sun, X., Song, X., Ren, Y., & Shan, P. F. (2020). Global, regional, and national burden and trend of diabetes in 195 countries and territories: an analysis from 1990 to 2025. *Scientific Reports*, 10(1), 14790.

International Association of Diabetes and Pregnancy Study Groups Consensus Panel, Metzger, B. E., Gabbe, S. G., Persson, B., Buchanan, T. A., Catalano, P. A., Damm, P., Dyer, A. R., Leiva, A.d, Hod, M., Kitzmiler, J. L., Lowe, L. P., McIntyre, H. D., Oats, J. J., Omori, Y., & Schmidt, M. I. (2010). International association of diabetes and pregnancy study groups recommendations on the diagnosis and classification of hyperglycemia in pregnancy. *Diabetes Care*, 33(3), 676–682.

Nowrouzi-Sohrabi, P., Tabrizi, R., Rezaei, S., Jafari, F., Hessami, K., Abedi, M., Jalali, M., Keshavarzi, P., Shahabi, S., Kolahi, A. A., Carson-Chahhoud, K., Sahebkar, A., & Safiri, S. (2020). The effect of voglibose on metabolic profiles in patients with type 2 diabetes mellitus: A systematic review and meta-analysis of clinical trials. *Pharmacological Research*, 159, 104988.

Ogurtsova, K., da Rocha Fernandes, J. D., Huang, Y., Linnenkamp, U., Guariguata, L., Cho, N. H., Cavan, D., Shaw, J. E., & Makaroff, L. E. (2017). IDF Diabetes Atlas: Global estimates for the prevalence of diabetes for 2015 and 2040. *Diabetes Research and Clinical Practice*, 128, 40–50.

Puls, W. (1996). Pharmacology of glucosidase inhibitors. In *Oral Antidiabetics*, J. Kuhlmann & W. Puls (Eds.) (pp. 497–534). Springer.

Ren, F., Ji, N., & Zhu, Y. (2023). Research progress of α-glucosidase inhibitors produced by microorganisms and their applications. *Foods*, 12(18), 3344.

Salehi, M., Vella, A., McLaughlin, T., & Patti, M.-E. (2018). Hypoglycemia after gastric bypass surgery: Current concepts and controversies. *The Journal of Clinical Endocrinology & Metabolism*, 103(8), 2815–2826.

Scott, L. J., & Spencer, C. M. (2000). Miglitol: A review of its therapeutic potential in type 2 diabetes mellitus. *Drugs*, 59(3), 521–549.

Sherwani, S. I., Khan, H. A., Ekhzaimy, A., Masood, A., & Sakharkar, M. K. (2016). Significance of HbA1c Test in Diagnosis and Prognosis of Diabetic Patients. *Biomarker Insights*, 11, 95–104.

Tabák, A. G., Herder, C., Rathmann, W., Brunner, E. J., & Kivimäki, M. (2012). Prediabetes: a high-risk state for diabetes development. *Lancet*, 379(9833), 2279–2290.

Valderas, J. P., Ahuad, J., Rubio, L., Escalona, M., Pollak, F., & Maiz, A. (2012). Acarbose improves hypoglycaemia following gastric bypass surgery without increasing glucagon-like peptide 1 levels. *Obesity Surgery*, 22(4), 582–586.

Yeh, H. C., Duncan, B. B., Schmidt, M. I., Wang, N. Y., & Brancati, F. L. (2010). Smoking, smoking cessation, and risk for type 2 diabetes mellitus: a cohort study. *Annals of Internal Medicine*, 152(1), 10–17.

Zhang, X. L., Yuan, S. Y., Wan, G., Yuan, M. X., Yang, G. R., Fu, H. J., Zhu, L. X., Zhang, J. D., Li, Y. L., Gao, D. Y., Cui, X. L., Wang, Z. M., Xie, R. R., & Chen, Y. J. (2021). The effects of acarbose therapy on reductions of myocardial infarction and all-cause death in T2DM during 10-year multifactorial interventions (The Beijing Community Diabetes Study 24). *Scientific Reports*, 11(1), 4839.

Chapter 20

Melatonin Receptors in Diabetes: Bridging Chronobiology and Metabolic Health

Prabhjot Kaur[1,*]
Monia Sharma[2]
Kumar Guarve[1]
Geeta Deswal[1]
and Ajmer Singh Grewal[1]
[1]Guru Gobind Singh College of Pharmacy, Yamuna Nagar, Haryana, India
[2]Department of Periodontology, J. N. Kapoor D.A.V. (C) Dental College, Yamuna Nagar, Haryana, India

Abstract

Diabetes mellitus (DM) and its associated complications are the leading causes of mortality worldwide. By 2035, the International Diabetes Federation (IDF) predicts that 592 million people globally will be affected by DM. Melatonin receptors (MT1 and MT2) play a crucial role in regulating insulin secretion. By inhibiting the cAMP and cGMP pathways, melatonin reduces insulin release. Genome-wide association studies have identified a strong genetic link between the MT2 receptor gene (MTNR1B) and type 2 diabetes, particularly with the rs10830963 (G allele) variant. Experimental studies have shown that melatonin promotes the synthesis of insulin-like growth factors and enhances the tyrosine phosphorylation of the insulin receptor. Additionally, clinical research indicates that diabetic patients with low melatonin levels experience an increase in blood glucose levels when melatonin treatment stimulates insulin secretion. Therefore, melatonin receptors in human pancreatic islets may influence the treatment of type 2 diabetes.

Keywords: diabetes mellitus, melatonin, circadian rhythm, MT1 and MT2, MTNR1B gene, insulin, type 2 diabetes.

---

* Corresponding Author's Email: prabhjotkaur102001@gmail.com

In: Receptor-Targeted Therapies in Diabetes Mellitus
Editors: Ajmer Singh Grewal, Neelam Singh, Swati Verma et al.
ISBN: 979-8-89530-587-4

Abbreviations

AMP	Adenosine monophosphate
ARNT	Aryl Hydrocarbon Receptor Nuclear Translocator
cAMP	cyclic Adenosine Monophosphate
cGMP	Cyclic guanosine monophosphate
CLOCK	Circadian Locomotor Output Cycles Kaput
CNG	Cyclic nucleotide-gated
CREB	Cyclic AMP-Responsive Element-Binding Protein
DAG	Diacyl Glycerol
DM	Diabetes Mellitus
Gi	Guanine nucleotide binding protein
GLUT 4	Glucose transporter 4
GPx	Glutathione Peroxidase
Gq	Guanine nucleotide binding protein
GSH	Glutathione
GSK3β	Glycogen synthase kinase 3 beta
GTP	Guanosine-5'-trisphosphate
GWA	Genome-wide association
HepG2	Hepatoblastoma cell line
IDF	International Diabetes Federation
iNOS	Inducible nitric oxide synthase
IP3	Inositol triphosphate
IRS-1	Insulin receptor substrate-1
MAPK	Mitogen Activated Protein Kinase
MDA	Malondialdehyde
mRNA	Messenger Ribo Nucleic Acid
MSK1	Mitogen- and stress-activated protein kinase-1
MT1	Melatonin Receptor Type 1
MT2	Melatonin Receptor Type 2
NO	Nitric oxide
Nrf-2-HO-1 p	Nuclear factor erythroid 2-heme oxygenase-1
PACAP	Pituitary adenylate cyclase-activating polypeptide
PGC1α	Peroxisome proliferator-activated receptor- gamma coactivator 1-alpha
PI-3	Phosphoinositide 3
PI3K	Phosphoinositide 3-kinases
PKA	Protein Kinase-A
PKC	Protein Kinase-C
PKCζ-Akt	Atypical Protein Kinase C zeta
ROS	Reactive oxygen species
SCN	Supra Chiasmatic Nucleus
SIRT1	Sirtuin (silent mating type information regulation 2 homolog) 1
SOD	Superoxide dismutase
T2DM	Type 2 diabetes mellitus.

Introduction

A compromised circadian rhythm results from our modern lifestyle's shift toward excessive nighttime activity and daytime inactivity. Nearly ninety percent of individuals with diabetes suffer from type 2 diabetes mellitus (T2DM) (Karthikeyan et al. 2014). According to Zhu et al. (2023), T2DM is a multifaceted metabolic condition that arises from a combination of genetic predisposition and lifestyle risk factors. Several factors contribute to an increased risk of T2DM, including pancreatic β-cell dysfunction, abnormal adipogenesis, insufficient insulin responsiveness, genetic factors, excessive food intake or high-calorie diets, and a sedentary lifestyle (Karthikeyan et al. 2014). In addition to these risk factors, growing evidence suggests that disruptions in circadian rhythm play a role in the development of T2DM. Impaired glucose tolerance and elevated complications of T2DM are closely associated with a disrupted circadian rhythm. While there have been conflicting reports on how the pineal hormone melatonin affects blood glucose levels, insulin release, and carbohydrate metabolism, the pathogenesis of T2DM is increasingly linked to sleep disturbances and disruptions in the circadian system. These disturbances are more common in individuals with irregular lifestyles, such as night shift workers, those exposed to light at night, or those with irregular meal times (Mühlbauer & Peschke, 2006). Therefore, combining melatonin's cytoprotective and chronobiotic properties could provide a novel approach to managing T2DM. The suprachiasmatic nucleus (SCN) in the hypothalamus regulates the release of melatonin, the primary hormone responsible for inducing sleep, which peaks at night. Melatonin is synthesized from tryptophan through a four-step process (Patel et al. 2022). Due to its broad range of antioxidant properties, melatonin may be applied in various pathological conditions. Specifically, it regulates endoplasmic reticulum stress, autophagy, and oxidative stress, making it a valuable therapeutic agent (Boga et al. 2019). Figure 1 illustrates a signaling pathway involved in maintaining circadian rhythm within the cell (Sharma et al. 2015).

Pancreatic islets have garnered significant attention in the study of melatonin's role in glucose metabolism. Although more research is needed, exogenous melatonin is considered a safe treatment option based on the limited available data. According to Doğanlar et al. (2019), melatonin administration in adolescents, children, and preterm newborns with various disorders has not been associated with major adverse effects, provided it is not administered excessively or too frequently. In addition to its well-known ability to promote sleep, melatonin has other physiological effects. For instance, it can induce hypothermia and heat loss in healthy individuals and those with disrupted circadian rhythms. In T2DM, elevated melatonin synthesis and decreased insulin production due to β-cell loss ultimately led to hyperglycemia. Insulin resistance in T2DM causes β-cell fatigue, resulting in increased glucagon levels and higher blood glucose levels. Melatonin depletion increases the mRNA expression of the melatonin membrane receptor (Karthikeyan et al. 2014). Moreover, it has been shown that insulin's primary target, adipocytes, express MT2 receptors. Upon melatonin stimulation, these receptors reduce the expression of glucose transporter 4 (GLUT4), an insulin-dependent glucose transporter (Sharma et al. 2015). Additionally, melatonin signaling through MT2 receptors enhances glucose uptake by muscle cells by phosphorylating insulin receptor substrate-1 (Brydon et al. 2001). Over time, genetic variations in melatonin receptors have been linked to various metabolic disorders, including T2DM, gestational diabetes mellitus, and obesity

(Owino et al. 2019). This chapter compiles the current understanding of melatonin's functions and its receptor interactions in the treatment and management of T2DM.

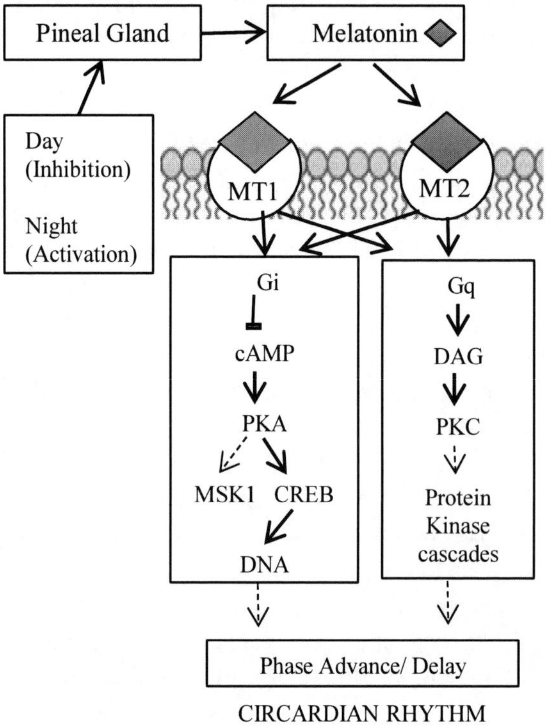

Figure 1. Mechanism of melatonin signaling in maintenance of circadian rhythm within cells.

Classification of Melatonin Receptors

Mammals respond to melatonin through interactions with intracellular proteins, such as calmodulin and orphan nuclear receptors, as well as plasma membrane receptors. These receptors, which are often high-affinity G protein-coupled receptors, mediate melatonin's actions in both central and peripheral organs, including human islet cells, where they are abundantly distributed (Zhu et al. 2023). Membrane receptors serve as sites for melatonin's high-affinity and specific binding. Different species possess various receptor subtypes, with the most well-characterized being the mammalian MT1 and MT2 receptors (Okamoto et al. 2024). The MT1 and MT2 receptors are the primary receptors in humans, sharing a sequence similarity of 55% for the entire region and 70% for the transmembrane portion (Wang et al. 2022). Functionally, MT1, which has a higher affinity for melatonin, has been shown to acutely suppress neuronal activation, while MT2 plays a critical role in effective phase-shifting (de Lima Menzes et al. 2024). Both receptors signal through Gi/o proteins, which inhibit adenylyl cyclase and decrease intracellular levels of cAMP (Wang et al. 2024). According to Karamitri et al. (2019), MT2 is functionally significant for T2DM, as indicated by single nucleotide polymorphisms. Experimental studies using the melatonin antagonist luzindole and the GTP analogue guanosine 5'-O-(3-thiotrisphosphate) have shown that melatonin influences the exocytosis of insulin by pancreatic β-cells. Both agents inhibit melatonin's effect on insulin secretion from islets of neonatal rats. Furthermore, melatonin treatment induces the MT2 receptor on pancreatic β-cells, which shifts the insulin rhythm phase in isolated rat islets (Sharma et al. 2015). Molecular and immunocytochemical research also confirms the presence of MT1 and MT2 in human pancreatic cells, including the islets of Langerhans (Mühlbauer & Peschke, 2006).

Melatonin and Chronobiology

The circadian system has evolved to generate rhythms in physiological and behavioral processes that typically last around 24 hours. Acting as a pacemaker, the circadian rhythm in the SCN synchronizes the metabolic activities of peripheral clocks and regulates daily cycles of eating, fasting, and sleep (Chao et al. 2016). In both diurnal and nocturnal species, melatonin production begins in the evening, peaks around midnight, and gradually decreases by morning. Due to its production pattern, melatonin is often referred to as the „hormone of darkness." Notably, melatonin levels decrease with age, with a significant decline observed during the 6th and 7th decades of life (de Lima Menzes et al. 2024). This decline affects neuronal sensitivity to endogenous clock phase shifts. Additionally, the pituitary adenylate cyclase-activating polypeptide (PACAP), a retinohypothalamic transmitter that induces phosphorylation of the cAMP response element-binding protein (CREB), is inhibited by rhythmic melatonin synthesis in SCN cells (Patel et al. 2022). Recent advancements in circadian rhythm regulation have revealed that Period genes are controlled by a combination of transcriptional factors, including the aryl hydrocarbon receptor nuclear translocator (ARNT) and the circadian locomotor output cycles kaput (CLOCK). This regulatory system counteracts oscillating feedback loops in transcription and translation, leading to 24-hour periodic waves of gene expression. While light is the most prominent external stimulus for this machinery, metabolism also plays a crucial role, with CLOCK activity being influenced by the cellular redox status (Espino et al. 2011).

The Relationship between T2DM and Melatonin Receptor

The growing recognition of the impact of circadian rhythm disturbances on glucose tolerance, complications, and treatment in T2DM highlights the importance of understanding these disruptions in the disease's pathophysiology. Disrupted circadian rhythms adversely affect glucose metabolism, and recent studies have identified polymorphisms in the MTNR1B gene as significant risk factors for T2DM, reinforcing the connection between melatonin and diabetes (Espino et al. 2011). Melatonin, which primarily regulates sleep-wake cycles, is increasingly linked to glucose homeostasis and appetite regulation. Sleep disturbances and reduced melatonin levels play a central role in the development of T2DM (Garaulet et al. 2020). Genome-wide association (GWA) studies, along with replicated cohort studies, have robustly associated the MT2 gene with glycemic traits, such as elevated fasting glucose levels, insulin resistance, and impaired β-cell function. The rs10830963 G allele is particularly associated with a higher risk of T2DM (Dupuis et al. 2010). Additionally, studies in pinealectomized mice, which show reduced GLUT4 gene expression, highlight the role of melatonin in glucose uptake and insulin sensitivity. Melatonin therapy has been shown to alleviate insulin resistance and glucose intolerance (Sun et al. 2018). Furthermore, diminished melatonin levels can increase the expression of the melatonin membrane receptor, exacerbating insulin resistance, raising insulin levels, and leading to hyperglycemia and β-cell exhaustion. This underscores the critical role of melatonin receptors in the development and management of T2D.

Melatonin in Glucose Homeostasis

The regulation of glucose metabolism is influenced by the endogenous circadian rhythm, which is coordinated by both central and peripheral clocks. The sleep-wake cycle, in synergy with feeding and fasting rhythms, complements glucose metabolism. Evidence suggests that melatonin plays a significant role in glucose regulation. For instance, glucose tolerance in healthy individuals is lower in the late afternoon or overnight compared to the morning when consuming the same meal. Due to the influence of circadian rhythm, glucose tolerance and β-cell responsiveness decrease at night. Disrupted endogenous rhythms and irregular eating patterns, such as those seen in long-term shift work, may contribute to the gradual decline in glucose tolerance and insulin sensitivity (Anothaisintawee et al. 2016). The hypothalamic SCN may exert an excitatory-inhibitory effect on the neuronal response in the arcuate nucleus to hypoglycemia, influenced by food intake. Melatonin also plays a role in enhancing glucose uptake by muscle cells through specific signaling pathways. It activates the phosphoinositide 3-kinase (PI3K) and insulin receptor substrate-1 (IRS-1) signaling cascades, which in turn stimulate protein kinase C (PKC) zeta via the MT2 receptor in rats. Furthermore, melatonin enhances glucose utilization and regulates glycogen levels in HepG2 cells by activating the PKC zeta-Akt-glycogen synthase kinase 3 beta (GSK3β) pathway (Chao et al. 2016).

Melatonin and Insulin Secretion

Melatonin is known to regulate insulin production in pancreatic β-cells through signaling pathways involving cAMP, cGMP, and inositol triphosphate (IP3) (Table 1). When melatonin binds to MT1 and MT2 receptors, it inhibits the cAMP and cGMP pathways, subsequently reducing insulin production in β-cells. Melatonin also briefly increases intracellular $Ca2+$ levels, leading to IP3 release and $Ca2+$-dependent insulin secretion. Studies suggest that melatonin therapy may benefit glucose metabolism. Sun et al. (2018) found that obese individuals with *Acanthosis nigricans* showed improved insulin sensitivity and reduced inflammation after a 12-week melatonin regimen (3 mg/day). Additionally, prolonged exposure to melatonin (>12 hours) has been associated with enhanced glucose-stimulated insulin secretion in cultured non-diabetic human islets (Costes et al. 2015). Melatonin supplementation has also been shown to reduce diabetes markers, including insulin resistance, compared to a placebo (Delpino et al. 2021). In patients with low melatonin levels, melatonin treatment can enhance insulin production, thereby increasing glucose levels in the body (Dhankhar et al. 2023). As a supplement, melatonin is generally safe, well-absorbed via all administration routes, and can cross physiological barriers, including the placenta and blood-brain barrier (Xie et al. 2017; Donga et al. 2010). However, acute daytime administration of melatonin has been shown to decrease insulin sensitivity by 10%-25% (Kampmann et al. 2021; Lauritzen et al.

2022). These findings suggest an antagonistic relationship between insulin and melatonin, where elevated insulin levels suppress melatonin production by the pineal gland. Historically, insulin levels are higher during the day, when melatonin is lower, while at night, insulin levels are typically low, but blood glucose is high (Espino et al. 2011).

Table 1. Regulation of insulin secretion via melatonin in β-cells of pancreas *via* cAMP, cGMP, and IP3

Signaling pathway	Receptor involved	Effect on insulin secretion	Mechanism in brief
cAMP	M1	Decreased	Activating protein kinase A, thereby inhibiting calcium dependent insulin secretion
cGMP	M2	Decreased	Binds to cyclic nucleotide- gated (CNG) ion channels, inhibiting Calcium-dependent insulin secretion
IP3	M1	Increased	Signals from phospholipase C leads to activation of calcium dependent insulin secretion

Melatonin and Glycaemic Variability

In individuals with T2DM, melatonin supplementation has been associated with increased glycemic variability. This effect may be due to melatonin's lingering impact throughout the day, which can interfere with its potential benefits and even exacerbate blood glucose fluctuations. One hypothesis is that melatonin, typically produced at night, influences the circadian rhythm of hormones that regulate glucose, such as insulin and counter-regulatory hormones like catecholamines and cortisol. Consequently, elevated melatonin levels at night might have residual effects that disrupt glycemic control into the following day, especially if taken in high doses. When melatonin is elevated during the day or around meals, it can further complicate glycemic management by increasing insulin resistance and reducing insulin secretion, leading to larger positive fluctuations in morning blood glucose (Martorina et al. 2023). As a result, caution is advised when considering melatonin for T2DM patients, taking into account factors such as dosage, duration of use, and genetic predispositions (Martorina et al. 2019). Despite research suggesting potential benefits of melatonin on glycemic control, controlled trials and genetic studies highlight its possible adverse effects on glucose regulation in T2DM. For instance, human pancreatic islets release somatostatin, an insulin-inhibitory hormone, in response to melatonin (Zibolka et al. 2018). Additionally, acute melatonin administration has been shown in placebo-controlled studies to impair glucose tolerance in both young and older adults, whether taken in the morning or evening (Rubio-Sastre et al. 2014; Garaulet et al. 2015). This effect is more pronounced in carriers of the MTNR1B rs10830963 T2DM risk variant, suggesting a genetic basis for melatonin's impact on glucose metabolism. Garaulet et al. (2020) further described this relationship in a timing model (Table 2), examining how melatonin influences glucose levels in both fasting and postprandial states. Low melatonin can result from factors such as inhibition by the SCN during the circadian day, light exposure that suppresses endogenous production, or exogenous supplementation (Garaulet et al. 2020).

Table 2. Effect of melatonin level with fasting or feed state on glucose metabolism

Conditions	Effect on Glucose Metabolism	
	High Melatonin	Low Melatonin
Fast state	Increased β- cells rest	Decreased β-cells rest
Feed State	Decreased function of β- cells and insulin sensitivity	Increased function of β- cells and insulin sensitivity

Role of Melatonin in Diabetic Complications

Melatonin therapy has been shown to mitigate oxidative stress, prevent apoptosis triggered by caspase activation and endoplasmic reticulum stress, reduce pro-inflammatory cytokines, and enhance steroidogenesis, providing protective effects against diabetes-induced reproductive damage, as demonstrated in both *in vivo* and *in vitro* studies (Armandeh et al. 2022; Boga et al. 2019). Additionally, in T2DM patients, melatonin levels in tooth pulp tissue are reduced. Therapeutic melatonin concentrations appear to protect dental pulp tissue in hyperglycemic conditions by boosting iNOS and SOD activity, which counters hyperglycemia-induced oxidative damage. Melatonin's antioxidant properties are crucial in lowering oxidative stress, a major risk factor in diabetes and other illnesses (Espino et al. 2019). Diabetes also correlates with higher incidences of anxiety and depression. In diabetic rats, melatonin has shown anxiolytic and antidepressant effects (Ergenc et al. 2022). While glycemic control helps delay diabetic microvascular complications, it has a limited impact on reducing diabetic cardiomyopathy-related mortality in T2DM patients. Melatonin contributes to cardiomyopathy management by activating the SIRT1-PGC1α pathway, reducing mitochondrial fission, and thus ameliorating cardiomyopathy (Wang et al. 2018). Moreover, melatonin lowers oxidative stress, reducing levels of ROS, MDA, and NO, and activating pathways like CAT and PI3K/Akt-Nrf2, which can alleviate diabetic retinopathy (Maniadakis et al. 2019). It also improves diabetic neuropathy by enhancing levels of antioxidants like GSH, CAT, SOD, and GPx, and activating the Nrf2-HO-1 pathway, which collectively reduces oxidative stress (Hazam et al. 2017).

Conclusion

Examining effective treatments for diabetes and its consequences is crucial given the substantial rise in the prevalence of diabetes mellitus (DM) worldwide. Recent studies have shown that melatonin may regulate a variety of signaling pathways and can both prevent and treat several disorders, including diabetes mellitus. Numerous modes of action for melatonin have been demonstrated in preclinical and clinical research, including decreased glucose production, enhanced pro-inflammatory pathways, and improved oxidative stress states in diabetic patients. It may be possible to reduce the prevalence of insulin resistance and hyperglycemia by focusing on the circadian clock. Although the impact of endogenous melatonin on human glucose metabolism remains unclear, research on human genetics and animal behavior indicates that diminished melatonin signaling or low melatonin production may worsen insulin sensitivity and contribute to T2DM. However, the finding that the MT2 receptor is related to T2DM highlights the importance of biological rhythms in controlling metabolism. Since multiple animal studies suggest that melatonin may have beneficial effects on glucose homeostasis and obesity management under certain conditions, human clinical trials should be encouraged to evaluate the hormone's therapeutic potential in diabetes.

References

Anothaisintawee, T., Reutrakul, S., Van Cauter, E., & Thakkinstian, A. (2016). Sleep disturbances compared to traditional risk factors for diabetes development: systematic review and meta-analysis. *Sleep Medicine Reviews*, 30, 11-24.

Armandeh, M., Bameri, B., Haghi-Aminjan, H., Foroumadi, R., Ataei, M., Hassani, S., Samadi, M., Shayesteh, M. R. H., & Abdollahi, M. (2022). A systematic review on the role of melatonin and its mechanisms on diabetes-related reproductive impairment in non-clinical studies. *Frontiers in Endocrinology*, 13, 1022989.

Boga, J. A., Caballero, B., Potes, Y., Perez-Martinez, Z., Reiter, R. J., Vega-Naredo, I., & Coto-Montes, A. (2019). Therapeutic potential of melatonin related to its role as an autophagy regulator: A review. *Journal of Pineal Research*, 66(1), e12534.

Brydon, L., Petit, L., Delagrange, P., Strosberg, A. D., & Jockers, R. (2001). Functional expression of MT2 (Mel1b) melatonin receptors in human PAZ6 adipocytes. *Endocrinology*, 142(10), 4264-4271.

Cagnacci, A., Arangino, S., Renzi, A., Paoletti, A. M., Melis, G. B., Cagnacci, P., & Volpe, A. (2001). Influence of melatonin administration on glucose tolerance and insulin sensitivity of postmenopausal women. *Clinical Endocrinology*, 54(3), 339-346.

Chao, D., León-Mercado, L., Foppen, E., Guzmán-Ruiz, M., Basualdo, M. C., Escobar, C., & Buijs, R. M. (2016). The suprachiasmatic nucleus modulates the sensitivity of arcuate nucleus to hypoglycemia in the male rat. *Endocrinology*, 157(9), 3439-3451.

Costes, S., Boss, M., Thomas, A. P., & Matveyenko, A. V. (2015). Activation of melatonin signaling promotes β-cell survival and function. *Molecular Endocrinology*, 29(5), 682-692.

de Lima Menezes, G., Sales Bezerra, K., Nobre Oliveira, J. I., Fontenele Araújo, J., Soares Galvão, D., Alves da Silva, R., Vogel Saivish, M & Laino Fulco, U. (2024). Quantum mechanics insights into melatonin and analogs binding to melatonin MT1 and MT2 receptors. *Scientific Reports*, 14(1), 10922.

Delpino, F. M., Figueiredo, L. M., & Nunes, B. P. (2021). Effects of melatonin supplementation on diabetes: A systematic review and meta-analysis of randomized clinical trials. *Clinical Nutrition*, 40(7), 4595-4605.

Dhankhar, S., Chauhan, S., Mehta, D. K., Nitika, Saini, K., Saini, M., Das, R., Gupta, S., & Gautam, V. (2023). Novel targets for potential therapeutic use in Diabetes mellitus. *Diabetology & Metabolic Syndrome*, 15(1), 17.

Doğanlar, Z. B., Güçlü, H., Öztopuz, Ö., Türkön, H., Dogan, A., Uzun, M., & Doğanlar, O. (2019). The role of melatonin in oxidative stress, DNA damage, apoptosis and angiogenesis in fetal eye under preeclampsia and melatonin deficiency stress. *Current Eye Research*, 44(10), 1157-1169.

Donga, E., Van Dijk, M., Van Dijk, J. G., Biermasz, N. R., Lammers, G. J., Van Kralingen, K., Hoogma, R. P., Corssmit, E. P., & Romijn, J. A. (2010). Partial sleep restriction decreases insulin sensitivity in type 1 diabetes. *Diabetes Care*, 33(7), 1573-1577.

Dupuis, J., Langenberg, C., Prokopenko, I., Saxena, R., Soranzo, N., Jackson, A. U., Wheeler, E., Glazer, N. L., Bouatia-Naji, N., Gloyn, A. L., & Lindgren, C. M. (2010). New genetic loci implicated in fasting glucose homeostasis and their impact on type 2 diabetes risk. *Nature Genetics*, 42(2), 105-116.

Ergenc, M., Ozacmak, H. S., Turan, I., & Ozacmak, V. H. (2022). Melatonin reverses depressive and anxiety like-behaviours induced by diabetes: involvement of oxidative stress, age, rage and S100B levels in the hippocampus and prefrontal cortex of rats. *Archives of Physiology and Biochemistry*, 128(2), 402-410.

Espino, J., Pariente, J. A., & Rodríguez, A. B. (2011). Role of melatonin on diabetes-related metabolic disorders. *World Journal of Diabetes*, 2(6), 82.

Espino, J., Rodríguez, A. B., & Pariente, J. A. (2019). Melatonin and oxidative stress in the diabetic state: clinical implications and potential therapeutic applications. *Current Medicinal Chemistry*, 26(22), 4178-4190.

Garaulet, M., Gómez-Abellán, P., Rubio-Sastre, P., Madrid, J. A., Saxena, R., & Scheer, F. A. (2015). Common type 2 diabetes risk variant in MTNR1B worsens the deleterious effect of melatonin on glucose tolerance in humans. *Metabolism*, 64(12), 1650-1657.

Garaulet, M., Qian, J., Florez, J. C., Arendt, J., Saxena, R., & Scheer, F. A. (2020). Melatonin effects on glucose metabolism: time to unlock the controversy. *Trends in Endocrinology & Metabolism*, 31(3), 192-204.

Hajam, Y. A., Rai, S., Roy, A., Basheer, M., & Ghosh, H. (2017). Research Article Repossession of Brain Complications in a Streptozotocin Induced Diabetic Rat by Exogenous Melatonin Administration. *International Journal of Zoological Research*, 13 (2): 64-73.

Kampmann, U., Lauritzen, E. S., Grarup, N., Jessen, N., Hansen, T., Møller, N., & Støy, J. (2021). Acute metabolic effects of melatonin—a randomized crossover study in healthy young men. *Journal of Pineal Research*, 70(2), e12706.

Karamitri, A., & Jockers, R. (2019). Melatonin in type 2 diabetes mellitus and obesity. *Nature Reviews Endocrinology*, 15(2), 105-125.

Karthikeyan, R., Marimuthu, G., Spence, D. W., Pandi-Perumal, S. R., BaHammam, A. S., Brown, G. M., & Cardinali, D. P. (2014). Should we listen to our clock to prevent type 2 diabetes mellitus? *Diabetes Research and Clinical Practice*, 106(2), 182-190.

Lauritzen, E. S., Kampmann, U., Pedersen, M. G., Christensen, L. L., Jessen, N., Møller, N., & Støy, J. (2022). Three months of melatonin treatment reduces insulin sensitivity in patients with type 2 diabetes—A randomized placebo-controlled crossover trial. *Journal of Pineal Research*, 73(1), e12809.

Maniadakis, N., & Konstantakopoulou, E. (2019). Cost effectiveness of treatments for diabetic retinopathy: a systematic literature review. *Pharmacoeconomics*, 37, 995-1010.

Martorina, W., & Tavares, A. (2019). Real-world data in support of short sleep duration with poor glycemic control, in people with type 2 diabetes mellitus. *Journal of Diabetes Research*, 2019(1), 6297162.

Martorina, W., & Tavares, A. (2023). Glycemic variability in patients with type 2 diabetes mellitus (T2DM): the role of melatonin in a crossover, double-blind, placebo-controlled, randomized study. *Nutrients*, 15(16), 3523.

Mühlbauer, E., & Peschke, E. (2006). Evidence for the expression of both the MT1- and, in addition, the MT2-melatonin receptor, in the rat pancreas, islet, and β-cell. Journal of Pineal Research, 42(1), 105-106.

Okamoto, H. H., Cecon, E., Nureki, O., Rivara, S., & Jockers, R. (2024). Melatonin receptor structure and signaling. *Journal of Pineal Research*, 76(3), e12952.

Owino, S., Buonfiglio, D. D., Tchio, C., & Tosini, G. (2019). Melatonin signaling a key regulator of glucose homeostasis and energy metabolism. *Frontiers in Endocrinology*, 10, 488.

Patel, R., Parmar, N., Palit, S. P., Rathwa, N., Ramachandran, A. V., & Begum, R. (2022). Diabetes mellitus and melatonin: Where are we? *Biochimie*, 202, 2-14.

Rubio-Sastre, P., Scheer, F. A., Gómez-Abellán, P., Madrid, J. A., & Garaulet, M. (2014). Acute melatonin administration in humans impairs glucose tolerance in both the morning and evening. *Sleep*, 37(10), 1715-1719.

Sharma, S., Singh, H., Ahmad, N., Mishra, P., & Tiwari, A. (2015). The role of melatonin in diabetes: therapeutic implications. *Archives of Endocrinology and Metabolism*, 59(5), 391-399.

Sun, H., Wang, X., Chen, J., Gusdon, A. M., Song, K., Li, L., & Qu, S. (2018). Melatonin treatment improves insulin resistance and pigmentation in obese patients with Acanthosis nigricans. *International Journal of Endocrinology*, 2018(1), 2304746.

Wang, Q., Lu, Q., Guo, Q., Teng, M., Gong, Q., Li, X., Du, Y., Liu, Z., & Tao, Y. (2022). Structural basis of the ligand binding and signaling mechanism of melatonin receptors. *Nature Communications*, 13(1), 454.

Wang, S., Zhao, Z., Feng, X., Cheng, Z., Xiong, Z., Wang, T., Lin, J., Zhang, M., Hu, J., Fan, Y., & Reiter, R. J. (2018). Melatonin activates Parkin translocation and rescues the impaired mitophagy activity of diabetic cardiomyopathy through Mst1 inhibition. *Journal of Cellular and Molecular Medicine*, 22(10), 5132-5144.

Xie, Z., Chen, F., Li, W. A., Geng, X., Li, C., Meng, X., & Yu, F. (2017). A review of sleep disorders and melatonin. *Neurological Research*, 39(6), 559-565.

Zhu, H., Zhao, Z. J., Liu, H. Y., Cai, J., Lu, Q. K., Ji, L. D., & Xu, J. (2023). The melatonin receptor 1B gene links circadian rhythms and type 2 diabetes mellitus: An evolutionary story. *Annals of Medicine*, 55(1), 1262-1286.

Zibolka, J., Bazwinsky-Wutschke, I., Mühlbauer, E., & Peschke, E. (2018). Distribution and density of melatonin receptors in human main pancreatic islet cell types. *Journal of Pineal Research*, 65(1), e12480.

Chapter 21

Pyruvate Kinase M2 Inhibition

Ajay Bilandi[1,*]
Maninderjeet Kaur[2]
and Naina[2]
[1]Bhai Gurdas College of Pharmacy, Sangrur, Punjab, India
[2]GHG Khalsa College, Gurusar Sudhar, Ludhiana, Punjab, India

Abstract

Pyruvate kinase M2 (PKM2) is a crucial enzyme that plays a central role in cellular metabolism and development, adapting to various physiological conditions. PKM2's primary function in metabolism involves catalyzing the final step of glycolysis, where it converts phosphoenolpyruvate (PEP) into pyruvate, simultaneously generating ATP. Beyond this metabolic activity, PKM2 exerts regulatory influence by phosphorylating key proteins involved in cellular signaling pathways, significantly contributing to redox balance, particularly in cancer cells. Elevated PKM2 expression has been observed in various cancers and inflammatory responses, prompting interest in its potential as a therapeutic target. This chapter explores the molecular mechanisms and therapeutic implications of targeting PKM2, with a focus on cancer metabolism, redox regulation, inflammation, and metabolic disorders. Both the metabolic and non-metabolic roles of PKM2 are analyzed, highlighting its importance in health and disease, as well as its potential in therapeutic applications.

Keywords: Warburg effect, pyruvate kinase, glycolysis, cancer, redox homeostasis, inflammation, metabolic disease

Abbreviations

ACL	ATP-citrate lyase
AKI	Acute kidney injury
ALDOA	Aldose A

* Corresponding Author's Email: ajaybilandi2031@gmail.com

In: Receptor-Targeted Therapies in Diabetes Mellitus
Editors: Ajmer Singh Grewal, Neelam Singh, Swati Verma et al.
ISBN: 979-8-89530-587-4

ATP	Adenosine triphosphate
BFGF	Basic fibroblast growth factor
CARM	Co-activator-associated arginine methyltransferase
CCI	Chronic construction injury
DHAP	Dihydroxyacetone phosphate
eNOS	Endothelial NO synthase
ERK	Extracellular signal-regulated protein kinase
FBP	Fructose 1,6-biphosphate
GLUT	Glucose transporter
HIF-1α	Hypoxia-inducible factor 1-alpha
JAK	Janus kinase
NPC	Nuclear pore complex
PEP	Phosphoenolpyruvate
PHD	Pyruvate dehydrogenase
PKC	Protein kinase C
PK	Pyruvate kinase
PKM2	Pyruvate kinase M2
PTB	Polypyrimidine tract binding protein
PTP	Protein-tyrosine phosphatase
SIR	Systematic inflammatory responses
SIRT	Sirtuins
STAT	Signal transducer and activator of transcription
TNF-α	Tumor necrosis factor alpha

Introduction

Pyruvate kinase (PK) is a crucial regulatory enzyme in glucose catabolism, with mammalian PK existing in several isoforms that exhibit differences in allosteric regulation and tissue distribution. This diversity is vital for meeting the distinct energy requirements of various cell types. The M2 isoform is particularly abundant in rapidly proliferating cells, such as cancer cells, where it promotes the accumulation of glycolytic intermediates that fuel tumor growth (Yang et al. 2014). Moreover, pyruvate kinase M2 plays a direct role in metabolic reprogramming, especially in the Warburg effect (aerobic glycolysis), which is linked to both cancer progression and inflammatory responses (Christofk et al. 2008). Unlike other PK isoforms, PKM2 also regulates gene expression and acts as a kinase that phosphorylates proteins essential for cellular growth and survival (Jiang et al. 2014). A deeper understanding of PKM2's role in cancer, inflammation, and metabolic diseases could pave the way for novel therapeutic strategies to address the harmful health consequences and mortality associated with these conditions (Yang et al. 2012).

PKM2: The Journey from Gene to Protein

In humans, the pyruvate kinase M (PKM) gene is located on chromosome 15, while in nonhuman primates it is found on chromosome 7, and in mice, it is located on chromosome 9 (Benson et al. 2017). Both the M1 and M2 isoforms are encoded by this gene. There is an 82% sequence similarity between the mouse and human PKM2 transcripts and a 99% sequence identity between the nonhuman primate and human PKM2 transcripts. The PKM gene consists of 12 exons and 11 introns, spanning approximately 32 kilobases. The differences observed in the final transcript are attributed to the similar length of exons 9 and 10. The mRNA transcripts of the PKM gene are located on chromosomes 15 and 9 in humans, nonhuman primates, and mice, respectively. The PK protein is composed of four identical subunits: N (43 amino acids), A (244 amino acids), B (102 amino acids), and C (142 amino acids), which together form the 531-amino acid PKM2 monomer. A specific region of 22 amino acids separates PKM1 and PKM2, which is encoded by exons 9 and 10. The A domain, located near the center of the PKM2 monomer, is crucial for promoting subunit interaction and facilitating dimer formation. The C domain contains the nuclear localization signal sequence as well as the allosteric binding pocket for fructose 1,6-bisphosphate (FBP). The active site of PKM2 is found in the region bounded by domains A and B, with domain B regulating the size of the active site by shifting its location relative to domain A. The N-terminal of the PKM2 monomer is its smallest domain (Dombrauckas et al. 2005).

Distribution of PK Isoforms in Tissues

wo distinct genes encode the four isoforms of the PK family: PKM1 (muscle), PKM2 (liver), PKL (liver), and PKR (erythrocytes). The PKLR gene produces both the L and R isoforms, including the M1 and M2 isoforms. Multiple isoforms can be expressed at the protein level in a single tissue. For example, PKM2 is predominantly expressed in the kidneys, whereas PKL and PKM1 are present in much lower amounts. Based on the metabolic needs of specific tissues, the PK isoforms exhibit tissue specificity and vary in their kinetic properties. The sole isoform present in erythrocytes is PKR, while PKM1 is mainly found in differentiated skeletal muscle, heart, and brain tissues. In contrast, PKL is the predominant isoform in the liver. PKM2 is present in a variety of adult organs and is the only isoform detectable during embryonic development. It is mainly found in the kidneys but can also be detected in various adult tissues such as the lungs, intestines, ovaries, testes, white and brown adipose tissues, and pancreatic islets (Imamura & Tanaka, 1972). Importantly, PKM2 is expressed at higher levels in proliferating cells, including tumor cells and stem cells. Its expression varies throughout development; for example, it is found in skeletal muscle in newborns but decreases as the muscle matures, causing the differentiated muscle to switch from PKM2 to PKM1 (Osterman et al. 1973). Phosphoenolpyruvate (PEP) and the glycolytic intermediates FBP or F-2,6-P2 (fructose 2,6-bisphosphate) often trigger its activation. PKM2 plays a key role in glycolysis by transferring a phosphate group from PEP to ADP, generating pyruvate and ATP. Both monovalent (K^+) and divalent (Mg^{2+} or Mn^{2+}) cations facilitate the binding of PEP and ATP to the active site. The glycolytic process is typically irreversible and crucial for regulating the flow of glycolysis. A significant conformational shift occurs between the T state (low enzyme activity) and the R state (high enzyme activity), which is key to PKM2's function.

PKM2 Post-Transnational Modifications

PKM2 undergoes various post-translational modifications that significantly regulate its activity, stability, and subcellular localization (Liu et al. 2017). Oxidation, acetylation, and methylation of PKM2 play crucial roles in modulating its enzymatic activity, with different oxidants, such as nitric oxide, hydrogen peroxide, and diamide, influencing its function. Nitric oxide, for example, regulates cancer metabolism by increasing cell proliferation, enhancing oxidative defense, and promoting glycolysis at low concentrations. However, at high concentrations, nitric oxide blocks glycolysis and induces cell death. Furthermore, nitric oxide induces S-nitrosylation of PKM2, inhibiting its tetramer formation, particularly in the context of acute kidney injury. PKM2's enzymatic activity can also be reduced by oxidative stress, as seen in lung cancer cells, where cysteine-358 undergoes oxidation, leading to the enzyme's dissociation from its tetrameric form. Additionally, oxidative stress activates the desuccinylation of PKM2 at lysine-498, resulting in decreased enzymatic activity and increased oxidative damage, which may impact tumor formation. Shikonin, a PKM2 inhibitor, increases oxidant levels, reduces PKM2 expression, and induces cell death—a process that can be mitigated by antioxidants like N-acetyl-L-cysteine (Siragusa et al. 2019). Regarding phosphorylation, PKM2 is phosphorylated at several sites by kinases such as JAK2, ERK1/2, and AKT, particularly in response to oncogenic stimuli. Phosphorylation at tyrosine-105 inhibits tetramer formation, promoting the Warburg effect, while phosphorylation at serine-37 and threonine-454 enhances nuclear accumulation and tumor growth. Dephosphorylation by low molecular weight protein tyrosine phosphatases (LMW-PTPs) restores PKM2 activity and prevents its nuclear translocation, which has been linked to reduced melanoma cell proliferation and invasiveness. Acetylation of PKM2 at lysine-433 promotes its nuclear import, while deacetylation by SIRT6 results in its export, with nuclear entry facilitating tumor cell proliferation and migration. PKM2 is also methylated at several arginine residues (R-445/447/455) by co-activator-associated arginine methyltransferase 1 (CARM1), which can either facilitate or inhibit its tetramerization, depending on the context (Lori et al. 2018). Interestingly, some studies suggest that methylation enhances PKM2 tetramerization and enzymatic activity, highlighting the complex role of CARM1 in cancer metabolism. Lastly, prolyl hydroxylase 3 mediates hydroxylation at proline-403/408, promoting PKM2's interaction with hypoxia-inducible factor 1-alpha (HIF-1α) and the transcriptional activation of HIF-1α-regulated genes, underlining the significance of PKM2's multiple post-translational modifications in cancer cell metabolism and survival (Abeywardana et al. 2018; Luo et al. 2011).

PKM2 in Health and Disease

PKM2, primarily a glycolytic enzyme located in the cytosol, exhibits additional functions when translocated to the nucleus under specific conditions, where it plays a critical role in cell division by regulating gene expression. The interaction between PKM2 and the peptidyl-proline isomerase (PIN1) protein is facilitated when PKM2 is phosphorylated at serine-37 (S-37), leading to cis-trans isomerization. This modification enables the binding of PKM2's nuclear localization signal (NLS) to importin α5, which then mediates its translocation through the nuclear pore complex (NPC) into the nucleus. This suggests that PKM2 has functions beyond glycolysis, particularly in controlling cell survival and proliferation. In neoplastic cells, PKM2 regulates the cell cycle by phosphorylating Bub3 and inhibiting cyclin D, thereby promoting the transition from the G1 to the S phase, which is crucial for tumor growth and survival (Jiang et al. 2014a). Additionally, PKM2 plays a significant role in regulating hypoxia-inducible factor 1-alpha (HIF-1α), a key regulator of the cellular response to hypoxia. PKM2 enhances HIF-1α's ability to bind to hypoxia-responsive elements (HREs) and control the expression of genes involved in tumor metabolism and survival. This nuclear migration is unique to PKM2, as no prior research has shown that PKM1, another isoform of pyruvate kinase, translocates to the nucleus. PKM2's dimeric form possesses kinase activity that extends beyond glycolysis to regulate gene expression. Furthermore, PKM2 may use phosphoenolpyruvate (PEP) as a phosphate source to phosphorylate key proteins involved in cancer metabolism and pathophysiology, including nuclear sterol regulatory element-binding protein 1a (SREBP1a), histone H3, Bub3, myosin regulatory light chain 1 (MLC-2), and signal transducer and activator of transcription 3 (STAT3) (Zhao et al. 2018).

Significance of PKM2 in Cancer Metabolism

Cancer cells consume more glucose and produce significant amounts of lactate, even in the presence of oxygen, a phenomenon known as the Warburg effect. This oxygen-dependent glycolysis occurs despite aerobic glycolysis generating less ATP compared to oxidative phosphorylation in mitochondria. Cancer cells preferentially use this pathway to rapidly produce ATP to meet their increased energy demands. PKM2 is integral in controlling this metabolic shift, with its elevated levels correlating with increased glucose consumption and alterations in redox balance. These metabolic changes not only provide ATP for malignant cells but also supply essential substrates for various anabolic processes. For instance, dihydroxyacetone phosphate (DHAP), an intermediate in glycolysis, is utilized in the synthesis of membrane lipids, which are vital for the creation of new membranes required for cell division. Additionally, other glycolytic metabolites serve as precursors for the synthesis of amino acids and nucleotides, which are essential for cell growth and proliferation. This altered metabolic pathway is commonly found in nearly all types of cancer and is often inhibited, leading to the accumulation of citrate in the mitochondria. The citrate is subsequently released into the cytosol, where ATP-citrate lyase (ACL) converts it into acetyl-CoA and oxaloacetate (OAA). OAA is further converted into pyruvate, while acetyl-CoA is utilized for de novo lipogenesis and histone acetylation, supporting the biosynthesis processes necessary for cancer cell proliferation (Fisher et al. 1976).

PKM2 in Inflammation-Related Disorders

Inflammation is a complex process that attracts neutrophils and leukocytes by activating neighboring immune cells. However, when systemic inflammatory responses (SIRs) become overactive or untreated, they can lead to severe health issues, such as sepsis and septic shock. These inflammatory responses require significant energy to meet the demands of immune cells. Metabolic programming, which involves a shift from a resting state to increased metabolic activity, plays a crucial role in providing immune cells with ATP and metabolic intermediates necessary for the production of pro-inflammatory cytokines. This metabolic change is similar to the Warburg effect seen in cancer cells. Consequently, glycolytic enzymes, particularly PKM2, are critical for facilitating this metabolic shift (Fox et al. 2005).

Research suggests that PKM2 may significantly impact the inflammatory responses associated with neuropathic pain. Pro-inflammatory cytokines, which attract leukocytes to the site of injury, are key players in the development of neuropathic pain after nerve damage. Notably, in the absence of PKM2, spinal cord levels of TNF-α and IL-1β decreased, and pain sensitivity was reduced following CCI. These findings suggest that PKM2 plays a crucial role in the development of neuropathic pain and warrants further investigation to fully understand its mechanisms of action. Chronic inflammation is a key factor in the development of various conditions, including metabolic disorders like diabetes and diabetic neuropathy. PKM2 plays an essential role in the pathogenesis of these diseases by regulating genes involved in chronic inflammation, glycolysis, and inflammatory processes. Through its interactions with metabolic pathways, including those involving GLUT, AKT, and HIF-1α, PKM2 may contribute to the development of metabolic diseases. These findings highlight the potential of PKM2 as a critical regulator of inflammation and metabolic dysfunction (Duran-Salgado et al. 2014).

Conclusion

While there is compelling evidence of PKM2's critical role in cancer, inflammation, and metabolic disorders, most of the research on its potential therapeutic benefits has been conducted in cell and animal models. Furthermore, many PKM2 modulatory inhibitors are not selective for the M2 isoform, which could lead to toxicity in non-target organs by affecting other PK isoforms essential for normal physiological function. Additionally, these compounds often lack tissue specificity, which may interfere with PKM2 activity in healthy tissues and result in adverse clinical outcomes. Therefore, further research is needed to fully understand the clinical relevance of PKM2 activators and inhibitors, as well as their short- and long-term health effects.

References

Abeywardana, T., Oh, M., Jiang, L., Yang, Y., Kong, M., Song, J., & Yang, Y. (2018). CARM1 suppresses de novo serine synthesis by promoting PKM2 activity. *The Journal of Biological Chemistry*, 293(39), 15290–15303.

Christofk, H. R., Vander Heiden, M. G., Harris, M. H., Ramanathan, A., Wei, R., Fleming, M. D., Schreiber, S. L., & Cantley, L. C. (2008). The M2 splice isoform of pyruvate kinase is important for cancer metabolism and tumour growth. *Nature*, 452(7184), 230–233.

Dombrauckas, J. D., Santarsiero, B. D., & Mesecar, A. D. (2005). Structural basis for tumor pyruvate kinase M2, allosteric regulation and catalysis. *Biochemistry*, 44(27), 9417–9429.

Duran-Salgado, M. B., & Rubio-Guerra, A. F. (2014). Diabetic nephropathy and inflammation. *World Journal of Diabetes*, 5(3), 393–398.

Fisher, A. B., Huber, G. A., Furia, L., Bassett, D., & Rabinowitz, J. L. (1976). Evidence for lipid synthesis by the dihydroxyacetone phosphate pathway in rabbit lung subcellular fractions. *The Journal of Laboratory and Clinical Medicine*, 87(6), 1033–1040.

Fox, C. J., Hammerman, P. S., & Thompson, C. B. (2005). Fuel feeds function: energy metabolism and the T-cell response. *Nature Reviews Immunology*, 5(11), 844–852.

Imamura, K., & Tanaka, T. (1972). Multimolecular forms of pyruvate kinase from rat and other mammalian tissues. I. Electrophoretic studies. *Journal of Biochemistry*, 71(6), 1043–1051.

Jiang, Y., Li, X., Yang, W., Hawke, D. H., Zheng, Y., Xia, Y., Aldape, K., Wei, C., Guo, F., Chen, Y., & Lu, Z. (2014). PKM2 regulates chromosome segregation and mitosis progression of tumor cells. *Molecular Cell*, 53(1), 75–87.

Jiang, Y., Wang, Y., Wang, T., Hawke, D. H., Zheng, Y., Li, X., Zhou, Q., Majumder, S., Bi, E., Liu, D. X., Huang, S., & Lu, Z. (2014a). PKM2 phosphorylates MLC2 and regulates cytokinesis of tumour cells. *Nature Communications*, 5, 5566.

Liu, F., Ma, F., Wang, Y., Hao, L., Zeng, H., Jia, C., Wang, Y., Liu, P., Ong, I. M., Li, B., Chen, G., Jiang, J., Gong, S., Li, L., & Xu, W. (2017). PKM2 methylation by CARM1 activates aerobic glycolysis to promote tumorigenesis. *Nature Cell Biology*, 19(11), 1358–1370.

Lori, G., Gamberi, T., Paoli, P., Caselli, A., Pranzini, E., Marzocchini, R., Modesti, A., & Raugei, G. (2018). LMW-PTP modulates glucose metabolism in cancer cells. *Biochimica et Biophysica Acta - General Subjects*, 1862(12), 2533–2544.

Luo, W., Hu, H., Chang, R., Zhong, J., Knabel, M., O'Meally, R., Cole, R. N., Pandey, A., & Semenza, G. L. (2011). Pyruvate kinase M2 is a PHD3-stimulated coactivator for hypoxia-inducible factor 1. *Cell*, 145(5), 732–744.

Masoud, G. N., & Li, W. (2015). HIF-1α pathway: role, regulation and intervention for cancer therapy. *Acta Pharmaceutica Sinica B*, 5(5), 378–389.

Osterman, J., Fritz, P. J., & Wuntch, T. (1973). Pyruvate kinase isozymes from rat tissues: developmental studies. *The Journal of Biological Chemistry*, 248(3), 1011–1018.

Siragusa, M., Thole, J., Bibli, S. I., Luck, B., Loot, A. E., de Silva, K., Wittig, I., Heidler, J., Stingl, H., Randriamboavonjy, V., Kohlstedt, K., Brune, B., Weigert, A., Fisslthaler, B., & Fleming, I. (2019). Nitric oxide maintains endothelial redox homeostasis through PKM2 inhibition. *The European Molecular Biology Organization Journal*, 38(17), e100938.

Yang, L., Xie, M., Yang, M., Yu, Y., Zhu, S., Hou, W., Kang, R., Lotze, M. T., Billiar, T. R., Wang, H., Li, L., & Tang, D. (2014). PKM2 regulates the Warburg effect and promotes HMGB1 release in sepsis. *Nature Communications*, 5, 4436.

Yang, W., Xia, Y., Hawke, D., Li, X., Liang, J., Xing, D., Aldape, K., Hunter, T., Yung, W. K. A., & Lu, Z. (2012). PKM2 phosphorylates histone H3 and promotes gene transcription and tumorigenesis. *Cell*, 150(4), 685–696.

Zhao, X., Zhao, L., Yang, H., Li, J., Min, X., Yang, F., Liu, J., & Huang, G. (2018). Pyruvate kinase M2 interacts with nuclear sterol regulatory element-binding protein 1a and thereby activates lipogenesis and cell proliferation in hepatocellular carcinoma. *The Journal of Biological Chemistry*, 293(17), 6623–6634.

Chapter 22

11β-Hydroxysteroid Dehydrogenase Type 1 (11β-HSD1): A Novel Therapeutic Target in Diabetes Mellitus

N. L. Swathi[1]
Riya Dave[2,*]
Muhammad Usama Saeed[3]
Anuj Barot[4]
Sakshi Roy[5]
and Litinkumar Sardhara[6]

[1]Jawaharlal Nehru Technological University, Anantapur, Andhra Pradesh, India
[2]Dental Practitioner, Ahmedabad, Gujarat, India
[3]National Institute of Health, Islamabad, Pakistan
[4]B. J. Medical College, Ahmedabad, Gujarat, India
[5]School of Medicine, Queen's University Belfast, United Kingdom
[6]Government Medical College, Surat, Gujarat, India

Abstract

Diabetes mellitus, a prevalent global health challenge characterized by chronic hyperglycemia, often defies optimal glycemic control despite advancements in treatment. Therefore, innovative therapeutic targets are essential. Among these, the 11β-hydroxysteroid dehydrogenase type 1 (11β-HSD1) enzyme emerges as a promising candidate due to its role in glucocorticoid metabolism and its link to insulin resistance, which significantly contributes to the pathophysiology of diabetes and its complications. This chapter provides an in-depth analysis of 11β-HSD1 as a novel therapeutic target for diabetes mellitus, examining its molecular mechanisms, tissue-specific functions, and genetic regulation. It thoroughly evaluates the development, efficacy, and safety of 11β-HSD1 inhibitors, comparing these agents with other antidiabetic treatments to assess their clinical potential. Additionally, it explores the genetic and epigenetic factors that influence 11β-HSD1 expression and activity, offering insights into pharmacogenomics and personalized medicine approaches.

* Corresponding Author's Email: riadave334@gmail.com

In: Receptor-Targeted Therapies in Diabetes Mellitus
Editors: Ajmer Singh Grewal, Neelam Singh, Swati Verma et al.
ISBN: 979-8-89530-587-4

Keywords: 11β-Hydroxysteroid dehydrogenase type 1, 11β-HSD1, diabetes mellitus, glucose metabolism, insulin resistance, antidiabetic therapy

Abbreviations

11β-HSD1	11 Beta-Hydroxysteroid Dehydrogenase Type 1
ACTH	Adrenocorticotropic Hormone
AZD	AstraZeneca Drug
CAD	Coronary artery disease
cAMP	Cyclic Adenosine Monophosphate
CBG	Corticosteroid-Binding Globulin
CpG	Cytosine-phosphate-Guanine (a sequence in DNA)
DM	Diabetes Mellitus
DNA	Deoxyribonucleic Acid
DPP-4	Dipeptidyl Peptidase-4
FFARs	Free Fatty Acid Receptors
G6Pase	Glucose-6-Phosphatase
GC	Glucocorticoid
GLP-1	Glucagon-Like Peptide-1
GPCRs	G Protein-Coupled Receptors
GR	Glucocorticoid Receptor
HbA1c	Hemoglobin A1c
HF	Heart Failure
HPA	Hypothalamic-Pituitary-Adrenal
INCB	Incyte Drug
LDL	Low-Density Lipoprotein
MI	Myocardial Infarction
PEPCK	Phosphoenolpyruvate Carboxykinase
ROS	Reactive Oxygen Species
SGLT-2	Sodium-Glucose Cotransporter-2
SNPs	Single Nucleotide Polymorphisms
T2DM	Type 2 Diabetes Mellitus
TNF	Tumor Necrosis Factor

Introduction

Diabetes mellitus is a chronic condition marked by elevated blood glucose levels due to impaired insulin secretion, insulin resistance, or both. It affects millions globally and imposes a significant burden on healthcare systems. Diabetes is generally classified into two main types: type 1 diabetes, an autoimmune disorder that leads to the destruction of pancreatic β-cells, and type 2 diabetes (T2DM), which results from a combination of insulin resistance and inadequate insulin production (Kupczyk et al. 2022). The rising prevalence of type 2 diabetes is largely attributed to poor diet, physical inactivity, and genetic factors. The increasing rates of obesity, metabolic syndrome, and Type 2 diabetes have become urgent public health challenges worldwide, with type 2 diabetes characterized by chronic hyperglycemia affecting individuals of all ages and genders, though it is more common with advancing age (American Diabetes Association, 2020). Uncontrolled diabetes can result in serious long-term complications that are often advanced by the time they are diagnosed. Key microvascular complications include retinopathy, a leading cause of blindness in adults, neuropathy, which can lead to diabetic foot ulcers and, in severe cases, amputation, and nephropathy, which may progress to renal failure (Habtemariam, 2019; Srinivasan & Davies, 2019). Macrovascular complications, primarily associated with atherosclerosis, may present as angina or coronary artery disease and, in advanced cases, lead to myocardial infarction and hypertension (Björntorp et al. 1999). Diagnostic criteria for type 2 diabetes include a random blood glucose measurement of 200 mg/dL or more, fasting glucose levels of 126 mg/dL or higher on multiple occasions, or a hemoglobin A1c level of at least 6.5% (Almeida et al. 2021). Treatment options cover a wide range of pharmacological agents, such as biguanides, sulfonylureas, thiazolidinediones, acarbose, GLP-1 agonists, DPP-4 inhibitors, SGLT-2 inhibitors, and insulin, each aimed at managing blood glucose levels and reducing the risk of complications (Feingold, 2024).

Biology and Function of 11β-HSD1

11β-HSD1 is an enzyme dependent on nicotinamide adenine dinucleotide phosphate (NADPH), primarily found in adipose and liver tissues. This enzyme converts cortisone into cortisol, an active glucocorticoid essential for regulating homeostasis. Glucocorticoids, including cortisol, have several functions, one of which is opposing insulin's effects (Byun et al. 2015). In the liver, cortisol supports the expression of key gluconeogenic enzymes such as phosphoenolpyruvate carboxykinase (PEPCK) and glucose-6-phosphatase (G6Pase), which catalyze the hydrolysis of glucose-6-phosphate to free glucose, a critical step in gluconeogenesis. This cortisol-driven upregulation of PEPCK and G6Pase can contribute to hyperglycemia, a common feature in metabolic disorders like diabetes (Cain & Cidlowski, 2017). Once produced, glucocorticoids are metabolized in the liver, where they are converted into metabolites that are excreted through urine. The liver uses specific enzymes to achieve this: 5β-reductase converts cortisone into tetrahydrocortisone (THE), while 5α-reductase converts cortisol into tetrahydrocortisol (THF) (Ye et al. 2017).

Functions of Glucocorticoids

Glucocorticoids (GCs), the primary representatives of corticosteroids in humans, play a critical role in regulating various physiological processes to maintain homeostasis, particularly in response to stress. They are essential in the metabolism of proteins, lipids, and carbohydrates (Samuel et al. 2017). Additionally, glucocorticoids are involved in controlling electrolyte and water balance, distributing adipose tissue, and supporting cardiovascular and central nervous system functions. GCs are also vital in modulating inflammatory and immune responses (Sapolsky et al. 2000). The production of cortisol begins when hypothalamic neurohormones stimulate the synthesis of the proopiomelanocortin peptide. This peptide undergoes proteolytic cleavage to produce adrenocorticotropic hormone (ACTH), which then enters the bloodstream and stimulates the adrenal cortex to produce cortisol. Consequently, cortisol levels in plasma are closely tied to ACTH levels, with both hormones being released in a pulsatile manner. Cortisol follows a circadian rhythm, typically peaking in the early morning within the first hour of waking, declining gradually throughout the day, and reaching its lowest levels in the evening and early nighttime (Gross et al. 2009). Circadian patterns can vary due to factors such as stress, diet, or altered sleep patterns. During the day, additional secretory bursts of cortisol are associated with physical activity and food intake. In the bloodstream, cortisol binds primarily to corticosteroid-binding globulin (CBG), also known as transcortin, which transports 70-90% of glucocorticoids in plasma (Kokkinopoulou et al. 2021). Cortisol also acts through the human glucocorticoid receptor, a member of the hormone receptor superfamily that includes receptors for thyroid hormones and vitamin D. In addition to genomic actions, glucocorticoids can initiate non-genomic signaling pathways by activating secondary messengers such as cGMP, cAMP, inositol triphosphate, and diacylglycerol. By limiting glucose uptake in muscle and adipose tissue, glucocorticoids also play a role in raising blood glucose levels, thus ensuring an energy supply during periods of stress (Akalestou et al. 2020).

Glucose Homeostasis and Pathophysiological Role in Diabetes

Glucose Homeostasis

The processes that maintain blood glucose levels within a specific range, essential for normal body functions, are known as glucose homeostasis. Insulin, produced by pancreatic beta cells, is the primary hormone that lowers blood glucose levels. It suppresses glucose production in the liver and enhances glucose uptake by tissues, particularly muscle and adipose tissue. In contrast, glucagon, released by pancreatic alpha cells, raises blood glucose levels by promoting gluconeogenesis and glycogenolysis in the liver (Heitaku et al. 2023; Hunter & Bailey, 2015).

Mechanism of Glucose Homeostasis

Insulin Resistance and Hyperglycemia

In a healthy individual, the pancreatic hormone insulin aids in transporting glucose from the bloodstream into cells for energy production. In T2DM, however, insulin resistance occurs, meaning the body's cells become less responsive to insulin. This resistance is often associated with obesity, especially the accumulation of visceral fat, which releases free fatty acids and inflammatory cytokines that disrupt insulin signaling pathways. Insulin resistance prompts the pancreas to overproduce insulin in an effort to compensate, resulting in hyperinsulinemia. Over time, however, pancreatic beta cells become exhausted and can no longer produce sufficient insulin (Gilon, 2020).

Glucose Production and Regulation

The liver plays a central role in maintaining glucose homeostasis. Under normal conditions, insulin suppresses hepatic glucose production (gluconeogenesis) while promoting glycogen synthesis. However, in diabetes, this regulatory mechanism is disrupted. Despite high insulin levels, the liver may continue to produce glucose, which further elevates blood glucose levels. Additionally, glucose homeostasis is partially managed by the kidneys, which reabsorb glucose from urine. In diabetes, the renal threshold for glucose reabsorption may be altered, causing excess glucose to leak into the urine (glycosuria) once blood glucose levels exceed a certain limit (Janssen, 2021).

Pathophysiological Role of 11β-HSD1 in Diabetes

11β-HSD1 plays a significant role in the pathophysiology of diabetes, particularly in glucocorticoid metabolism and insulin sensitivity. This enzyme primarily converts inactive cortisone to active cortisol in organs such as adipose tissue and the liver, where it is essential for regulating metabolic processes (Kupczyk et al. 2022).

Mechanism of Action

Glucocorticoid Activation

11β-HSD1 plays a crucial role in locally activating glucocorticoids. Elevated cortisol levels can lead to insulin resistance, as 11β-HSD1 increases local cortisol concentrations in target tissues such as adipose tissue and the liver. This mechanism contributes to hyperglycemia and impaired glucose metabolism (Kokkinopoulou et al. 2021; Li & Cummins, 2022).

Adipose Tissue Function

11β-HSD1 influences the distribution and storage of fat in adipose tissue. An increase in the activity of this enzyme is associated with the accumulation of visceral fat, which is closely linked to T2DM and metabolic syndrome. Furthermore, 11β-HSD1 exacerbates insulin resistance through its role in promoting adipogenesis and modulating adipose tissue inflammation (Blaschke et al. 2021).

Hepatic Glucose Production

11β-HSD1 promotes liver gluconeogenesis, a process in which glucose is produced from non-carbohydrate sources. Elevated glucocorticoid levels, often seen during stress or obesity, enhance this effect, leading to increased blood glucose levels (Polyzos & Targher, 2024).

11β-HSD1 as a Biomarker in Diabetes

11β-HSD1 plays a critical role in converting inactive cortisone to active cortisol within cells, influencing glucocorticoid levels and metabolic processes. Its activity is particularly significant in diabetes and its complications, as it regulates intracellular glucocorticoid levels, rather than plasma levels. In diabetes, altered glucocorticoid metabolism increases 11β-HSD1 activity in various tissues, which contributes to insulin resistance and glucose intolerance through glucocorticoid receptors. Experiments with tissue-specific 11β-HSD1 transgenic mice have demonstrated that increased enzyme expression leads to insulin resistance, elevated blood sugar, lipids, and blood pressure. Conversely, inhibition of this enzyme reduces weight, blood sugar levels, and cholesterol, suggesting potential therapeutic benefits (Zou et al. 2017). However, there are concerns that inhibiting tissue-level cortisol synthesis could trigger compensatory cortisol production by the adrenal glands (Harno & White, 2010). In individuals with T2DM and obesity, as well as in rodent models, the expression and activity of enzymes regulating cortisol metabolism are significantly elevated in muscle and adipose tissues. This localized glucocorticoid production contributes to obesity and metabolic syndrome. Increased 11β-HSD1 activity in the liver and fat tissues is associated with T2DM, impairing glucose tolerance, promoting insulin resistance, fat accumulation, and weight gain. In adipose tissue, elevated glucocorticoid levels reduce adiponectin and increase TNFα and fasting glucose. In the liver, overexpression of 11β-HSD1 leads to increased insulinemia, LDL cholesterol, and serum glucose levels (Anil et al. 2014). Morgan et al. (2009) demonstrated a link between increased 11β-HSD1 activity and impaired insulin signaling in dexamethasone-treated myotubes. In a 4-week trial by Heise et al. (2014), two inhibitors (RO-151 and RO838) were used alongside metformin in 110 participants. The inhibitors were well-tolerated, with adverse effects occurring in both placebo and treatment groups. Results showed improvements in body weight, HbA1c levels, and insulin sensitivity, although RO-151 caused increased ACTH plasma levels. The study suggested that further research is needed to assess the long-term benefits and risks of these inhibitors (Heise et al. 2014). A 12-week, randomized, double-blind, placebo-controlled study by Feig et al. (2011) evaluated the 11β-HSD1 inhibitor MK-0916 in 154 patients with diabetes and metabolic syndrome. Doses of 10 mg, 50 mg, or 100 mg improved body weight and blood pressure but showed only minimal changes in glycated hemoglobin and no significant changes in fasting plasma glucose levels. MK-0916 was well-tolerated, with no serious adverse effects reported, highlighting its potential for further exploration in diabetes treatment.

Development of 11β-HSD1 Inhibitors

11β-HSD1 inhibitors exhibit a range of pharmacokinetic and pharmacodynamic properties that make them promising candidates for therapeutic applications. These properties include the modulation of cortisol levels, improvements in metabolic and cognitive outcomes, and their potential use as biomarkers for therapeutic monitoring. Such diverse effects significantly enhance the therapeutic potential of 11β-HSD1 inhibitors, positioning them as an appealing subject for research, particularly in preclinical efficacy studies. One notable example is the inhibitor 11b-0048, which has demonstrated the ability to effectively modulate cortisol levels in both cultured keratinocytes and diabetic murine skin. This modulation leads to enhanced skin barrier function and a reduction in inflammation, which are critical aspects of skin health and function (Chen et al. 2024). 11β-HSD1 inhibitors play a significant role in regulating hepatic gluconeogenesis by reducing cortisol levels. Cortisol upregulates the expression of key enzymes involved in gluconeogenesis, and by inhibiting cortisol conversion, 11β-HSD1 inhibitors decrease hepatic glucose production, leading to lower hepatic glucose output. This reduction is particularly beneficial for patients with type 2 diabetes, as it helps control fasting blood glucose levels and improves overall glycemic control. Studies have demonstrated that therapy with 11β-HSD1 inhibitors leads to improvements in hyperglycemia and insulin sensitivity, primarily through the reduction of hepatic glucose production. In addition to their effects on the liver, 11β-HSD1 inhibitors also influence adipose tissue and muscle. In adipose tissue, cortisol promotes lipogenesis and inhibits lipolysis, which results in increased fat storage and adipocyte hypertrophy. By reducing cortisol levels, 11β-HSD1 inhibitors help decrease adiposity, particularly in visceral adipose tissue, thereby improving metabolic health. Additionally, when cortisol levels are reduced in muscle tissue, insulin sensitivity and glucose uptake are enhanced, further contributing to the overall improvement in metabolic health (Chen et al. 2024; Lagos et al. 2014).

Clinical Trials

11β-HSD1 activates cortisol from cortisone, influencing glucose metabolism and insulin sensitivity, making it a key target for T2DM therapies (Table 1) (Walker et al. 1995). A study found that in a study of 616 South Indian participants, the HSD11B1 SNP rs12086634 G allele increased the risk of T2DM (OR = 1.91, $p = 0.0005$) and metabolic syndrome (MetS) (OR = 2.37, $p = 0.0015$), while the rs846910 A allele was linked to higher T2DM risk (OR = 1.62, $p = 0.03$) (Shukla et al. 2019).

Efficacy in Lowering Blood Glucose and Improving Insulin Sensitivity

11β-HSD1 inhibitors BVT-2733 and BVT-116429 have been shown to reduce fasting glucose levels and increase adiponectin. INCB-13739 has demonstrated the ability to lower HbA1c in patients with high BMI and poorly controlled diabetes. Specifically, BVT-116429 lowers fasting glucose but does not improve insulin sensitivity, while PF-00915275 reduces 11β-HSD1 activity without enhancing glucose disposal (Labrie et al. 1997).

Safety and Tolerability

11β-HSD1 inhibitors require thorough safety assessments due to issues observed in early trials, including high blood pressure and hypokalemia. New compounds have been tolerated for up to three months, but monitoring of the HPA axis and androgen levels is crucial. Selective inhibition may lead to increased adrenal androgens, posing a risk for women, as well as potential glucocorticoid deficiency, which increases susceptibility to infections. Long-term effects on immune response, stress, and androgen levels must be carefully evaluated to ensure safety and efficacy (Puig & Pellitero, 2015).

Table 1. Summary of outcomes from clinical and genetic studies on T2DM

Study	Disease	Participants	Study Design	Outcomes
Feig et al. (2011)	T2DM	154 participants, 54% male	Randomized trial (12 weeks)	Reduction in A1C, body weight, BP; Increase in LDL; No significant differences in fasting plasma glucose
Walker et al. (1995)	T2DM	7 healthy males	Crossover trial (7 days)	Increased sensitivity to insulin
Andrews et al. (2003)	T2DM	12 participants	Crossover trial (7 days)	Reduced glucose production and increased cholesterol
Sandeep, Andrew, et al. (2005)	T2DM	6 obese and 6 lean men	Crossover trial (7 days)	No improvement in insulin sensitivity; No alteration in glucose disposal rate
Sandeep, Yau, et al. (2004)	T2DM	12 participants	Crossover trial (6 weeks)	Enhanced verbal and cognitive abilities
Devang et al. (2017)	T2DM	616 South Indian participants	SNP association study	Increased risks of T2DM
Valsamakis et al. (2004)	T2DM and obesity	33 diabetics, 38 healthy participants	Analysis of 11β-HSD1 activity	No significant differences
Heise et al. (2014)	T2DM	110 participants	Randomized trial (28 days)	Changes in cholesterol, LDL, Apolipoprotein B, body weight; No difference in glucose measures
Jang et al. (2007)	T2DM	24 participants (12 diabetic, 12 controls)	Analysis of mRNA expression in muscle	Higher activity and expression
Nair et al. (2004)	T2DM	800 Pima Indians	SNP association study	Significant associations with SNP1 and SNP5; Significant associations with glucose uptake and insulin levels
Rosenstock et al. (2010)	T2DM	302 participants (on metformin)	Randomized trial (12 weeks)	Significant reduction in A1C (100 mg, 200 mg); Changes in weight, LDL, triglycerides
Shukla et al. (2019)	T2DM	60 participants (30 diabetic, 30 controls)	Analysis of 11β-HSD1 activity	Higher 11β-HSD1 activity in diabetes group; Variations based on age, physical activity, calorie intake, BMI

Combination Therapies Involving 11β-HSD1 Inhibitors

11β-HSD1 inhibitors, such as AZD4017, have shown promise in enhancing wound healing and epidermal integrity in diabetic patients, making them potential therapeutic agents for managing chronic wounds associated with diabetes (Ajjan et al. 2022). By blocking 11β-HSD1, these inhibitors improve skin barrier function and reduce inflammatory cytokines in diabetic animal models, suggesting a novel approach to addressing diabetes-related skin complications (Lee et al. 2024). In addition to their effects on skin health, 11β-HSD1 inhibitors have shown promise in improving blood glucose regulation without worsening atherosclerosis, a common concern in diabetes (Lloyd et al. 2009). This supports the potential for combining these inhibitors with other diabetes treatments, as they appear to have a favorable safety profile. Clinical trials have demonstrated that 11β-HSD1 inhibitors can contribute to better management of blood glucose, lipid levels, and blood pressure, albeit with modest impacts compared to other antidiabetic medications (Anderson & Walker, 2013). This indicates that when used in combination with other therapies, 11β-HSD1 inhibitors could offer synergistic effects, enhancing overall treatment outcomes. Notably, the specific inhibitor INCB13739 has shown impressive reductions in blood and plasma glucose levels in individuals with Type 2 diabetes, particularly in those with higher body mass indexes. This highlights the significant role of 11β-HSD1 activity in adipose tissue and its impact on the metabolic and cardiovascular consequences of obesity (Hollis & Huber, 2011).

Genetic and Epigenetic Regulation of 11β-HSD1

Epigenetic modifications play a crucial role in modulating gene expression and influencing physiological processes. In vertebrates, DNA methylation predominantly occurs at CpG dinucleotides, often located in the promoter regions of genes. The HSD11B1 gene, which encodes the enzyme 11β-HSD1, has two transcription start sites with corresponding promoters, P1 and P2 (Inder et al. 2012). Research has shown that elevated levels of 11β-HSD1 mRNA and enzyme activity are linked to a marked decrease in DNA methylation at the CpG region of the HSD11B1 P1 promoter (Inder et al. 2012). Environmental factors, diet, and stress are all potential modulators of epigenetic changes, influencing gene expression and metabolic outcomes. Studies have highlighted several SNPs, rs2235543, rs12565406, and rs4844880, that show a strong association with liver fat content. The major alleles of these SNPs are linked to increased fat accumulation, and individuals homozygous for these alleles are nearly twice as likely to develop non-alcoholic fatty liver disease compared to those carrying the minor alleles (Ahmed et al. 2012; Lutz et al. 2016). The association between HSD11B1 gene expression and metabolic disorders such as T2DM, insulin sensitivity, and metabolic syndrome remains inconclusive. Some studies have found that SNPs rs846910 and rs3334312 are linked to T2DM and insulin sensitivity, but not obesity, in Pima Indians (Nair et al. 2004). Other research has shown that SNPs rs846910 and rs12086634 are only associated with metabolic syndrome (Gambineri et al. 2011), while a third study reported a correlation solely with glucose levels and HDL cholesterol (Turek et al. 2014).

11β-HSD1 and Cardiovascular Risk in Diabetes

Impact on Blood Pressure Regulation

11β-HSD1 plays a crucial role in blood pressure regulation, primarily through its influence on glucocorticoid metabolism. Glucocorticoids are known to increase the sensitivity of blood vessels to vasoconstrictors, such as catecholamines, which can lead to elevated blood pressure. In rat kidneys, 11β-HSD1 is expressed in the convoluted tubules and cells, while in human kidneys, it is localized to the S3 segment of the proximal convoluted tubule and the medullary interstitium (Hunter & Bailey, 2015). Although the precise mechanism linking systemic blood pressure with 11β-HSD1 activity is not yet fully understood, it is hypothesized that increased 11β-HSD1 activity in the renal medulla leads to the production of active glucocorticoids. These glucocorticoids may stimulate renal sodium retention, contributing to the development of hypertension, which is commonly seen in patients with diabetes and metabolic syndrome. Clinical trials have shown that 11β-HSD1 inhibitors result in a modest reduction in blood pressure in individuals with type 2 diabetes or metabolic syndrome (Feig et al. 2011; Shah et al. 2011). These findings suggest that targeting 11β-HSD1 could provide a novel therapeutic strategy for managing hypertension, particularly in patients with metabolic disorders where both hypertension and glucocorticoid dysregulation are prevalent.

Correlation with Cardiovascular Events

The dysregulation of 11β-HSD1 in diabetic patients is a significant factor contributing to an increased risk of cardiovascular events. 11β-HSD1 expression and activity are closely linked to key cardiovascular risk factors such as hypertension, dyslipidemia, and obesity, all of which independently contribute to the development of cardiovascular diseases. Elevated glucocorticoid levels, often seen with 11β-HSD1 overactivity, are associated with endothelial dysfunction, which is considered a critical early step in the formation of atherosclerotic plaque. This dysfunction ultimately leads to various vascular diseases, further exacerbating cardiovascular risk in diabetic individuals (Gathercole et al. 2013). Studies have shown that 11β-HSD1 plays a role in myocardial injury and subsequent heart failure (HF) progression. White et al. (2016) demonstrated that after myocardial infarction (MI) in male mice, increased 11β-HSD1 activity led to myocardial hypertrophy and worsened heart failure progression, while other studies by McSweeney et al. (2010) and Gordon et al. (2014) reported similar findings. These results underscore the involvement of 11β-HSD1 in the development of coronary artery disease (CAD) and the myocardial response following MI. Given its significant role in cardiovascular pathophysiology, targeted therapies aimed at regulating 11β-HSD1 activity could hold promise in reducing cardiovascular risks, especially in diabetic patients. These treatments could help mitigate the negative effects of 11β-HSD1 dysregulation, improving both vascular and myocardial outcomes in this high-risk population.

Conclusion

Receptor-targeted therapies represent a significant advancement in the treatment of diabetes mellitus, offering the potential for more effective and individualized treatment strategies. While progress has been made, challenges such as specificity, novel target identification, combination strategies, personalization, and safety must be addressed. Future research and technological advancements will play a critical role in overcoming these challenges and improving patient outcomes.

References

Ahmed, A., Rabbitt, E., Brady, T., Brown, C., Guest, P., Bujalska, I. J., Doig, C., Newsome, P. N., Hubscher, S., Elias, E., Adams, D. H., Tomlinson, J. W., & Stewart, P. M. (2012). A switch in hepatic cortisol metabolism across the spectrum of non alcoholic fatty liver disease. *PloS one*, 7(2), e29531.

Ajjan, R. A., Hensor, E. M. A., Del Galdo, F., Shams, K., Abbas, A., Fairclough, R. J., Webber, L., Pegg, L., Freeman, A., Taylor, A. E., Arlt, W., Morgan, A. W., Tahrani, A. A., Stewart, P. M., Russell, D. A., & Tiganescu, A. (2022). Oral 11β-HSD1 inhibitor AZD4017 improves wound healing and skin integrity in adults with type 2 diabetes mellitus: a pilot randomized controlled trial. *European journal of endocrinology*, 186(4), 441–455.

Akalestou, E., Genser, L., & Rutter, G. A. (2020). Glucocorticoid Metabolism in Obesity and Following Weight Loss. *Frontiers in endocrinology*, 11, 59.

Almeida, C., Monteiro, C., & Silvestre, S. (2021). Inhibitors of 11β-hydroxysteroid dehydrogenase type 1 as potential drugs for type 2 diabetes mellitus—a systematic review of clinical and *in vivo* preclinical studies. *Scientia Pharmaceutica*, 89(1), 5.

American Diabetes Association (2020). 2. Classification and Diagnosis of Diabetes: Standards of Medical Care in Diabetes-2020. *Diabetes care*, 43(Suppl 1), S14–S31.

Anderson, A., & Walker, B. R. (2013). 11β-HSD1 inhibitors for the treatment of type 2 diabetes and cardiovascular disease. *Drugs*, 73(13), 1385–1393.

Andrews, R. C., Rooyackers, O., & Walker, B. R. (2003). Effects of the 11 beta-hydroxysteroid dehydrogenase inhibitor carbenoxolone on insulin sensitivity in men with type 2 diabetes. *The Journal of clinical endocrinology and metabolism*, 88(1), 285–291.

Anil, T. M., Dandu, A., Harsha, K., Singh, J., Shree, N., Kumar, V. S., Lakshmi, M. N., Sunil, V., Harish, C., Balamurali, G. V., Naveen Kumar, B. S., Gopala, A. S., Pratibha, S., Sadasivuni, M., Anup, M. O., Moolemath, Y., Venkataranganna, M. V., Jagannath, M. R., & Somesh, B. P. (2014). A novel 11β-hydroxysteroid dehydrogenase type1 inhibitor CNX-010-49 improves hyperglycemia, lipid profile and reduces body weight in diet induced obese C57B6/J mice with a potential to provide cardio protective benefits. *BMC pharmacology & toxicology*, 15, 43.

Björntorp, P., Holm, G., & Rosmond, R. (1999). Hypothalamic arousal, insulin resistance and Type 2 diabetes mellitus. *Diabetic medicine*, 16(5), 373–383.

Blaschke, M., Koepp, R., Streit, F., Beismann, J., Manthey, G., Seitz, M. T., Kragl, A., & Siggelkow, H. (2021). The rise in expression and activity of 11β-HSD1 in human mesenchymal progenitor cells induces adipogenesis through increased local cortisol synthesis. *The Journal of steroid biochemistry and molecular biology*, 210, 105850.

Byun, S. Y., Shin, Y. J., Nam, K. Y., Hong, S. P., & Ahn, S. K. (2015). A novel highly potent and selective 11β-hydroxysteroid dehydrogenase type 1 inhibitor, UI-1499. *Life sciences*, 120, 1–7.

Cain, D. W., & Cidlowski, J. A. (2017). Immune regulation by glucocorticoids. *Nature reviews. Immunology*, 17(4), 233–247.

Chen, X., Liu, X., Zhang, L., Li, J., Liu, R., Shu, M., & Huang, K. (2024). Identify the Novel Potential 11β-HSD1 Inhibitors Based on Deep Learning, Molecular Modelling and Activity Evaluation. *SSRN*, https://dx.doi.org/10.2139/ssrn.4743752.

Devang, N., Satyamoorthy, K., Rai, P. S., Nandini, M., Rao, S., Phani, N. M., & Adhikari, P. (2017). Association of HSD11B1 gene polymorphisms with type 2 diabetes and metabolic syndrome in South Indian population. *Diabetes research and clinical practice*, 131, 142–148

Feig, P. U., Shah, S., Hermanowski-Vosatka, A., Plotkin, D., Springer, M. S., Donahue, S., Thach, C., Klein, E. J., Lai, E., & Kaufman, K. D. (2011). Effects of an 11β-hydroxysteroid dehydrogenase type 1 inhibitor,

MK-0916, in patients with type 2 diabetes mellitus and metabolic syndrome. *Diabetes, obesity & metabolism*, 13(6), 498–504.

Feingold, K. R. (2024). *Oral and Injectable (Non-Insulin) Pharmacological Agents for the Treatment of Type 2 Diabetes*. Endotext. MDText.com, Inc.

Gambineri, A., Tomassoni, F., Munarini, A., Stimson, R. H., Mioni, R., Pagotto, U., Chapman, K. E., Andrew, R., Mantovani, V., Pasquali, R., & Walker, B. R. (2011). A combination of polymorphisms in HSD11B1 associates with *in vivo* 11{beta}-HSD1 activity and metabolic syndrome in women with and without polycystic ovary syndrome. *European journal of endocrinology*, 165(2), 283–292.

Gathercole, L. L., Lavery, G. G., Morgan, S. A., Cooper, M. S., Sinclair, A. J., Tomlinson, J. W., & Stewart, P. M. (2013). 11β-Hydroxysteroid dehydrogenase 1: translational and therapeutic aspects. *Endocrine reviews*, 34(4), 525–555.

Gilon P. (2020). The Role of α-Cells in Islet Function and Glucose Homeostasis in Health and Type 2 Diabetes. *Journal of molecular biology*, 432(5), 1367–1394.

Gordon, O., He, Z., Gilon, D., Gruener, S., Pietranico-Cole, S., Oppenheim, A., & Keshet, E. (2014). A transgenic platform for testing drugs intended for reversal of cardiac remodeling identifies a novel 11βHSD1 inhibitor rescuing hypertrophy independently of re-vascularization. *PloS one*, 9(3), e92869.

Gross, K. L., Lu, N. Z., & Cidlowski, J. A. (2009). Molecular mechanisms regulating glucocorticoid sensitivity and resistance. *Molecular and cellular endocrinology*, 300(1-2), 7–16.

Habtemariam, S. (2019). Pathophysiology of type 2 diabetes complications. In *Medicinal Foods as Potential Therapies for Type-2 Diabetes and Associated Diseases*, Elsevier, (pp. 69–88).

Harno, E., & White, A. (2010). Will treating diabetes with 11β-HSD1 inhibitors affect the HPA axis? *Trends in endocrinology and metabolism*, 21(10), 619–627.

Heise, T., Morrow, L., Hompesch, M., Häring, H. U., Kapitza, C., Abt, M., Ramsauer, M., Magnone, M. C., & Fuerst-Recktenwald, S. (2014). Safety, efficacy and weight effect of two 11β-HSD1 inhibitors in metformin-treated patients with type 2 diabetes. *Diabetes, obesity & metabolism*, 16(11), 1070–1077.

Heitaku, S., Sasase, T., Sotani, T., Maki, M., Katsumi, S., Fukuda, S., Goto, H., Yamamoto, H., & Nishiu, J. (2023). An 11-Beta Hydroxysteroid Dehydrogenase Type 1 Inhibitor, JTT-654 Ameliorates Insulin Resistance and Non-obese Type 2 Diabetes. *Biological & pharmaceutical bulletin*, 46(7), 969–978.

Hollis, G., & Huber, R. (2011). 11β-Hydroxysteroid dehydrogenase type 1 inhibition in type 2 diabetes mellitus. *Diabetes, obesity & metabolism*, 13(1), 1–6.

Hunter, R. W., & Bailey, M. A. (2015). Glucocorticoids and 11β-hydroxysteroid dehydrogenases: mechanisms for hypertension. *Current opinion in pharmacology*, 21, 105–114.

Inder, W. J., Obeyesekere, V. R., Jang, C., & Saffery, R. (2012). Evidence for transcript-specific epigenetic regulation of glucocorticoid-stimulated skeletal muscle 11β-hydroxysteroid dehydrogenase-1 activity in type 2 diabetes. *Clinical epigenetics*, 4(1), 24.

Jang, C., Obeyesekere, V. R., Dilley, R. J., Krozowski, Z., Inder, W. J., & Alford, F. P. (2007). Altered activity of 11beta-hydroxysteroid dehydrogenase types 1 and 2 in skeletal muscle confers metabolic protection in subjects with type 2 diabetes. *The Journal of clinical endocrinology and metabolism*, 92(8), 3314–3320.

Janssen J. A. M. J. L. (2021). Hyperinsulinemia and Its Pivotal Role in Aging, Obesity, Type 2 Diabetes, Cardiovascular Disease and Cancer. *International journal of molecular sciences*, 22(15), 7797.

Kokkinopoulou, I., Diakoumi, A., & Moutsatsou, P. (2021). Glucocorticoid Receptor Signaling in Diabetes. *International journal of molecular sciences*, 22(20), 11173.

Kupczyk, D., Bilski, R., Kozakiewicz, M., Studzińska, R., Kędziora-Kornatowska, K., Kosmalski, T., Pedrycz-Wieczorska, A., & Głowacka, M. (2022). 11β-HSD as a New Target in Pharmacotherapy of Metabolic Diseases. *International journal of molecular sciences*, 23(16), 8984.

Labrie, F., Bélanger, A., Cusan, L., Gomez, J. L., & Candas, B. (1997). Marked decline in serum concentrations of adrenal C19 sex steroid precursors and conjugated androgen metabolites during aging. *The Journal of clinical endocrinology and metabolism*, 82(8), 2396–2402.

Lagos, C. F., Vecchiola, A., Allende, F., Fuentes, C. A., Tichauer, J. E., Valdivia, C., Solari, S., Campino, C., Tapia-Castillo, A., Baudrand, R., Villarroel, P., Cifuentes, M., Owen, G. I., Carvajal, C. A., & Fardella, C. E. (2014). Identification of novel 11β-HSD1 inhibitors by combined ligand- and structure-based virtual screening. *Molecular and cellular endocrinology*, 384(1-2), 71–82.

Lee, J. Y., Heo, Y. W., Hwang, H. J., Kim, E., Lee, J. Y., Kang, S., & Choi, E. H. (2024). A 11β-Hydroxysteroid dehydrogenase type 1 (11β-HSD1) inhibitor, 11b-0048, effectively suppresses the expression of 11β-HSD1 activated in cultured keratinocytes and in diabetic murine skin. Research Square.

Li, J. X., & Cummins, C. L. (2022). Fresh insights into glucocorticoid-induced diabetes mellitus and new therapeutic directions. *Nature reviews. Endocrinology*, 18(9), 540–557.

Lloyd, D. J., Helmering, J., Cordover, D., Bowsman, M., Chen, M., Hale, C., Fordstrom, P., Zhou, M., Wang, M., Kaufman, S. A., & Véniant, M. M. (2009). Antidiabetic effects of 11beta-HSD1 inhibition in a mouse model of combined diabetes, dyslipidaemia and atherosclerosis. *Diabetes, obesity & metabolism*, 11(7), 688–699.

Lutz, S. Z., Peter, A., Machicao, F., Lamprinou, A., Machann, J., Schick, F., Königsrainer, I., Königsrainer, A., Fritsche, A., Staiger, H., Häring, H. U., Stefan, N., & Kantartzis, K. (2016). Genetic Variation in the 11β-hydroxysteroid-dehydrogenase 1 Gene Determines NAFLD and Visceral Obesity. *The Journal of clinical endocrinology and metabolism*, 101(12), 4743–4751.

McSweeney, S. J., Hadoke, P. W., Kozak, A. M., Small, G. R., Khaled, H., Walker, B. R., & Gray, G. A. (2010). Improved heart function follows enhanced inflammatory cell recruitment and angiogenesis in 11betaHSD1-deficient mice post-MI. *Cardiovascular research*, 88(1), 159–167.

Morgan, S. A., Sherlock, M., Gathercole, L. L., Lavery, G. G., Lenaghan, C., Bujalska, I. J., Laber, D., Yu, A., Convey, G., Mayers, R., Hegyi, K., Sethi, J. K., Stewart, P. M., Smith, D. M., & Tomlinson, J. W. (2009). 11beta-hydroxysteroid dehydrogenase type 1 regulates glucocorticoid-induced insulin resistance in skeletal muscle. *Diabetes*, 58(11), 2506–2515.

Nair, S., Lee, Y. H., Lindsay, R. S., Walker, B. R., Tataranni, P. A., Bogardus, C., Baier, L. J., & Permana, P. A. (2004). 11beta-Hydroxysteroid dehydrogenase Type 1: genetic polymorphisms are associated with Type 2 diabetes in Pima Indians independently of obesity and expression in adipocyte and muscle. *Diabetologia*, 47(6), 1088–1095.

Polyzos, S. A., & Targher, G. (2024). Role of Glucocorticoids in Metabolic Dysfunction-Associated Steatotic Liver Disease. *Current obesity reports*, 13(2), 242–255.

Puig-Domingo, M., & Pellitero, S. (2015). Nuevos agentes terapéuticos para la diabetes tipo 2 [New therapies for type 2 diabetes mellitus]. *Medicina clinica*, 144(12), 560–565.

Rosenstock, J., Banarer, S., Fonseca, V. A., Inzucchi, S. E., Sun, W., Yao, W., Hollis, G., Flores, R., Levy, R., Williams, W. V., Seckl, J. R., Huber, R., & INCB13739-202 Principal Investigators (2010). The 11-beta-hydroxysteroid dehydrogenase type 1 inhibitor INCB13739 improves hyperglycemia in patients with type 2 diabetes inadequately controlled by metformin monotherapy. *Diabetes care*, 33(7), 1516–1522.

Samuel, S., Nguyen, T., & Choi, H. A. (2017). Pharmacologic characteristics of corticosteroids. *Journal of Neurocritical care*, 10(2), 53-59.

Sandeep, T. C., Andrew, R., Homer, N. Z., Andrews, R. C., Smith, K., & Walker, B. R. (2005). Increased *in vivo* regeneration of cortisol in adipose tissue in human obesity and effects of the 11beta-hydroxysteroid dehydrogenase type 1 inhibitor carbenoxolone. *Diabetes*, 54(3), 872–879.

Sandeep, T. C., Yau, J. L., MacLullich, A. M., Noble, J., Deary, I. J., Walker, B. R., & Seckl, J. R. (2004). 11Beta-hydroxysteroid dehydrogenase inhibition improves cognitive function in healthy elderly men and type 2 diabetics. *Proceedings of the National Academy of Sciences of the United States of America*, 101(17), 6734–6739.

Sapolsky, R. M., Romero, L. M., & Munck, A. U. (2000). How do glucocorticoids influence stress responses? Integrating permissive, suppressive, stimulatory, and preparative actions. *Endocrine reviews*, 21(1), 55–89.

Shah, S., Hermanowski-Vosatka, A., Gibson, K., Ruck, R. A., Jia, G., Zhang, J., Hwang, P. M., Ryan, N. W., Langdon, R. B., & Feig, P. U. (2011). Efficacy and safety of the selective 11β-HSD-1 inhibitors MK-0736 and MK-0916 in overweight and obese patients with hypertension. *Journal of the American Society of Hypertension*, 5(3), 166–176.

Shukla, R., Basu, A. K., Mandal, B., Mukhopadhyay, P., Maity, A., Chakraborty, S., & Devrabhai, P. K. (2019). 11β Hydroxysteroid dehydrogenase - 1 activity in type 2 diabetes mellitus: a comparative study. *BMC endocrine disorders*, 19(1), 15.

Srinivasan, B. T., & Davies, M. (2019). Glycaemic management of type 2 diabetes. *Medicine*, 47(1), 32-39.

Turek, L. V., Leite, N., Rodrigues Souza, R. L., Lima, J. K., Milano, G. E., Timossi, L. daS., Osiecki, A. C., Osiecki, R., & Alle, L. F. (2014). Gender-dependent association of HSD11B1 single nucleotide polymorphisms with glucose and HDL-C levels. *Genetics and molecular biology*, 37(3), 490–495.

Valsamakis, G., Anwar, A., Tomlinson, J. W., Shackleton, C. H., McTernan, P. G., Chetty, R., Wood, P. J., Banerjee, A. K., Holder, G., Barnett, A. H., Stewart, P. M., & Kumar, S. (2004). 11beta-hydroxysteroid dehydrogenase type 1 activity in lean and obese males with type 2 diabetes mellitus. *The Journal of clinical endocrinology and metabolism*, 89(9), 4755–4761.

Walker, B. R., Connacher, A. A., Lindsay, R. M., Webb, D. J., & Edwards, C. R. (1995). Carbenoxolone increases hepatic insulin sensitivity in man: a novel role for 11-oxosteroid reductase in enhancing glucocorticoid receptor activation. *The Journal of clinical endocrinology and metabolism*, 80(11), 3155–3159.

White, C. I., Jansen, M. A., McGregor, K., Mylonas, K. J., Richardson, R. V., Thomson, A., Moran, C. M., Seckl, J. R., Walker, B. R., Chapman, K. E., & Gray, G. A. (2016). Cardiomyocyte and Vascular Smooth Muscle-Independent 11β-Hydroxysteroid Dehydrogenase 1 Amplifies Infarct Expansion, Hypertrophy, and the Development of Heart Failure After Myocardial Infarction in Male Mice. *Endocrinology*, 157(1), 346–357.

Ye, X. Y., Chen, S. Y., Wu, S., Yoon, D. S., Wang, H., Hong, Z., O'Connor, S. P., Li, J., Li, J. J., Kennedy, L. J., Walker, S. J., Nayeem, A., Sheriff, S., Camac, D. M., Ramamurthy, V., Morin, P. E., Zebo, R., Taylor, J. R., Morgan, N. N., Ponticiello, R. P., Harrity, T., Apedo, A., Golla, R., Seethala, R., Wang, M., Harper, T. W., Sleczka, B. G., He, B., Kirby, M., Leahy, D. K., Li, J., Hanson, R. L., Guo, Z., Li, Y. X., DiMarco, J. D., Scaringe, R., Maxwell, B., Moulin, F., Barrish, J. C., Gordon, D. A., & Robl, J. A. (2017). Discovery of clinical candidate 2-((2S,6S)-2-phenyl-6-hydroxyadamantan-2-yl)-1-(3'-hydroxyazetidin-1-yl)ethanone [BMS-816336], an orally active novel selective 11β-hydroxysteroid dehydrogenase type 1 inhibitor. *Journal of medicinal chemistry*, 60(12), 4932–4948.

Zou, C., Li, W., Pan, Y., Khan, Z. A., Li, J., Wu, X., Wang, Y., Deng, L., Liang, G., & Zhao, Y. (2017). 11β-HSD1 inhibition ameliorates diabetes-induced cardiomyocyte hypertrophy and cardiac fibrosis through modulation of EGFR activity. *Oncotarget*, 8(56), 96263–96275.

Chapter 23

Future Directions in Receptor Targeted Therapies for Diabetes Mellitus

Chirag Jain
Shikha Baghel Chauhan*
and Indu Singh
Amity Institute of Pharmacy, Amity University, Noida, Uttar Pradesh, India

Abstract

This chapter provides a comprehensive analysis of the latest advancements and future prospects in receptor-based therapeutic strategies for diabetes mellitus. It explores the current landscape of receptor-targeted treatments, including gene-editing technologies, GLP-1 receptor agonists, phosphoinositide 3-kinases (PI3Ks), adiponectin, GPR119 agonists, and other emerging receptor targets. The chapter discusses recent breakthroughs in receptor biology and drug development, highlighting innovations such as HbA1c-adjusted glycemic targets, preoperative carbohydrate loading, and the targeting of long non-coding RNAs. It also examines potential therapies targeting IL-2 cytokines, biologics, and gene therapies that hold promise for improving treatment efficacy and patient outcomes. Additionally, the chapter explains various CRISPR-Cas9 silencing investigations involving nanoparticles for the management of type 2 diabetes mellitus (T2DM) and the effects of GLP/GIP dual agonists on pancreatic β-cell function, glucagon secretion, and food intake. By synthesizing the latest research and emerging trends, this review aims to provide healthcare professionals, researchers, and clinicians with valuable insights to advance diabetes management through novel receptor-based therapeutics.

Keywords: diabetes mellitus, interleukin, hyperglycemia, glucose metabolism, adipose tissue, incretin, tyrosine kinase, hypertension, GLUT-4

* Corresponding Author's Email: shikha.pharma@gmail.com

In: Receptor-Targeted Therapies in Diabetes Mellitus
Editors: Ajmer Singh Grewal, Neelam Singh, Swati Verma et al.
ISBN: 979-8-89530-587-4

Abbreviations

CRISPR	Clustered Regularly Interspaced Short Palindromic Repeats
DM	Diabetes Mellitus
DPP-4	Dipeptidyl Peptidase-4
ERp44	Endoplasmic Reticulum Resident Protein 44
GIP	Glucose-Dependent Insulinotropic Polypeptide
IDF	International Diabetes Federation
JAK-STAT	Janus Kinase and Signal Transducers and Activators of Transcription
MOGAT1	Monoacylglycerol O-Acyltransferase 1
NAFLD	Non-Alcoholic Fatty Liver Disease
NF-κB	Nuclear Factor Kappa B
PAM	Protospacer Adjacent Motif
PEPCK	Phosphoenolpyruvate carboxykinase
T1DM	Type 1 Diabetes Mellitus
T2DM	Type 2 Diabetes Mellitus

Introduction

The global prevalence of diabetes mellitus (DM) has been steadily rising, presenting significant public health challenges. According to the International Diabetes Federation (IDF), the prevalence of DM in 2022 was projected to reach 10.5%, affecting approximately 536 million individuals aged 20 to 79 worldwide. Among surgical patients, diabetes mellitus is notably more prevalent than in the general population, as diabetes-related comorbidities increase the likelihood of requiring surgical interventions (Martin et al. 2020). Landmark randomized controlled trials (RCTs) have emphasized the critical role of insulin therapy in achieving tight glycemic control and reducing the risk of both microvascular and macrovascular complications. Insulin remains a cornerstone of diabetes treatment, with an estimated 150–200 million people worldwide requiring insulin therapy. However, insulin administration is often associated with challenges, including discomfort, weight gain, and hypoglycemia. Recent advancements, particularly the development and availability of insulin analogs, have significantly reduced the risk of hypoglycemia and improved the overall effectiveness of insulin therapy (Chadha et al. 2023).

Targeting IL-12 Cytokines Family

Blocking cytokine production or signaling pathways within the IL-12 family has been recognized as an effective therapeutic strategy for reducing islet inflammation in diabetes. Targeting cytokines at their primary sources has shown promising outcomes. For instance, empagliflozin has been demonstrated to improve T2DM-associated non-alcoholic fatty liver disease (NAFLD) by promoting autophagy in hepatocellular phagocytes, which are major sources of IL-23 (Meng et al. 2021; Luo et al. 2024). Similarly, sitagliptin has been reported to lower circulating Th17 cells, thereby reducing IL-23 production. Crucially, the therapeutic focus is not on eliminating source cells but rather on disrupting the synthetic signaling cascade. This can be effectively achieved by modulating toll-like receptors (TLRs), providing a targeted approach to mitigating inflammatory pathways while preserving essential cellular functions (Luo et al. 2024). For example, *Lactobacillus plantarum* OLL2712 enhances TLR-2 activation and decreases IL-12 and IL-23 production via bone marrow-derived DCs. TLR-2 antagonists have also been shown to reduce islet inflammation and decrease IL-27 production, highlighting the potential complexity due to the involvement of various TLR-2-expressing cell types. For example, quercetin inhibits IL-12 by blocking β-catenin in bone marrow-derived dendritic cells (DCs), though β-catenin is essential in monocyte-derived DCs for regulating IL-12 and inflammation, suggesting cell-type-specific effects (Zirnheld et al. 2019). Another approach to targeting IL-12 involves restricting IL-12 components IL-12p35 and IL-12p40 using Apilimod (STA-5326), which prevents C-Rel, a protein involved in NF-κB signaling, from entering the nucleus (Luo et al. 2024). Another area of interest is targeting the JAK-STAT pathway, as all IL-12 family cytokines activate JAK-STAT signaling. Baricitinib, a JAK2 inhibitor, has shown potential by inhibiting Th1 differentiation through IL-12 and Th17 differentiation through IL-23 (Luo et al. 2024). Clinical trials with baricitinib in patients with newly diagnosed T1DM (NCT04774224) are ongoing to explore its utility, including its potential to reduce insulin resistance by decreasing T-cell infiltration in skeletal muscle and adipose tissue (Waibel et al. 2022). Inhibiting STAT phosphorylation is also being investigated, with lisofylline, a drug that blocks STAT4 phosphorylation, demonstrating benefits in treating T1DM by reducing islet inflammation and potentially delaying disease onset and complications (Luo et al. 2024).

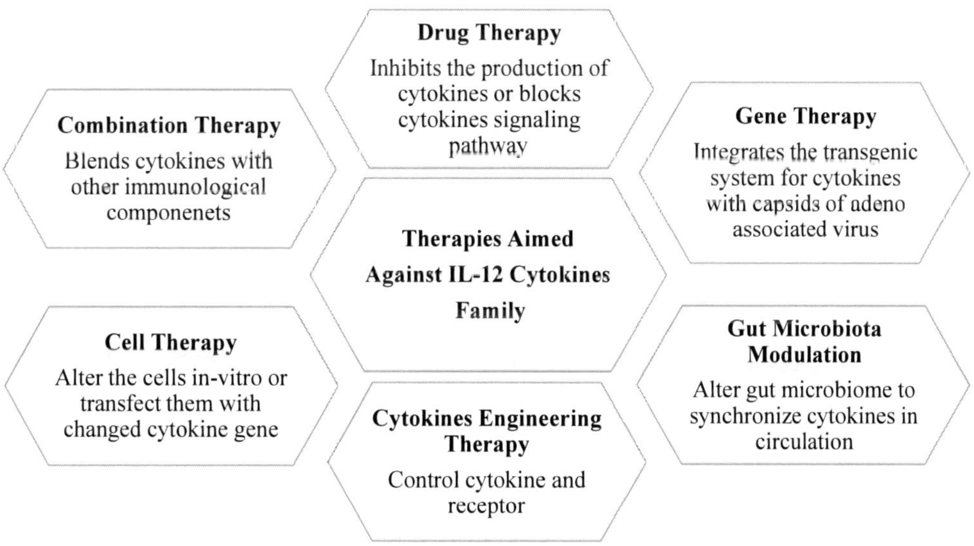

Figure 1. Potential therapies for targeting IL-2 cytokines.

CRISPR/Cas9 Gene Editing Technology

The CRISPR-Cas9 genome-editing technology, originally discovered in bacteria and archaea as an adaptive immune mechanism, is now widely applied in eukaryotic systems. By using single-guided RNAs (sgRNAs) with complementary sequences matching target genes, Cas9, an RNA-guided DNA endonuclease, induces targeted double-strand breaks. These breaks can lead to gene disruption via nonhomologous end-joining (NHEJ) or gene insertion through homologous directed recombination (HDR) when applicable (Cheng et al. 2023). In microbial defense, CRISPR-Cas9 provides an „acquired immune system" by integrating virus-specific protospacer adjacent motif (PAM) sequences into the CRISPR spacer region, enabling the bacterium to recognize and recall invasive DNA (Cheng et al. 2023; Roy et al. 2021). ViaCyte and CRISPR Therapeutics are conducting clinical trials with VCTX210, a stem cell therapy for T1DM that combines PEC210A pancreatic endoderm cells with CRISPR/Cas9-modified cells to enhance immune response and cell survival (Cheng et al. 2023; Roy et al. 2021). Although CRISPR-Cas9 demonstrates high precision in gene editing with minimal off-target effects, some limitations exist: (a) the need for a PAM sequence to target specific genes, and (b) the permanent deletion of essential genes, which may disrupt related signaling pathways. Moreover, CRISPR-Cas9 can either inhibit or enhance gene expression, such as by introducing an activating element in a genomic region. Recent studies suggest that nanoparticle-based delivery of CRISPR-Cas9 may offer an effective approach for silencing genes implicated in T2DM (Table 1) (Roy et al. 2021; Rohiwal et al. 2020).

Table 1. Various CRISPR-Cas9 silencing investigations based on nanoparticles in relation to T2DM management

Nature of the Nanoparticle	Integrated Gene	Effects	References
Polymer-based NP	BMP9, Ntn-1, DPP-4, PEPCK	Reduce hepatic PEPCK by 50%, lower blood sugar, and improve glucose tolerance. Enhance insulin sensitivity, inhibit hepatic gluconeogenesis, decrease insulin resistance and inflammation, and restore normal glucose levels while protecting the liver and kidneys.	(Roy et al. 2021)
Liquid NPs	TORC2, TNF α, MOGAT1, DPP-4, glucagon receptor	DPP-4 gene knockdown enhances hepatic lipid metabolism, reduces gluconeogenesis, significantly lowers blood glucose, downregulates TNF-α, accelerates wound healing in diabetic mice, and improves insulin signaling and glucose tolerance.	(Rohiwal et al. 2020; Roy et al. 2021)
Lipoproteoplex	Keap1	Greatly enhances the diabetic wound	(Lan et al. 2020)
Inorganic NPs	MIRR-155, GM3, SCCS3, STAT, PEPCK	Speeds up the healing of T2DM wounds. Enhance GLUT4 membrane translocation and preserve glucose homeostasis.	(Parashar et al. 2020)
Nanomicelle based on chitosan	TNF α, MCP-1, and adiponectin	Increase in insulin sensitivity, and lower levels of cytokines that promote inflammation.	(Roy et al. 2021)

Combination of GLP-1 Agonists and GIP Incretin

Incretins, specifically GLP-1 (glucagon-like peptide-1) and GIP (glucose-dependent insulinotropic polypeptide), are gut-derived hormones that enhance insulin secretion following nutrient absorption in the gut, a response known as the "incretin effect." This effect highlights the body's heightened insulin production in response to oral glucose compared to intravenous glucose, where similar blood glucose levels would not trigger the same insulin response. The insulinotropic action of incretins occurs only when plasma glucose levels are elevated, making them promising therapeutic targets for hyperglycemia without causing hypoglycemia (Haller

& Lutz, 2024; Campbell et al. 2023). GLP-1 is a post-translational product of the preproglucagon gene (Gcg) and is produced in multiple tissues: α cells of the pancreas, L cells in the gastrointestinal tract, and specific regions in the brainstem and hypothalamus. Interestingly, GLP-1 receptors (GLP-1R) are also found in human adipose tissue, where their expression in visceral fat has been linked to obesity and insulin resistance risks. GIP, on the other hand, is secreted primarily by enteroendocrine K cells located in the duodenum and jejunum, though co-localization of GLP-1 and GIP-producing cells occurs in the mid-small intestine. GLP-1 synthesis predominates in the distal intestine, whereas GIP is mainly produced in the proximal gut (Haller & Lutz, 2024; Campbell et al. 2023; McLean et al. 2020). These effects are comprehensively summarized in Table 2.

Table 2. Effects of GLP-1 and GLP/ GIP dual agonists

Target	Result	References
Effects on pancreatic beta cells	GLP-1 boosts insulin production via cAMP pathways, mobilizing insulin granules only when blood glucose is elevated, while also promoting β-cell growth and reducing cell death.	(Haller & Lutz, 2024; Campbell et al. 2023)
Effects on glucagon secretion	GLP-1 inhibits glucagon release from pancreatic α cells, a mechanism therapeutically significant as T1DM and T2DM involves impaired glucagon suppression, worsening postprandial hyperglycemia. This inhibition is lifted during hypoglycemia.	(Haller & Lutz, 2024: Campbell et al. 2023: McLean et al. 2020)
Affecting body weight and food consumption	GLP-1 decreases food intake in several animals, including rats, mice, and primates. GLP-1 and GLP-1RA-mediated reductions in food consumption and body weight are thought to be regulated by both peripheral (paracrine) and central signaling pathways.	(Haller & Lutz, 2024: Campbell et al. 2023: McLean et al. 2020)

GPR119 Agonists and Their Receptor Expression

The diagnosis of T2DM has spotlighted a receptor type called GPR119, which is associated with G-proteins and found primarily in intestinal L-cells and pancreatic β-cells. GPR119 regulates glucose homeostasis by monitoring and enhancing physiological processes such as GIP production, insulin synthesis by pancreatic β-cells, and levels of incretin hormones like GLP-1 (Manaithiya et al. 2021). Critical sites of GPR119 expression, such as the gastrointestinal tract and pancreas, have been identified based on GPR119 mRNA distribution in various rodent and mouse tissues, using real-time PCR and hybridization analyses (Matsumoto et al. 2018). GPR119 is primarily linked with the Gαs signal transducer, and receptor activation is known to increase intracellular cAMP and adenylate cyclase activity. GPR119 influences the actions of gastric inhibitory polypeptide, peptide YY 3-36, and GLP-1 (Li et al. 2018). Consequently, GPR119 analogues play a role in glucose homeostasis through enteroendocrine activity. Notably, intestinal sub-regions associated with gastric inhibitory polypeptide and GLP-1 exhibit significant levels of GPR119 mRNA, and in situ hybridization has shown that most GLP-1-producing cells co-express GPR119 mRNA (Matsumoto et al. 2018; Li et al. 2018). Interestingly, agonists significantly increase GIP plasma levels in a GPR119-dependent manner, even though duodenal GIP-producing cells express minimal levels of the receptor (Manaithiya et al. 2021; Li et al. 2018).

4-Thiazolidinone Derivatives as Potential Multi-Target Ligands

To manage glucose levels and prevent hyperglycemic complications in diabetes mellitus, a combination of medications is often required. Pancreatic α-amylase and intestinal α-glucosidase, enzymes linked to diabetes, have been investigated as potential inhibitors by 5-arylidene-4-oxo-2-thioxothiazolidin-3-yl) acetic acids (Kaas et al. 2024). Blocking these enzymes, which convert complex carbohydrates into monosaccharides, may help reduce postprandial hyperglycemia (Szabó et al. 2021; Gamal et al. 2024). Aldose reductase, an oxidoreductase, initiates the polyol pathway, converting glucose to sorbitol. Elevated activity in the polyol pathway, driven by high blood sugar levels typical of T2DM, disrupts the osmotic balance and redox states, leading to cardiovascular and nervous system complications (Szabó et al. 2021; Gamal et al. 2024). Protein tyrosine phosphatase 1B (PTP1B) also contributes to insulin resistance by dephosphorylating insulin receptors, impairing insulin signaling. Inhibiting PTP1B can improve insulin action and reduce resistance in diabetic patients. Pancreatic α-amylase and α-glucosidase, crucial for breaking down carbohydrates, are associated with postprandial hyperglycemia, a hallmark of diabetes. Blocking these enzymes prevents the conversion of oligo- and polysaccharides into glucose, making it a key strategy in diabetes treatment (Szabó et al. 2021; Gamal et al. 2024; Kaas et al. 2024; Maccari et al. 2023; Estrada et al. 2022; Sahiba et al. 2020; Maccari et al. 2018). The structure-activity relationship (SAR) of 4-thiazolidinone derivatives has highlighted their role in inhibiting PTP1B and aldose reductase (AR), both of which are involved in T2DM progression. A thioxo-thiazolidinyl acetic acid motif is essential for significant AR inhibition (Maccari et al. 2023; Estrada et al. 2022), leading to the discovery of inhibitors with low submicromolar IC50 values for human and bovine AR enzymes. Thiazolidinyl benzoic acid derivatives exhibit insulin-mimetic properties in cell cultures and inhibit PTP1B. Recently, new 4-thiazolidinone compounds have been developed as dual blockers for PTP1B and AR, exhibiting strong AR inhibition and moderate PTP1B effects (Gamal et al. 2024; Kaas et al. 2024; Maccari et al. 2023). These compounds can aggregate and inhibit target proteins through two mechanisms: (1) inhibitor molecules may form large aggregates that interact with protein sites, or (2) protein adsorption on aggregate surfaces may partially unfold the enzyme, altering its activity (Sahiba et al. 2020; Maccari et al. 2018). Aggregation-based promiscuous inhibitors often impair enzyme function through non-specific interactions (Szabó et al. 2021; Gamal et al. 2024).

HbA1c-Adjusted Glycaemic Targets and Preoperative Carbohydrate Loading (CHL)

Researchers have long sought to create universal guidelines for diabetes management, but patients with T2DM exhibit significant heterogeneity in their conditions. For example, a T2DM patient who is morbidly obese with low insulin tolerance differs greatly from a T2DM patient taking only metformin, or from a T1DM patient. In many cases, individualized treatment is the best approach for managing glycemic control. For instance, chronic essential hypertension can alter a patient's typical blood pressure equilibrium, and these patients may have higher thresholds for both low blood pressure and hypertension. In such cases, researchers may adjust the target mean arterial pressure (MAP) as a proportion of the individual's baseline MAP, particularly during the perioperative phase. Similarly, chronic hyperglycemia should influence perioperative glycemic management goals, adjusting the upper and lower limits of target ranges. Although randomized clinical trials may not directly support this approach, there is indirect evidence suggesting that it improves outcomes. Acute hyperglycemia is associated with worse outcomes, including higher mortality in intensive care units. However, this relationship is likely only a risk factor in patients with generally well-regulated glucose control. In patients with long-standing diabetes (HbA1c > 53 mmol/mol), the link between hyperglycemia and adverse outcomes appears to diminish (Polderman et al. 2024; Rayman et al. 2024; Jones et al. 2017). Preoperative carbohydrate loading (CHL) has been increasingly incorporated into surgical protocols to enhance postoperative recovery. The primary goal of CHL is to prevent the body from entering a fasting state, which triggers catabolic processes. Research suggests that CHL may reduce the inflammatory response associated with surgery by lowering cortisol, interleukin-6, and insulin resistance. However, concerns have been raised about the potential increased risk of aspiration due to delayed gastric emptying or reflux in diabetic patients. Small trials using ultrasonography to measure gastric volume two hours before surgery have found no significant differences between T2DM patients who underwent CHL and those without diabetes who underwent CHL. Additionally, limited studies in T2DM patients who were given insulin to supplement the carbohydrate load after CHL have shown encouraging results, including better glycemic control (Batchelor et al. 2018).

Adiponectin and Phosphoinositide 3-Kinases (PI3Ks)

PI3Ks play a crucial role in cellular signaling by phosphorylating phosphatidylinositol lipids, specifically targeting the 3-hydroxyl group of the inositol ring. The PI3K enzyme consists of a regulatory subunit (p85) and a catalytic subunit (p110). A key downstream participant in the PI3K signaling pathway is AKT (also known as protein kinase B, or PKB), a serine/threonine kinase. The recruitment of the p85 subunit to the cell membrane occurs after stimulation by G protein-coupled receptors or tyrosine kinase enzymes. This interaction leads to the conversion of phosphatidylinositol 4,5-bisphosphate (PIP2) to phosphatidylinositol 3,4,5-trisphosphate (PIP3) by p85 and p110. The generated PIP3 then facilitates the translocation of AKT to the membrane through its pleckstrin homology (PH) domain. Once at the membrane, AKT is activated, leading to various cellular effects, including the regulation of glucose transporters. Activated AKT promotes the movement of GLUT4, a key glucose transporter in skeletal muscles and adipocytes, to the cell membrane, thereby increasing insulin sensitivity. Targeting the PI3K signaling pathway pharmacologically holds therapeutic potential for enhancing insulin sensitivity (Dehghan et al. 2022; Aghaei-Zarch, 2024). Adiponectin, an endocrine protein produced and secreted by adipose tissue, plays a pivotal role in regulating insulin sensitivity and metabolic processes. Adiponectin levels are tightly regulated by various biological chaperones in the endoplasmic reticulum, including ERp44, DsbA-L, and ER oxidoreductase, which assist in the protein's synthesis, polymerization, and release. Adiponectin interacts with its receptors, AdipoR1 and AdipoR2, and the adaptor protein APPL1, which modulates the insulin receptor substrates. This interaction triggers the activation of PI3K and the generation of PIP3 at the plasma membrane, contributing to insulin signaling. Furthermore, adiponectin enhances the inhibition of phosphatase and tensin homolog (PTEN), nuclear factor kappa B (NFκB), and IκB kinase (IKK) through activation of AMPK and translocation of liver kinase B1 (LKB1) to the cytoplasm. These actions make adiponectin a critical factor in the defense against insulin resistance, diabetes, and atherosclerosis (Dehghan et al. 2022; Banerjee et al. 2020). In gestational diabetes mellitus (GDM), adiponectin levels are consistently lower, regardless of the patient's body mass index (BMI) or the degree of insulin resistance. Research suggests that early pregnancy adiponectin levels could predict GDM risk later in pregnancy, and its combination with other biomarkers could improve diagnostic accuracy. A meta-analysis has supported the potential of blood adiponectin levels as a reliable indicator of insulin resistance, aiding in estimating GDM risk. Therefore, adiponectin presents a promising therapeutic target for managing GDM (Achari & Jain, 2017; Banerjee et al. 2020).

Long Non-Coding RNAs (lncRNAs)

LncRNAs, typically smaller than 200 nucleotides, represent a diverse group of molecules involved in various cellular processes. A study using microarray analysis combined with gene ontology to investigate blood samples from individuals newly diagnosed with T2DM and normal controls identified 55 differentially expressed lncRNAs. These findings highlighted the association between dysregulated lncRNAs and immune modulation, inflammation, and insulin resistance—key factors in the pathophysiology of T2DM (Yan et al. 2023). The KCNQ1OT1/miR-214/caspase-1 signaling pathway, in particular, has been implicated in the progression of diabetes-related corneal endothelial keratopathy, suggesting that KCNQ1OT1 may serve as a potential therapeutic target. Furthermore, research on ob/ob mice has shown that depletion of the lncRNA MALAT1 in the liver improves insulin sensitivity. This suggests that targeting MALAT1 with antisense oligonucleotides or locked nucleic acid (LNA) GapmeRs could provide a novel therapeutic strategy for treating T2DM and obesity. In addition to their role in the pathophysiological mechanisms of diabetes, lncRNAs offer promising opportunities for therapeutic intervention, making them potential targets for clinical applications in the management and treatment of T2DM (Yan et al. 2023; Lu et al. 2022; Taheri et al. 2020).

Conclusion

The future of diabetes treatment looks promising with the development of new therapeutic techniques and a deeper understanding of molecular mechanisms. One of the key areas of innovation is the targeting of IL-12 cytokines, which can regulate immune responses and reduce inflammation, offering potential for improving autoimmune-related aspects of diabetes. The CRISPR/Cas9 gene-editing technology also holds promise for correcting genetic defects with high precision, which could provide long-term solutions to genetically driven forms of diabetes. Incretin-based therapies, such as GLP-1 agonists and GLP-1/GIP combination agonists, represent a novel approach to boosting insulin production and improving glycemic control. Additionally, GPR119 agonists offer another strategy to suppress glucagon release and stimulate insulin secretion, contributing to better glucose management. Another promising development involves derivatives of 4-thiazolidinone, which subtly regulate glucose metabolism, providing another layer of control over blood sugar levels. Furthermore, CHL is becoming an important strategy to improve surgical outcomes by enhancing metabolic stability and reducing the risk of stress-induced hyperglycemia during and after surgery. By combining immune modulation, genetic correction, incretin therapies, receptor targeting, enzyme inhibition, personalized glycemic goals, and perioperative care, these advancements form a multimodal approach to diabetes management. As these therapies progress through clinical trials, they have the potential to transform diabetes care, offering patients more effective, individualized, and comprehensive treatment options. These developments could significantly improve quality of life and outcomes for individuals with diabetes.

References

Achari, A., & Jain, S. (2017). Adiponectin, a Therapeutic Target for Obesity, Diabetes, and Endothelial Dysfunction. *International Journal of Molecular Sciences*, 18(6), 1321.

Aghaei-Zarch, S. M. (2024). Crosstalk between MiRNAs/lncRNAs and PI3K/AKT signaling pathway in diabetes mellitus: Mechanistic and therapeutic perspectives. *Non-coding RNA Research*, 9(2), 486–507.

Banerjee, A., Sharma, D., Trivedi, R., & Singh, J. (2020). Treatment of insulin resistance in obesity-associated type 2 diabetes mellitus through adiponectin gene therapy. *International Journal of Pharmaceutics*, 583, 119357.

Batchelor, T. J. P., Rasburn, N. J., Abdelnour-Berchtold, E., Brunelli, A., Cerfolio, R. J., Gonzalez, M., Ljungqvist, O., Petersen, R. H., Popescu, W. M., Slinger, P. D., & Naidu, B. (2018). Guidelines for enhanced recovery after lung surgery: recommendations of the Enhanced Recovery After Surgery (ERAS®) Society and the European Society of Thoracic Surgeons (ESTS). *European Journal of Cardio-thoracic Surgery*, 55(1), 91–115.

Bensellam, M., Jonas, J. C., & Laybutt, D. R. (2018). Mechanisms of β-cell dedifferentiation in diabetes: recent findings and future research directions. *Journal of Endocrinology*, 236(2), R109–R143.

Campbell, J. E., Müller, T. D., Finan, B., DiMarchi, R. D., Tschöp, M. H., & D'Alessio, D. A. (2023). GIPR/GLP-1R dual agonist therapies for diabetes and weight loss—chemistry, physiology, and clinical applications. *Cell Metabolism*, 35(9), 1519–1529.

Chadha, M., Jain, S. M., Chawla, R., Dharmalingam, M., Chaudhury, T., Talwalkar, P., Tripathi, S., Singh, S., Gutch, M., & Dasgupta, A. (2023). Evolution of guideline recommendations on insulin therapy in type 2 diabetes mellitus over the last two decades: a narrative review. *Current Diabetes Reviews*, 19(8), e160123212777.

Cheng, Y., Wang, H., & Li, M. (2023). The promise of CRISPR/Cas9 technology in diabetes mellitus therapy: How gene editing is revolutionizing diabetes research and treatment. *Journal of Diabetes and Its Complications*, 37(8), 108524.

Dehghan, M., Ghorbani, F., Najafi, S., Ravaei, N., Karimian, M., Kalhor, K., Movafagh, A., & Zarch, S. M. A. (2022). Progress toward molecular therapy for diabetes mellitus: A focus on targeting inflammatory factors. *Diabetes Research and Clinical Practice*, 189, 109945.

Estrada, A. K., Delgado-Maldonado, T., Lara-Ramírez, E. E., Martínez-Vázquez, A. V., Ortiz-Pérez, E., Paz-González, A. D., Bandyopadhyay, D., & Rivera, G. (2022). Recent Advances in the Development of Type 2 Sodium-Glucose Cotransporter Inhibitors for the Treatment of Type 2 Diabetes Mellitus. *Mini-Reviews in Medicinal Chemistry*, 22(4), 586–599.

Gamal, M. A., Fahim, S. H., Giovannuzzi, S., Fouad, M. A., Bonardi, A., Gratteri, P., Supuran, C. T., & Hassan, G. S. (2024). Probing benzenesulfonamide–thiazolidinone hybrids as multitarget directed ligands for efficient control of type 2 diabetes mellitus through targeting the enzymes: α-glucosidase and carbonic anhydrase II. *European Journal of Medicinal Chemistry*, 271, 116434.

Haller, N., & Lutz, T. A. (2024). Incretin therapy in feline diabetes mellitus – A review of the current state of research. *Domestic Animal Endocrinology*, 89, 106869.

Jones, C. E., Graham, L. A., Morris, M. S., Richman, J. S., Hollis, R. H., Wahl, T. S., Copeland, L. A., Burns, E. A., Itani, K. M. F., & Hawn, M. T. (2017). Association Between Preoperative Hemoglobin A1cLevels,

Postoperative Hyperglycemia, and Readmissions Following Gastrointestinal Surgery. *JAMA Surgery*, 152(11), 1031.

Kaas, S. A., Baara, F. T., Megrouss, Y., Yahiaoui, S., Djafri, A., Boudjenane, F. Z., Chouaih, A., Djafri, A., & Hatzidimitriou, A. (2024). Synthesis, crystal structure, hirshfeld surface analysis, computational investigations and molecular docking studies of (z)-3-N-(methyl)-2-N'-(4-methoxyphenylimino) thiazolidin-4-one dihydrate. *Journal of Molecular Structure*, 1308, 137964.

Lan, B., Wu, J., Li, N., Pan, C., Yan, L., Yang, C., Zhang, L., Yang, L., & Ren, M. (2020). Hyperbranched cationic polysaccharide derivatives for efficient siRNA delivery and diabetic wound healing enhancement. *International Journal of Biological Macromolecules*, 154, 855–865.

Li, N. X., Brown, S., Kowalski, T., Wu, M., Yang, L., Dai, G., Petrov, A., Ding, Y., Dlugos, T., Wood, H. B., Wang, L., Erion, M., Sherwin, R., & Kelley, D. E. (2018). GPR119 Agonism Increases Glucagon Secretion During Insulin-Induced Hypoglycemia. *Diabetes*, 67(7), 1401–1413.

Lu, X., Tan, Q., Ma, J., Zhang, J., & Yu, P. (2022). Emerging Role of LncRNA Regulation for NLRP3 Inflammasome in Diabetes Complications. *Frontiers in Cell and Developmental Biology*, 9, 792401.

Luo, J., Ning, T., Li, X., Jiang, T., Tan, S., & Ma, D. (2024). Targeting IL-12 family cytokines: A potential strategy for type 1 and type 2 diabetes mellitus. *Biomedicine & Pharmacotherapy*, 170, 115958.

Maccari, R., Del Corso, A., Paoli, P., Adornato, I., Lori, G., Balestri, F., Cappiello, M., Naß, A., Wolber, G., & Ottanà, R. (2018). An investigation on 4-thiazolidinone derivatives as dual inhibitors of aldose reductase and protein tyrosine phosphatase 1B, in the search for potential agents for the treatment of type 2 diabetes mellitus and its complications. *Bioorganic & Medicinal Chemistry Letters*, 28(23–24), 3712–3720.

Maccari, R., Wolber, G., Genovese, M., Sardelli, G., Talagayev, V., Balestri, F., Luti, S., Santi, A., Moschini, R., Del Corso, A., Paoli, P., & Ottanà, R. (2023). Designed multiple ligands for the treatment of type 2 diabetes mellitus and its complications: Discovery of (5-arylidene-4-oxo-2-thioxothiazolidin-3-yl) alkanoic acids active as novel dual-targeted PTP1B/AKR1B1 inhibitors. *European Journal of Medicinal Chemistry*, 252, 115270.

Manaithiya, A., Alam, O., Sharma, V., Naim, M. J., Mittal, S., & Khan, I. A. (2021). GPR119 agonists: Novel therapeutic agents for type 2 diabetes mellitus. *Bioorganic Chemistry*, 113, 104998.

Martin, L. D., Hoagland, M. A., Rhodes, E. T., Wolfsdorf, J. I., & Hamrick, J. L. (2020). Perioperative management of pediatric patients with type 1 diabetes mellitus, updated recommendations for anesthesiologists. *Anesthesia and Analgesia*, 130(4), 821–827.

Matsumoto, K., Yoshitomi, T., Ishimoto, Y., Tanaka, N., Takahashi, K., Watanabe, A., & Chiba, K. (2018). DS-8500a, an orally available G protein-coupled receptor 119 agonist, upregulates glucagon-like peptide-1 and enhances glucose-dependent insulin secretion and improves glucose homeostasis in type 2 diabetic rats. *The Journal of Pharmacology and Experimental Therapeutics*, 367(3), 509–517.

McLean, B. A., Wong, C. K., Campbell, J. E., Hodson, D. J., Trapp, S., & Drucker, D. J. (2020). Revisiting the Complexity of GLP-1 Action from Sites of Synthesis to Receptor Activation. *Endocrine Reviews*, 42(2), 101–132.

Meng, Z., Liu, X., Li, T., Fang, T., Cheng, Y., Han, L., Sun, B., & Chen, L. (2021). The SGLT2 inhibitor empagliflozin negatively regulates IL-17/IL-23 axis-mediated inflammatory responses in T2DM with NAFLD via the AMPK/mTOR/autophagy pathway. *International Immunopharmacology*, 94, 107492.

Parashar, D., Rajendran, V., Shukla, R., & Sistla, R. (2020). Lipid-based nanocarriers for delivery of small interfering RNA for therapeutic use. *European Journal of Pharmaceutical Sciences*, 142, 105159.

Polderman, J., Hermanides, J., & Hulst, A. (2024). Update on the perioperative management of diabetes mellitus. *BJA Education*, 24(8), 261-269.

Rayman, G., Page, E., Hodgson, S., Henley, W., Briggs, T. W., & Gray, W. K. (2024). Improving the outcomes for people with diabetes undergoing surgery: An observational study of the Improving the Peri-operative Pathway of People with Diabetes (IP3D) intervention. *Diabetes Research and Clinical Practice*, 207, 111062.

Rohiwal, S. S., Dvorakova, N., Klima, J., Vaskovicova, M., Senigl, F., Slouf, M., Pavlova, E., Stepanek, P., Babuka, D., Benes, H., Ellederova, Z., & Stieger, K. (2020). Polyethylenimine based magnetic nanoparticles mediated non-viral CRISPR/Cas9 system for genome editing. *Scientific Reports*, 10(1), 4619.

Roy, P., Saha, S., & Chakraborty, J. (2021). Looking into the possibilities of cure of the type 2 diabetes mellitus by nanoparticle-based RNAi and CRISPR-Cas9 system: A review. *Journal of Drug Delivery Science and Technology*, 66, 102830.

Sahiba, N., Sethiya, A., Soni, J., Agarwal, D. K., & Agarwal, S. (2020). Saturated Five-Membered Thiazolidines and Their Derivatives: From Synthesis to Biological Applications. *Topics in Current Chemistry*, 378(2).

Szabó, K., Maccari, R., Ottanà, R., & Gyémánt, G. (2021). Extending the investigation of 4-thiazolidinone derivatives as potential multi-target ligands of enzymes involved in diabetes mellitus and its long-term complications: A study with pancreatic α-amylase. *Carbohydrate Research*, 499, 108220.

Taheri, M., Eghtedarian, R., Ghafouri-Fard, S., & Omrani, M. D. (2020). Non-coding RNAs and type 2 diabetes mellitus. *Archives of Physiology and Biochemistry*, 129(2), 526–535.

Waibel, M., Thomas, H. E., Wentworth, J. M., Couper, J. J., MacIsaac, R. J., Cameron, F. J., So, M., Krishnamurthy, B., Doyle, M. C., & Kay, T. W. (2022). Investigating the efficacy of baricitinib in new onset type 1 diabetes mellitus (BANDIT)—study protocol for a phase 2, randomized, placebo-controlled trial. *Trials*, 23(1), 433.

Yan, S., Yao, N., Li, X., Sun, M., Yang, Y., Cui, W., & Li, B. (2023). The association between the differential expression of lncRNA and type 2 diabetes mellitus in people with hypertriglyceridemia. International *Journal of Molecular Sciences*, 24(5), 4279.

Zirnheld, A. L., Villard, M., Harrison, A. M., Kosiewicz, M. M., & Alard, P. (2019). β-Catenin stabilization in NOD dendritic cells increases IL-12 production and subsequent induction of IFN-γ-producing T cells. *Journal of Leukocyte Biology*, 106(6), 1349–1358.

About the Editors

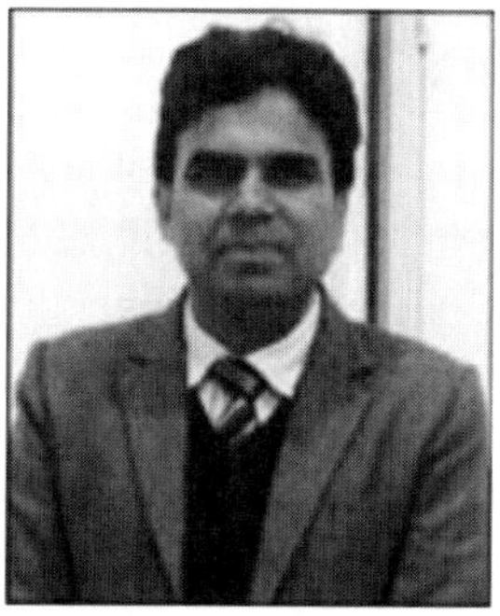

Dr. Ajmer Singh Grewal, Professor (Pharmaceutical Chemistry), Guru Gobind Singh College of Pharmacy, Yamuna Nagar, Haryana (India), has over 13 years of academic and research experience in medicinal chemistry. He completed a PhD in Pharmaceutical Sciences in the subject area of Computational and Medicinal Chemistry from I.K. Gujral Punjab Technical University, Jalandhar, Punjab (India) in 2020. His current research focuses on structure-based drug design and medicinal chemistry of MMP2 and MMP9 inhibitors as anticancer agents, antibacterial drug resistance (NDM-1), GK activators as anti-diabetic agents, AR inhibitors for diabetic complications, PPAR agonists for metabolic syndrome, multi-potent anti-Alzheimer's agents, selective PDE4 & 7 inhibitors as anti-inflammatory agents and environmental chemistry. He has more than 100 publications in national and international journals of repute, 23 book chapters, 15 books, 6 patents and 3 designs. He serves as a reviewer for reputed international journals published by Elsevier, Springer, Wiley, SAGE, and Frontiers. He is a life member of the Indian Society for Technical Education (ISTE). He had worked on various sophisticated analytical instruments including UV-Vis and FTIR spectrophotometer, Flash chromatography, and HPLC; and also, on various molecular modeling softwares including ChemSketch, ChemDraw and Marvin Sketch; Open Babel and Frog2 for structure optimization; PyMOL for molecular graphics, Glide (Schrodinger), AutoDock Tools, AutoDock Vina, Discovery Studio (Dassault Systemes BIOVIA), Omega and Open Eye for in silico molecular docking studies.

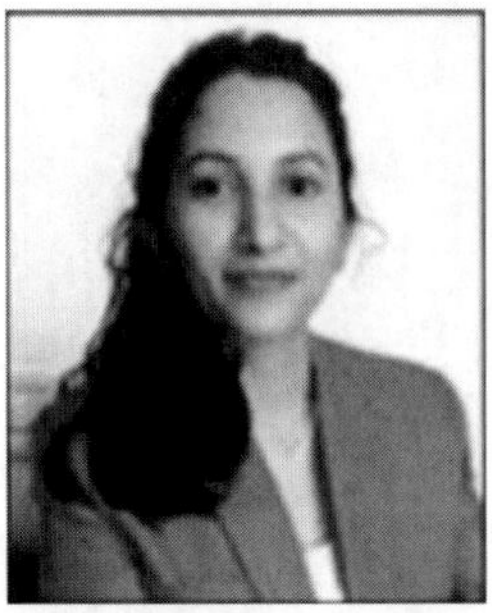

Dr. Neelam Singh is currently a Professor and HOD, HR Institute of Pharmacy, HRIT University, Ghaziabad, Uttar Pradesh, India. She is also an adjunct faculty member and a member of UIAP at Management and Science University, Shah Alam, Selangor, Malaysia. Dr. Singh completed her graduation, post-graduation, and doctorate in Pharmaceutical Sciences from Uttar Pradesh Technical University, Lucknow, Uttar Pradesh, India. With over 14 years of teaching and research experience in pharmacy and pharmaceutical nanotechnology, she has published numerous research and review articles in national and international journals of repute, book chapters, and books in journals of international repute. She has also been granted national patents. Additionally, she serves as an editor and reviewer for various journals. Her current research interests include the nano delivery of phyto-molecules as a therapeutic option for dermatological illnesses.

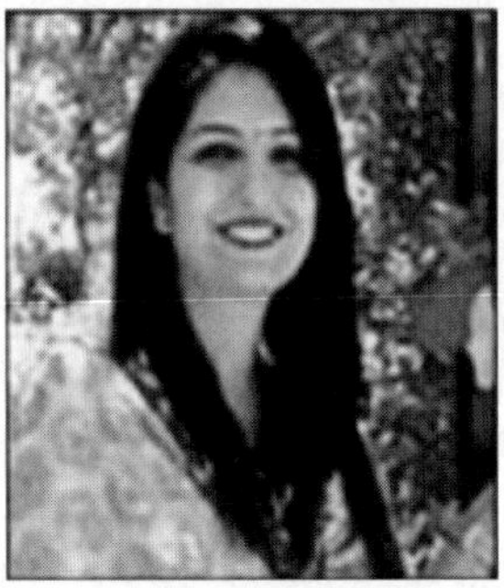

Ms. Swati Verma completed her B. Pharmacy from Dr. A.P.J. Abdul Kalam Technical University and her M. Pharmacy in Pharmaceutical Chemistry from Banasthali Vidyapith, Rajasthan, where she was awarded a Gold Medal in both her bachelor's and master's degrees. Her Ph.D. research focuses on neuro-disorders. She has been working in the Department of Pharmacy at I.T.S. College of Pharmacy for the past 1.5 years. Previously, she held the position of Assistant Professor at Galgotias University, Greater Noida, and BBDNIIT, Lucknow. Her areas of interest include Computer-Aided Drug Design, Analytical Chemistry, Targeted Drug Delivery, and Nanoformulations. She has authored numerous review and research papers published in international journals, six patents, various book chapters, and edited seven books with publishers such as Apple Academic Press, Taylor and Francis, River Publishers, Nova, and Elsevier.

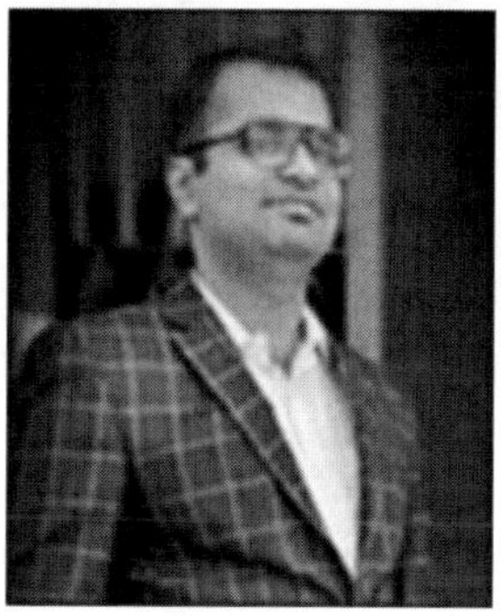

Mr. Chaitanay Vinayak Narayan completed his B. Pharmacy from PT. B. D. Sharma University of Health Sciences, Rohtak (Haryana) and M. Pharmacy (Pharmaceutical Chemistry) from Amity Institute of Pharmacy, Amity University, Noida, Uttar Pradesh (India). Presently he has been working in the Department of Pharmacy, I.T.S. College of Pharmacy, Ghaziabad for the past 2 years. His areas of research interest include computer-aided drug design, targeted drug delivery, and nanoformulation. He has authored many review papers, and research papers published in international journals. He has authored various book chapters.

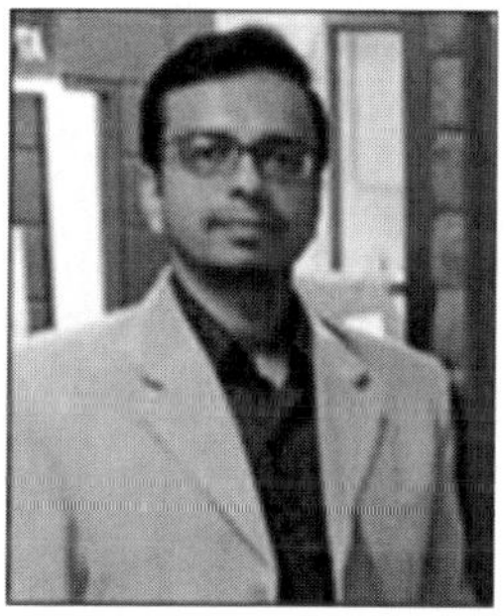

Mr. Ashutosh Kumar Verma is a lecturer in the Clinical Pharmacy and Practice Unit at Management and Science University, Shah Alam, Selangor, Malaysia. He holds a Bachelor of Pharmacy from Uttar Pradesh Technical University, Lucknow, India, and a Master's in Pharmacy Practice from Universiti Sains Malaysia, Penang, Malaysia. With a strong background in academia and research, he has collaborated on numerous projects and contributed to several publications in his field. He has also co-authored educational materials aimed at healthcare professionals, patients, and the general public. He has been actively involved in international initiatives, including the WHO-funded National Antimicrobial Mapping Study in Malaysia and the Antimicrobial Stewardship Program Implementation Study in the Kingdom of Saudi Arabia. His diverse research interests span rational and quality use of medicine, antimicrobial resistance, drug and patient safety, patient education, clinical and pharmacy practice, pharmacoepidemiology, health informatics, research protocol design, systematic reviews, and meta-analysis.

Index

#

β

A

B

C

D

E

F

G

H

N

P

R

S

T

V

W